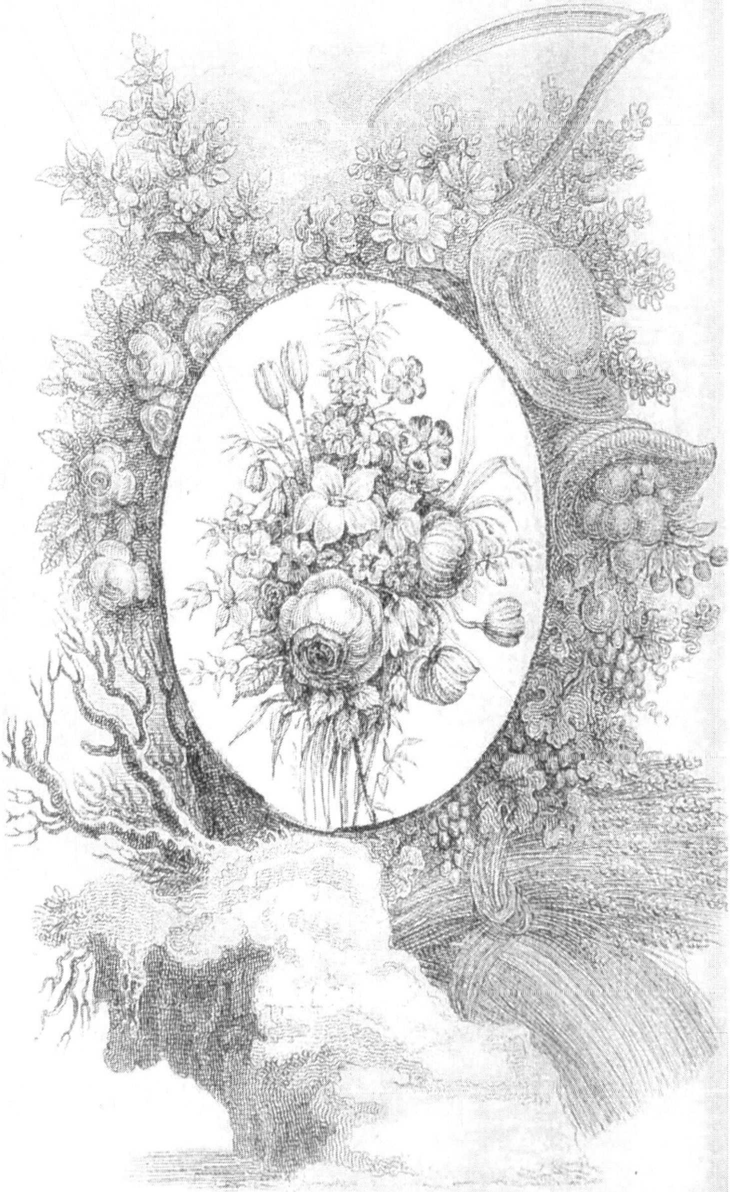

THE NEW
FAMILY HERBAL

THE NEW
FAMILY HERBAL:

COMPRISING

A DESCRIPTION, AND THE MEDICAL VIRTUES

OF

British and Foreign Plants,

FOUNDED ON THE

WORKS OF EMINENT MODERN ENGLISH AND

AMERICAN WRITERS

ON THE MEDICAL PROPERTIES OF HERBS:

TO WHICH IS ADDED,

THE BOTANIC FAMILY PHYSICIAN;

VALUABLE MEDICAL RECEIPTS;

AND

IMPORTANT DIRECTIONS REGARDING DIET, CLOTHING, BATHING, AIR, EXERCISE, &C., &C.

BY

MATTHEW ROBINSON

GYAN

Published by

Gyan Publishing House
5, Ansari Road
Daryaganj, New Delhi-110002
Phone: 011-47034999, 9811692060
E-mail: books@gyanbooks.com

Distribution Network
gyanbooks.com
India, USA, Canada, UK, Australia, France

ISBN : 978-81-212-6133-3 (PB)
First Published, 1912

2nd Impression 2022

Printed at: Gyan Press, Delhi.

THE NEW FAMILY HERBAL
Author: Matthew Robinson

THE NEW

FAMILY HERBAL:

COMPRISING

A DESCRIPTION, AND THE MEDICAL VIRTUES

OF

British and Foreign Plants,

FOUNDED ON THE

WORKS OF EMINENT MODERN ENGLISH AND AMERICAN WRITERS ON THE MEDICAL PROPERTIES OF HERBS:

TO WHICH IS ADDED,

THE BOTANIC FAMILY PHYSICIAN;

VALUABLE MEDICAL RECEIPTS;

AND

IMPORTANT DIRECTIONS REGARDING DIET, CLOTHING, BATHING, AIR, EXERCISE, &c., &c.

BY MATTHEW ROBINSON.

1872.

PREFACE.

SUCH works as Culpeper's Herbal, and those before his time, have been in great repute till of late; and they contain some really valuable information. But a great portion of their works is entirely useless.

The *government of Herbs by the sun, moon, and planets*, has been exploded by modern science; and is now regarded by persons of ordinary capacity to be absurd in the extreme. He who would now connect Astrology with Botany would stultify himself, and hold himself up to public contempt. Botanical knowledge has been greatly augmented of late years, and some Medical men and Herbalists have very ably written upon it. The properties of Herbs, by scientific study, and by Medical experience, are now better understood than they were in the days of Culpeper, and others. While, therefore, the Botanic System of Medicine is making rapid progress, it would be the greatest folly to perpetuate the ignorance and absurdities of ancient Herbalists.

Finally, whatever is valuable in former Herbals, I have adopted. But the *Astrological government* I have rejected with disgust, and also their laughable and ignorant descriptions of some Herbs—take *Culpeper's* description of *Wormwood* as a specimen. I have consulted the works of Hill, Woodville, Don, Thornton, and modern writers, and particularly some of the *great American Herbalists*.

Matthew Robinson

AN EXPLANATION

OF THE

TEMPERAMENTS OF THE HERBS.

I. All medicines simply considered in themselves are either hot, cold, moist, dry or temperate.

The qualities of medicines are considered in respect of man, not of themselves; for those simples are called hot, which heat our bodies; those cold, which cool them; and those temperate, which work no change at all in them, in respect to either heat, cold, dryness, or moisture. And these may be temperate, as being neither hot nor cold; yet may be moist or dry: or being neither moist nor dry, yet may be hot or cold; or lastly, being neither hot, cold, moist nor dry.

II. In temperature there is no degree or difference, the differences of the other qualities are divided into four degrees, beginning at temperature; so that a medicine may be said to be hot, cold, moist or dry, in the first, second, third or fourth degree.

The use of temperate medicines is in those cases where there is no apparent excess of the first qualities to preserve the body temperate, to conserve strength, and to repair decayed nature. And observe, that those medicines which we call cold, are not so called because that they are really cold in themselves, but because the degree of their heat falls below the heat of our bodies, and so only in respect of our temperature are said to be cold, while they are in themselves really hot; for without there could be no vegetation, nor life.

III. Such as are hot in the first degree, are of equal heat with our bodies, and they only add a natural heat to them, if it be cooled by nature or by accident thereby cherishing the natural heat when weak, and restoring it when it is wanting.

Their use is, 1. To make the offending humours thin, that they may be expelled by sweat or perspiration. 2. By outward application to abate inflammations and fevers by opening the pores of the skin. 3. To help concoction, and keep the blood in its just temperature.

IV. Such as are hot in the second degree, as much exceed the first, as our natural heat exceeds a temperature.

Their use is, to open the pores, and take away obstructions, by relaxing tough humours and by their essential force and strength, when nature cannot do it.

V. Such as are hot in the third degree, are more powerful in heating, because they tend to inflame and cause fevers.

Their use is to promote perspiration extremely, and soften tough humours; and therefore all of them resist poison.

VI. Such as are hot in the fourth degree, burn the body, if outwardly applied.

Their use is to cause inflammation, raise blisters, and corrode the skin.

VII. Such as are cold in the first degree, fall as much on the one side of temperature as hot doth on the other.

Their use is, 1. To qualify the heat of the stomach and cause digestion. 2. To abate the heat in fevers; and 3. To refresh the spirits being almost suffocated.

VIII. Such as are cold in the third degree, are, such as have a repercussive force.

And their use is, 1. to drive back the matter, and stop defluctions; 2. to make the humours thick; and 3. to limit the violence of choler, repress perspiration, and keep the spirits from fainting.

IX. Such as are cold in the fourth degree, are such as stupify the senses.

They are used, 1. In violent pains; and 2. in extreme watchings, and the like cases, where life is despaired of.

X. Drying medicines consume the humours, stop fluxes, stiffen the parts and strengthen nature.

But if the humidity be exhausted already, then those consume the natural strength.

XII. Such as are dry in the first degree strengthen; in the second degree bind; in the third, stop fluxes, but spoil the nourishment, and bring consumption; in the fourth, dry up the radical moisture, which being exhausted, the body must needs perish.

XIII. Moist medicines are opposed to drying; they are lenitive, and make slippery.

These cannot exceed the third degree; for all things are either hot or cold. Now heat dries up, and cold congeals; both which destroy moisture.

XIV. Such as are moist in the first degree, ease coughs and help the roughness of the windpipe; in the second, loosen the belly; in the third, make the whole habit of body watery and phlegmatic; filling it with dropsies, lethargies, and such like diseases.

XV. Thus medicines alter according to their temperature, whose active qualities are heat and cold, and whose passive are dryness and moisture.

XVI. The active qualities eradicate diseases, the passive are subservient to nature.

So hot medicines may cure the dropsy, by opening obstructions: and the same may also cure the yellow jaundice, by its attractive quality in sympathising with the humour abounding; and contrarywise cold medicines may compress or abate a fever by condensing the hot vapours, and the same may stop any defluxion or looseness.

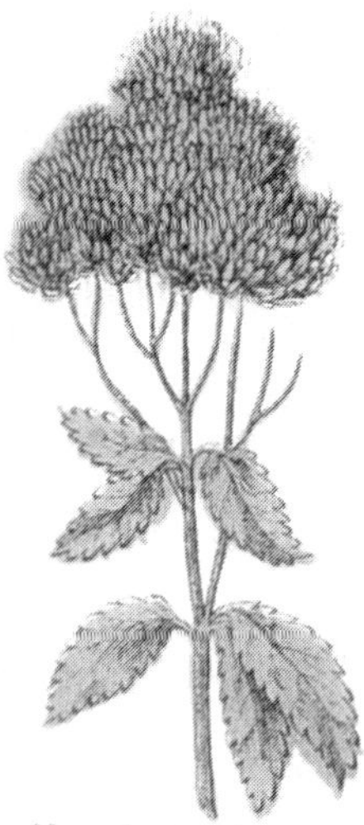

Hemp Agrimony

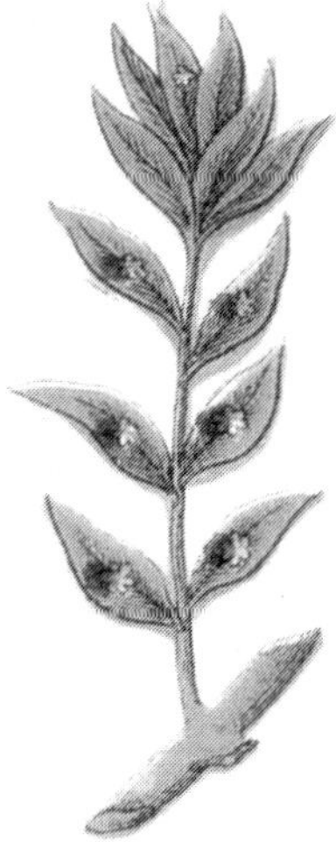

Butchers Broom

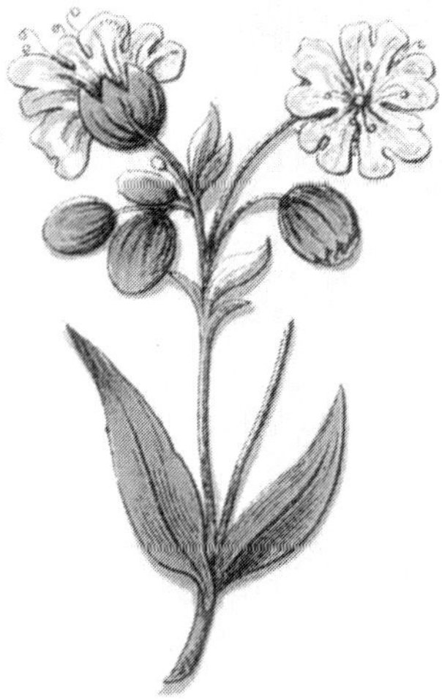

White Behen

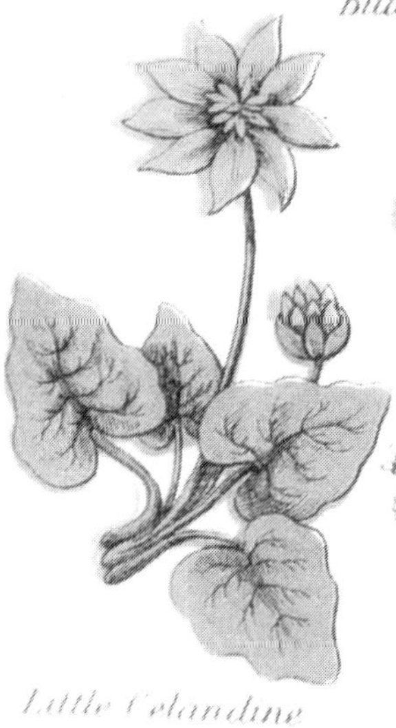

Little Celandine

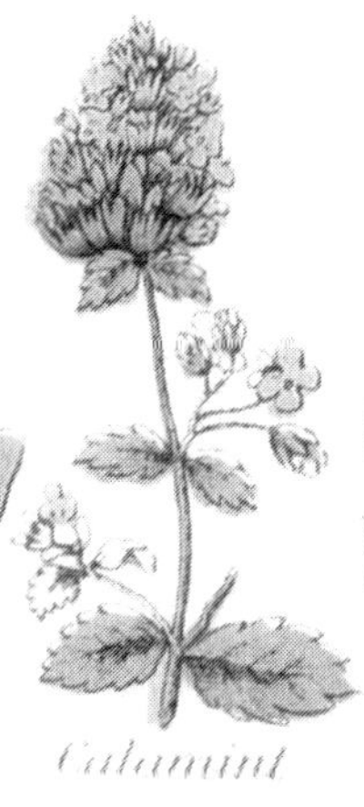

Calamint

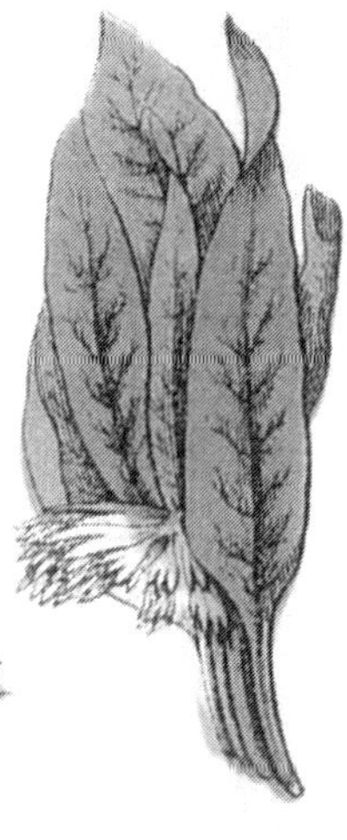

Comfrey

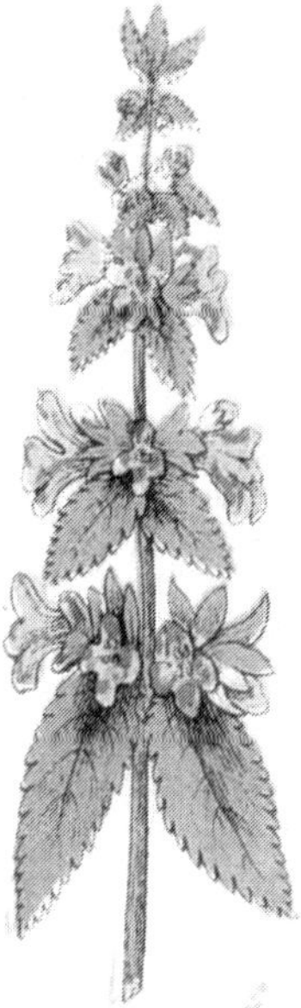

All Heal

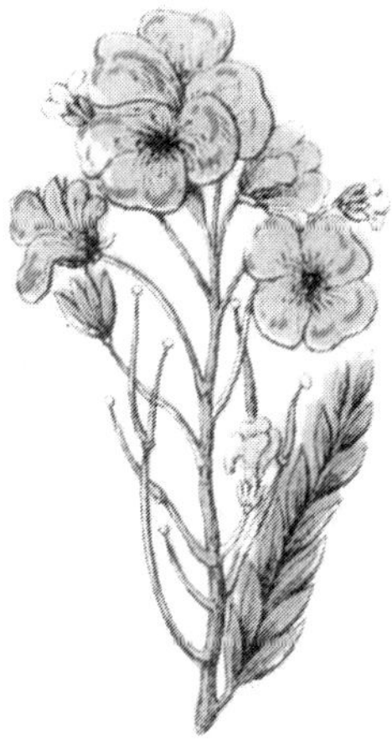

Cuckow Flower

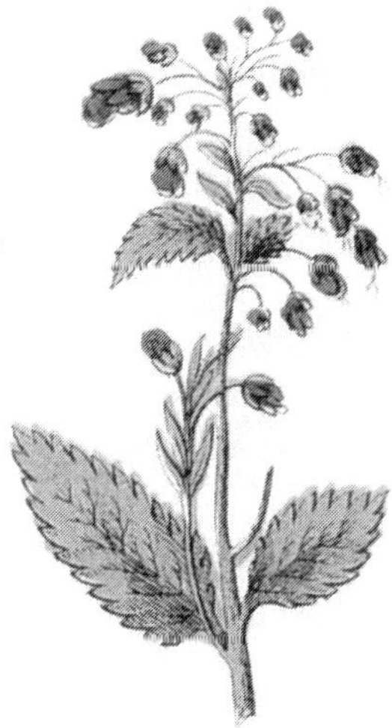

Fig Wort

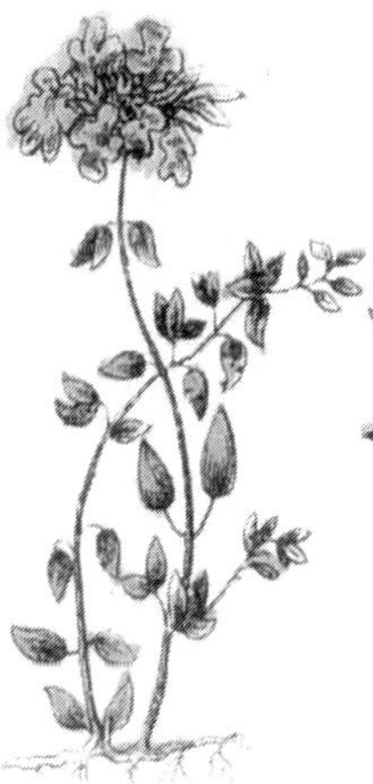

Mother of Thyme

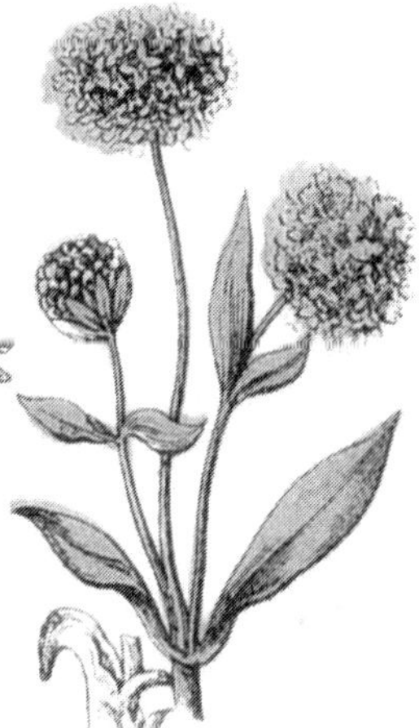

Devilsbit

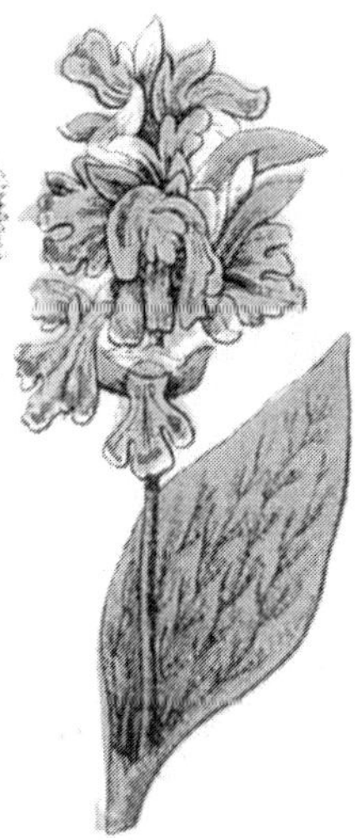

Orchis

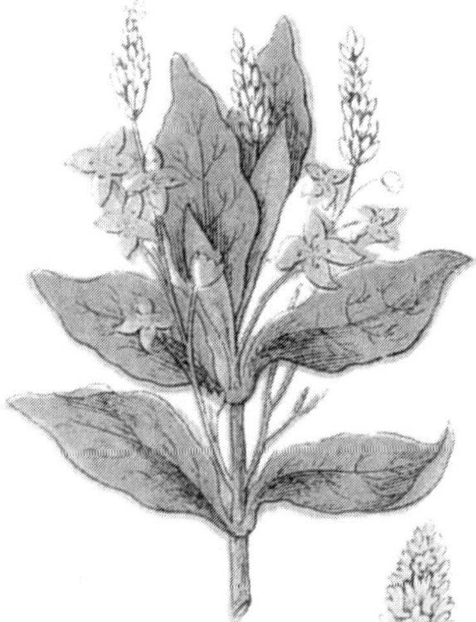

Brook Lime

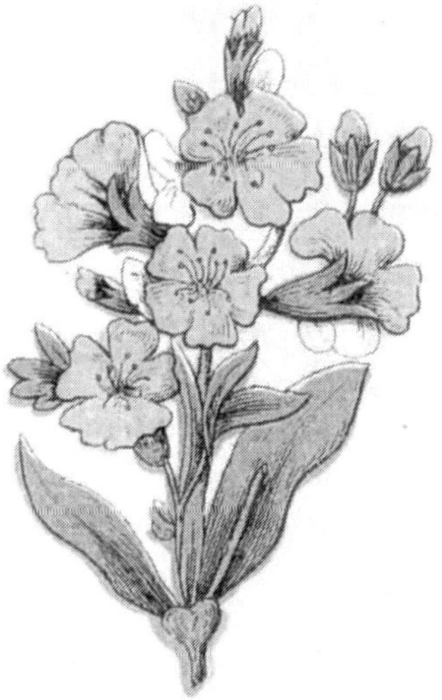

Soap Wort

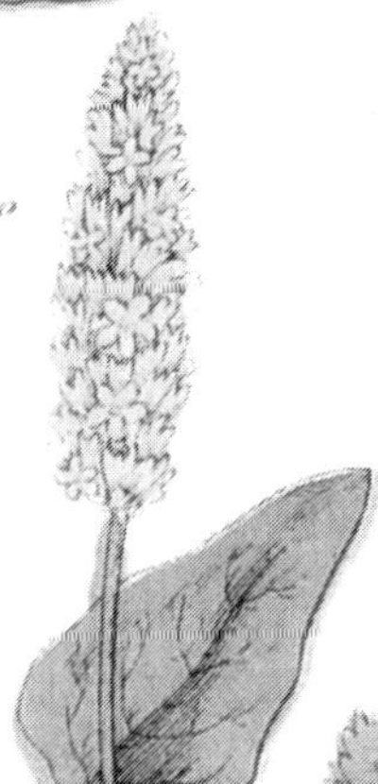

Bistort

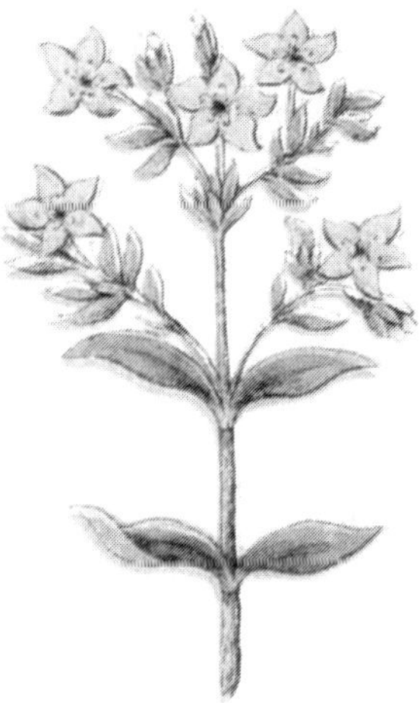

Centuary

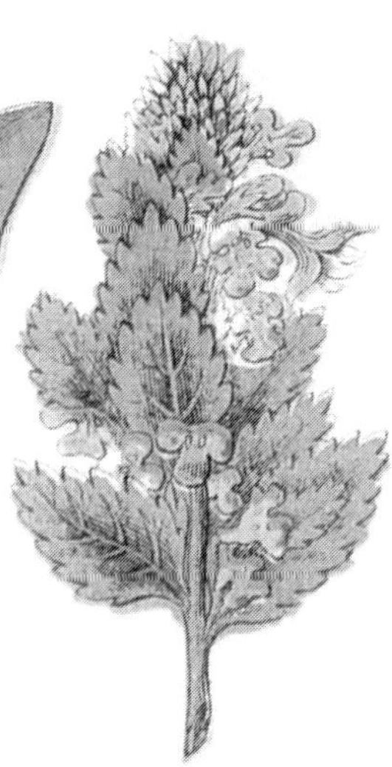

Bugle

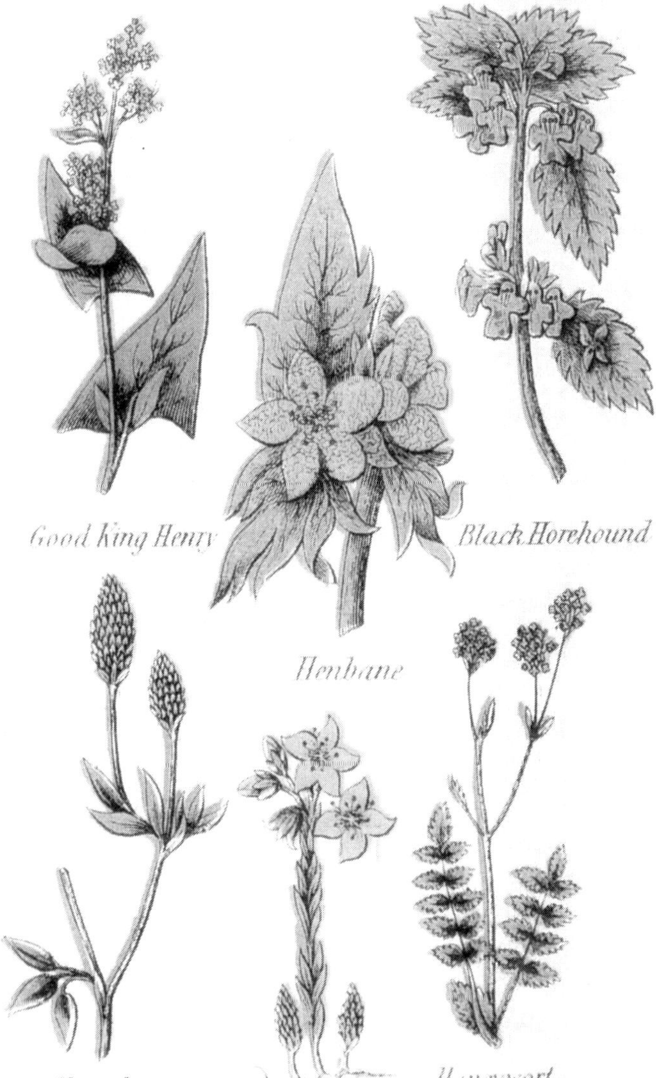
Good King Henry
Henbane
Black Horehound
Haresfoot
Least Houseleek
Honeywort

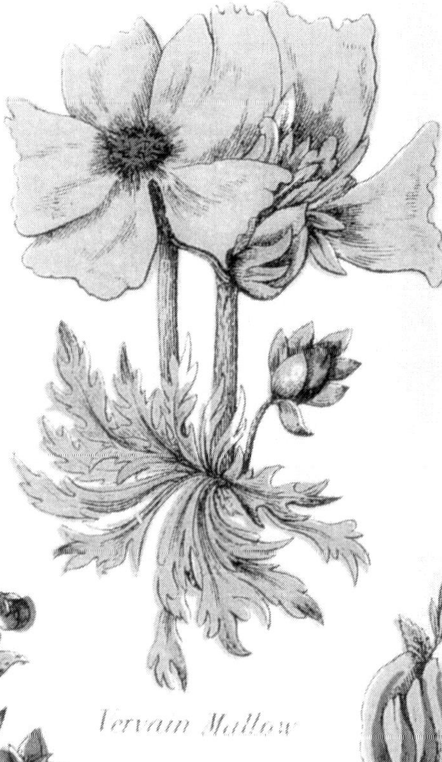

Vervain Mallow

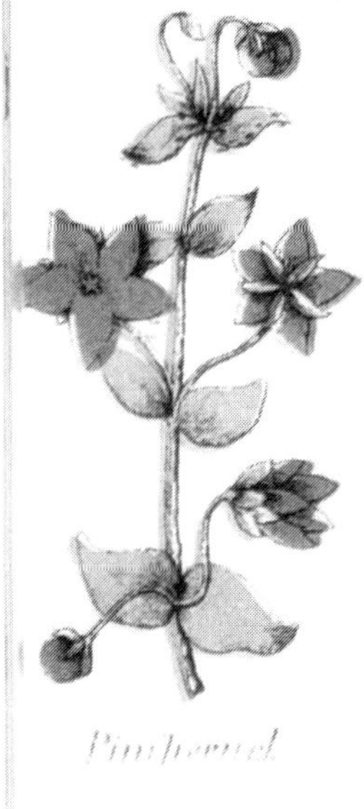

Pimpernel

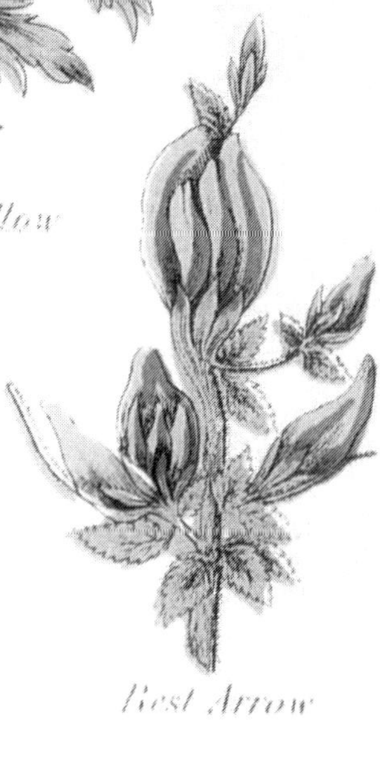

Rest Arrow

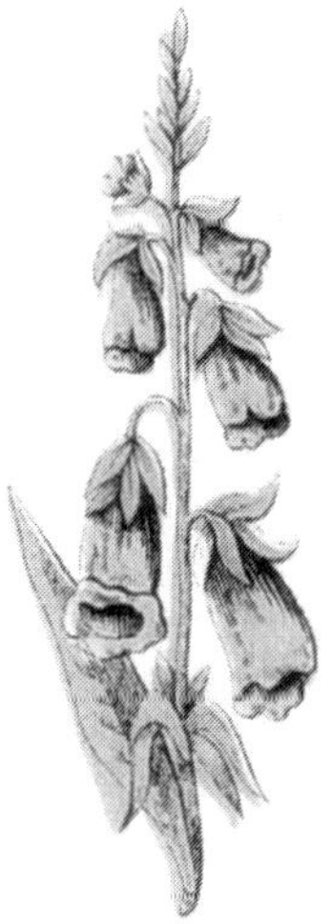

Fox Glove

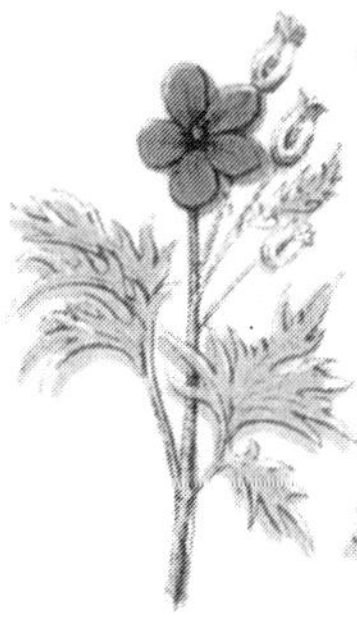

Cranesbill

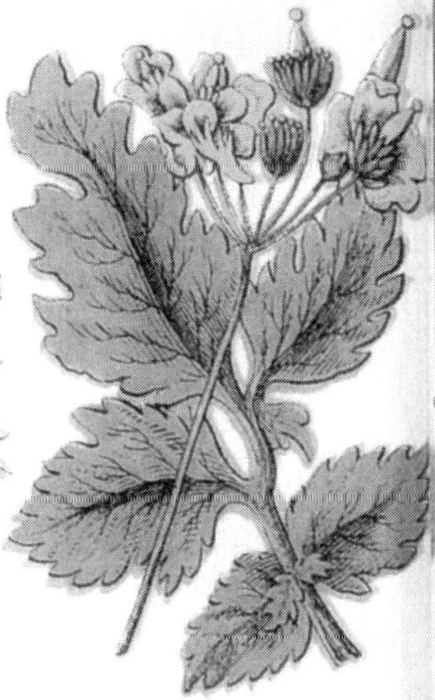

Great Celandine

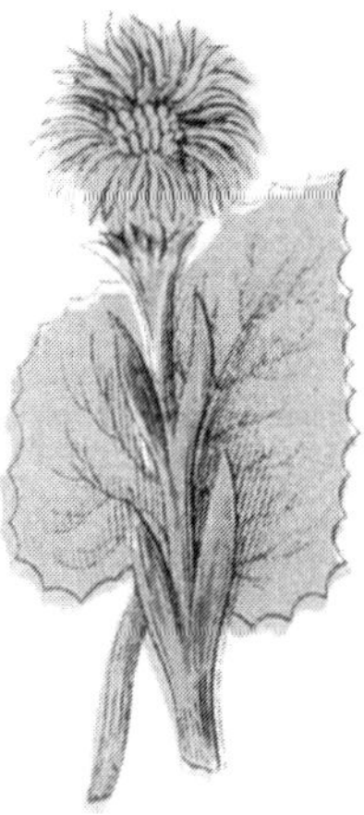

Coltsfoot

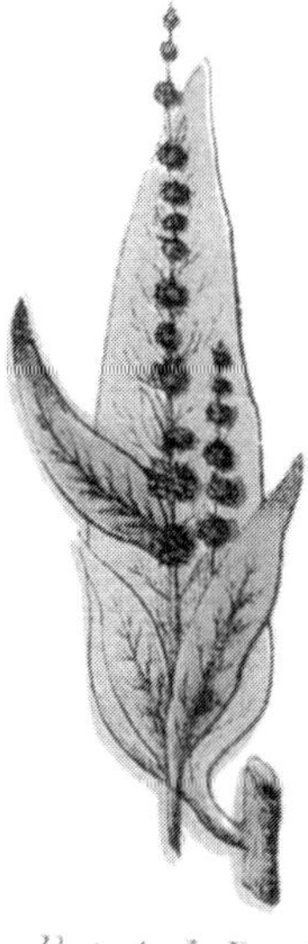

Pointed Dock

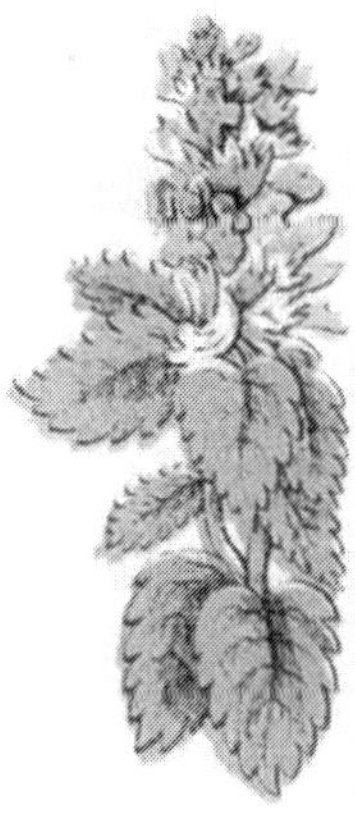

Cat Mint

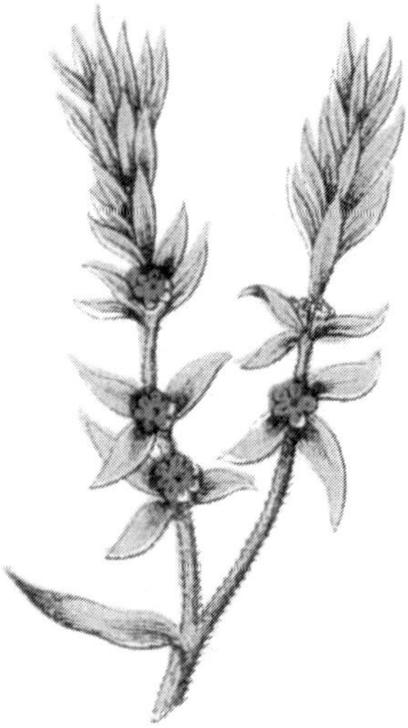

Glasswort

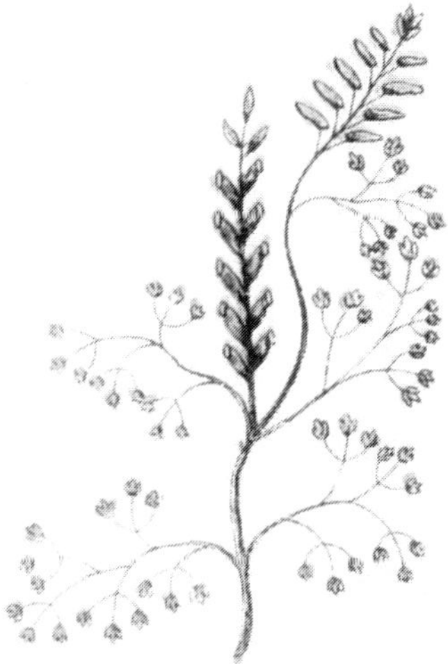

Fumitory

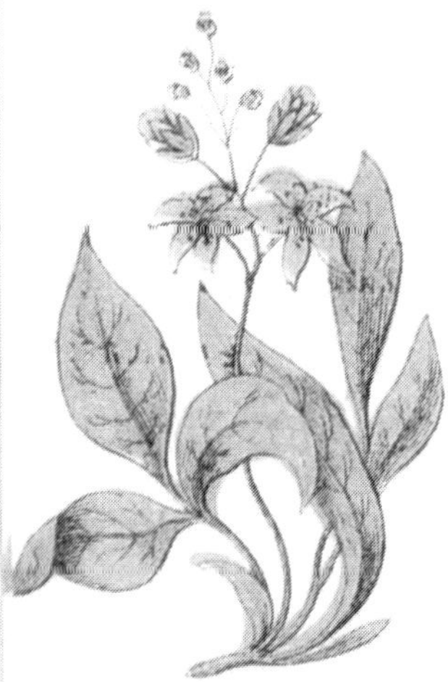

Buckbean

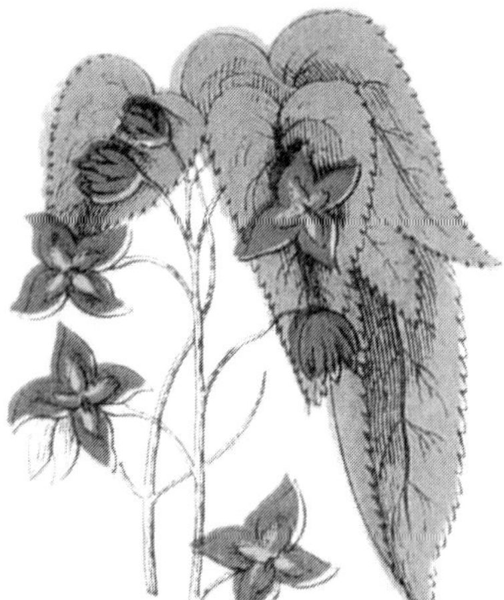

Baren Wort

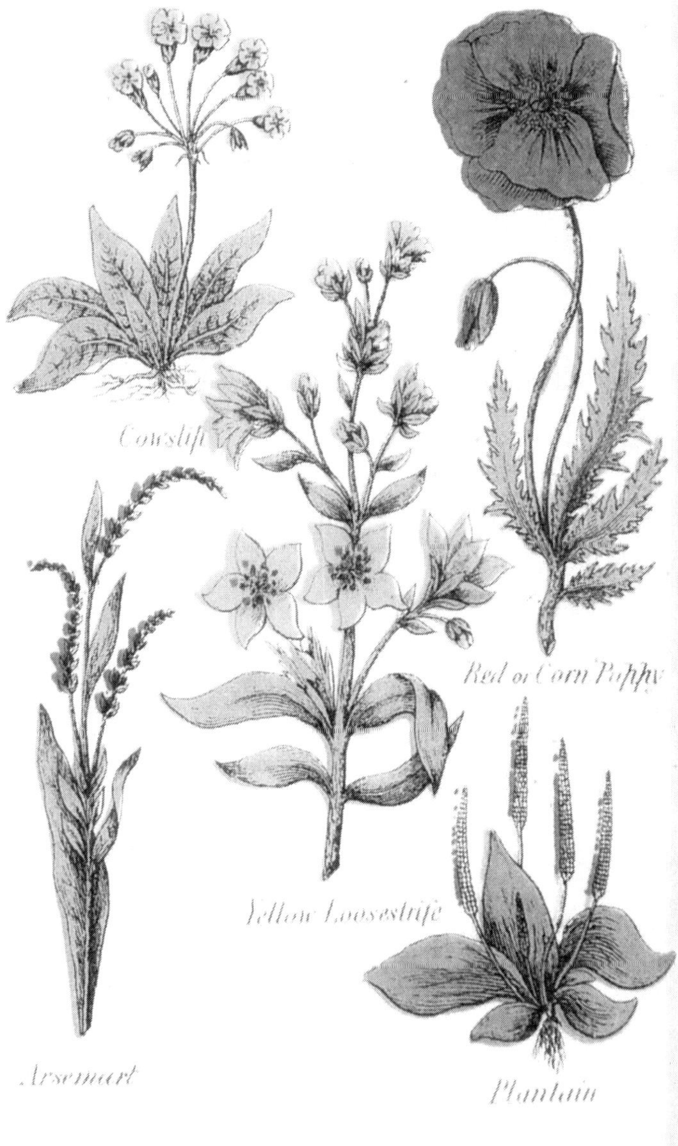
Cowslip
Red or Corn Poppy
Yellow Loosestrife
Arsemart
Plantain

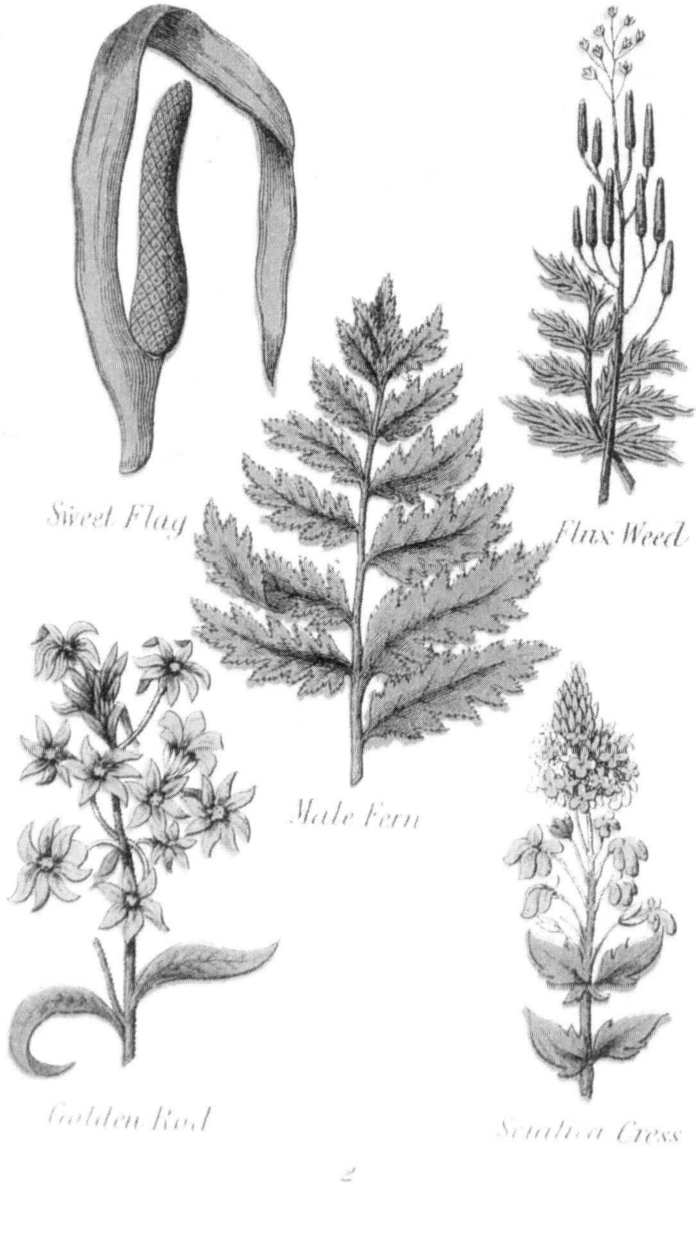
Sweet Flag
Flux Weed
Male Fern
Golden Rod
Sciatica Cress
2

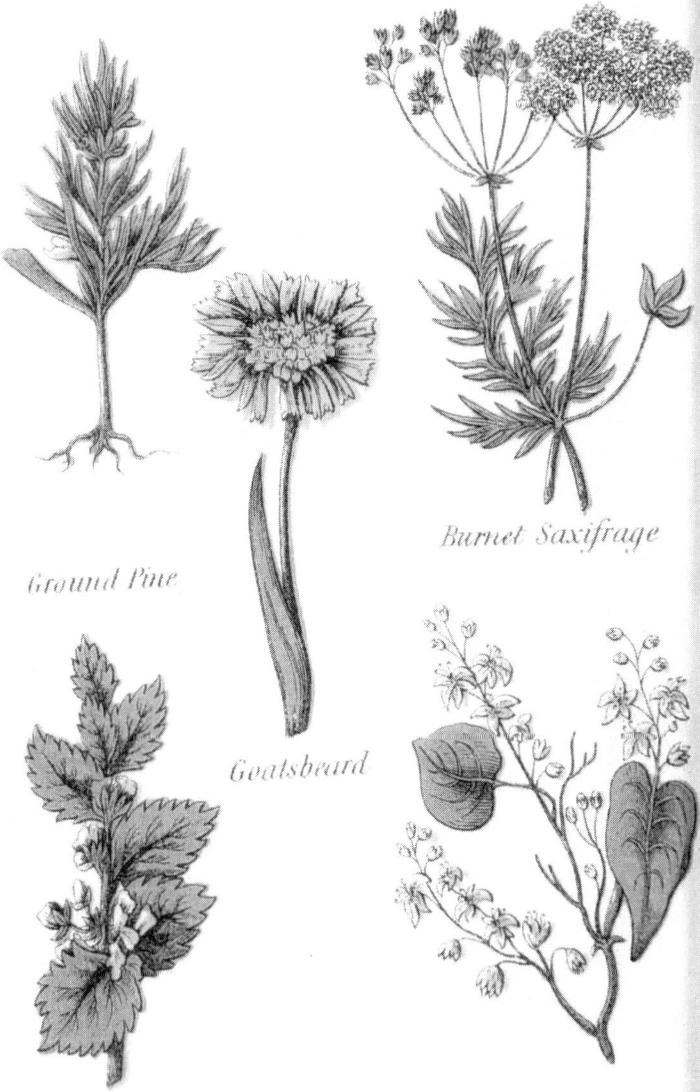
Ground Pine
Burnet Saxifrage
Goatsbeard
White Horehound
Bryony

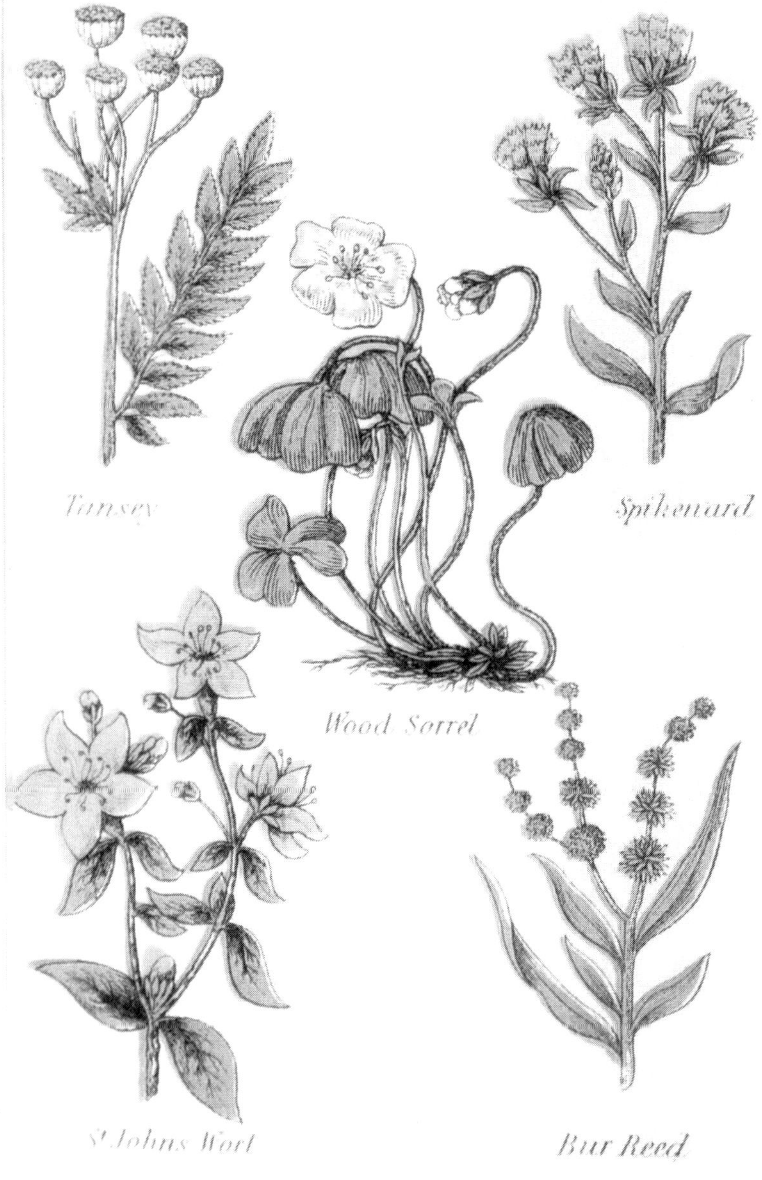
Tansey
Spikenard
Wood Sorrel
St Johns Wort
Bur Reed

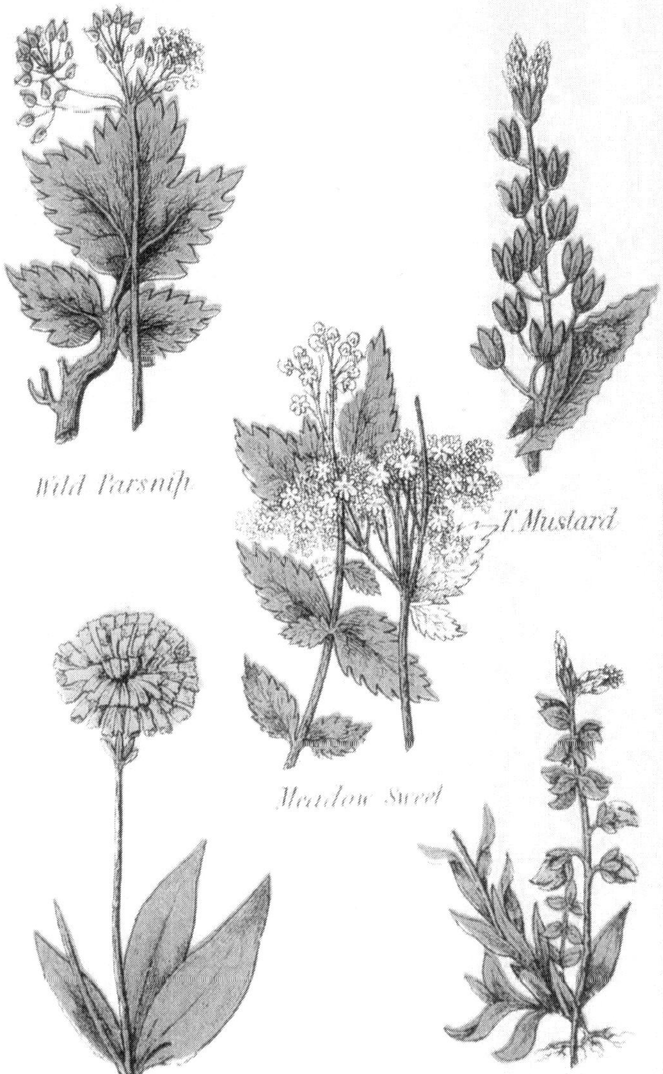
Wild Parsnip
T. Mustard
Meadow Sweet
Mouse Ear
Milk Wort

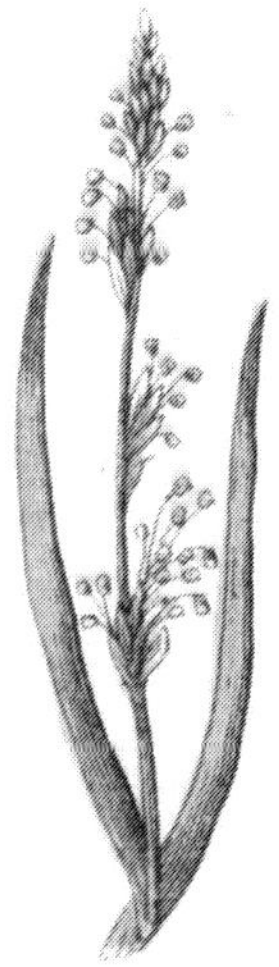

Red Darnel

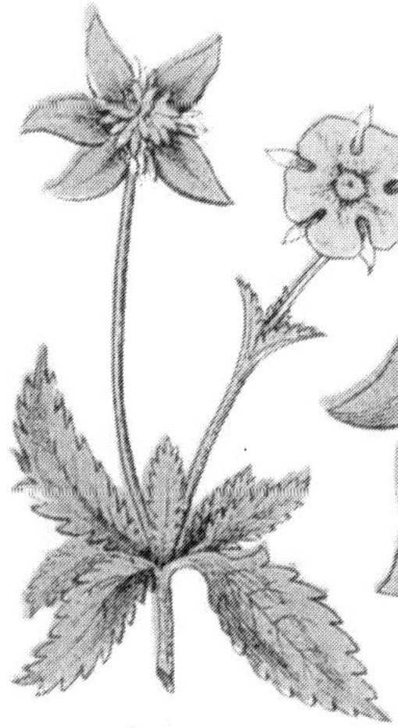

Avens

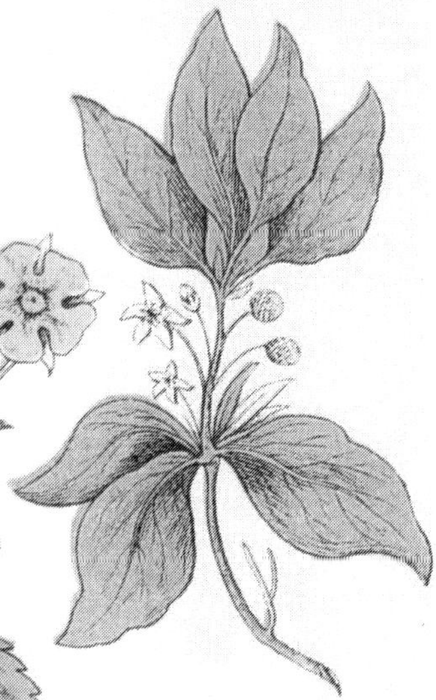

Black Alder

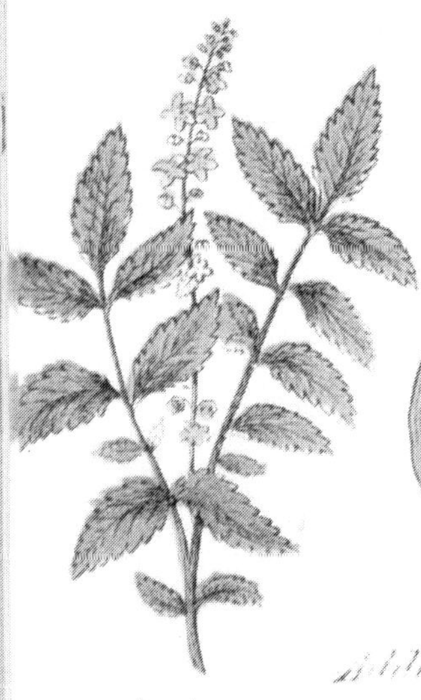

Agrimony

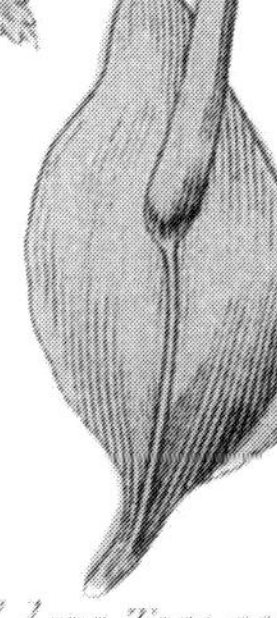

Adders Tongue

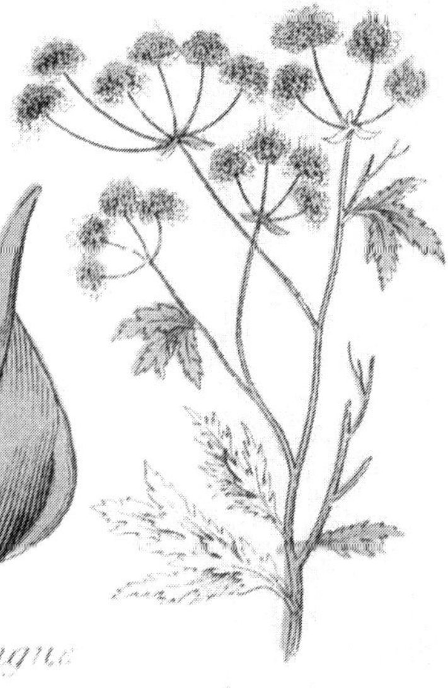

Amomum

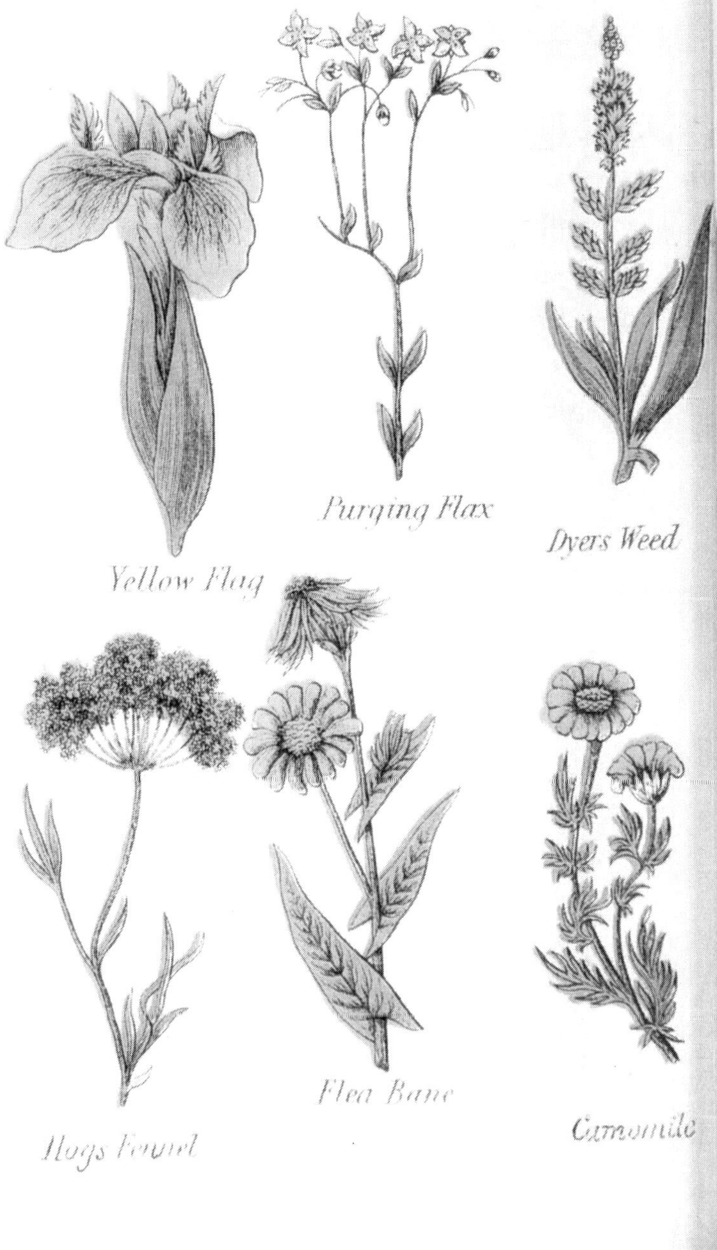
Purging Flax
Dyers Weed
Yellow Flag
Flea Bane
Camomile
Hogs Fennel

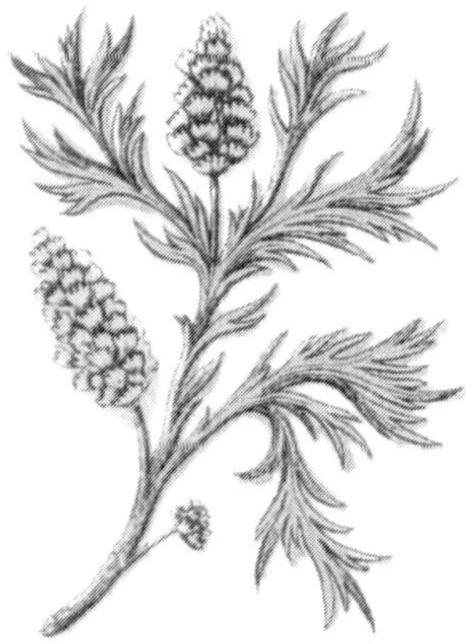

Wart Cress

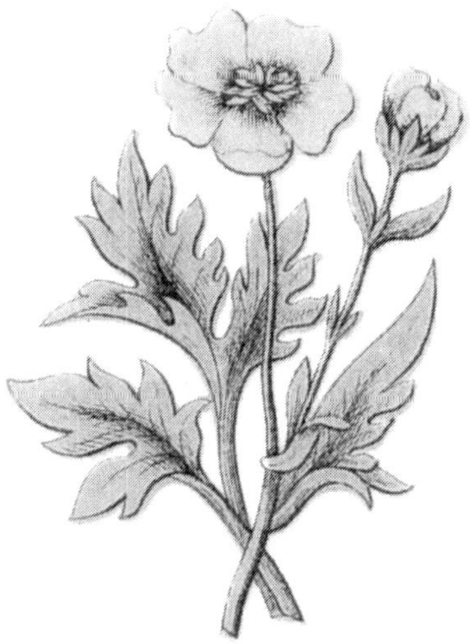

Crowfoot

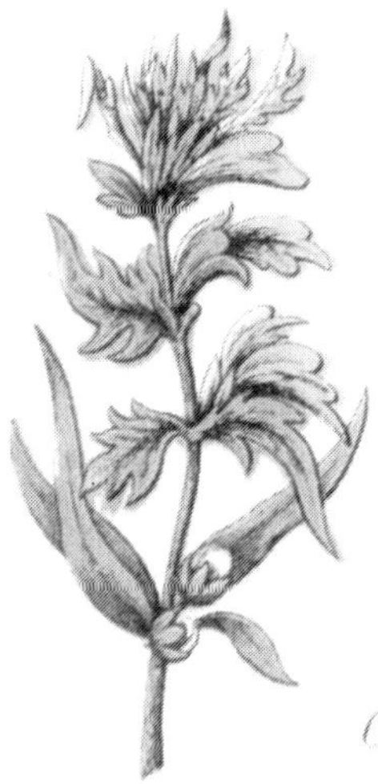

Cow Wheat

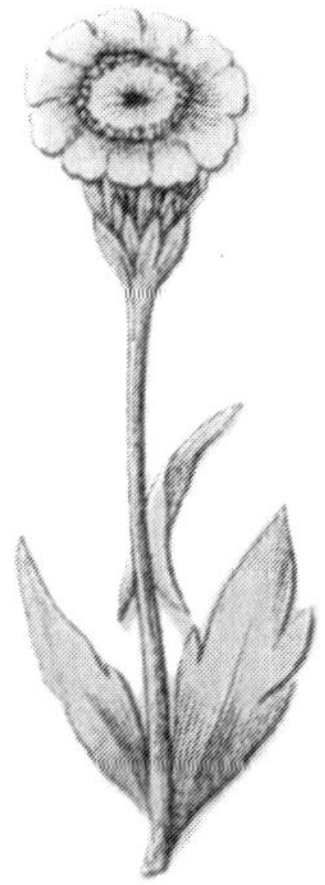

Corn Marygold

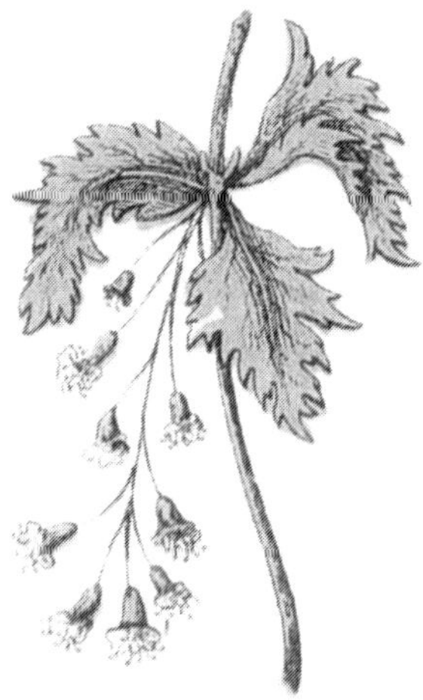

Black Currant

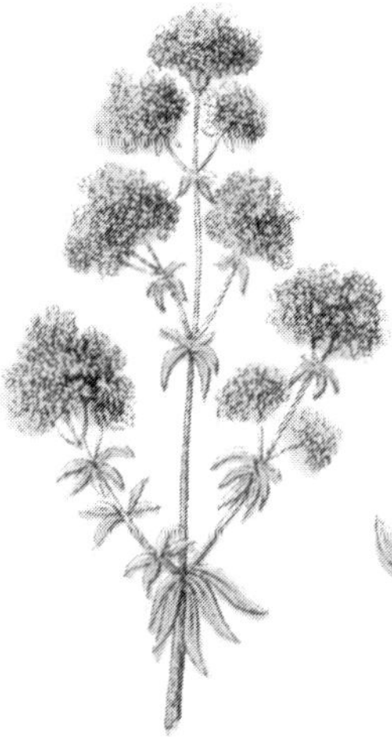

Bedstraw

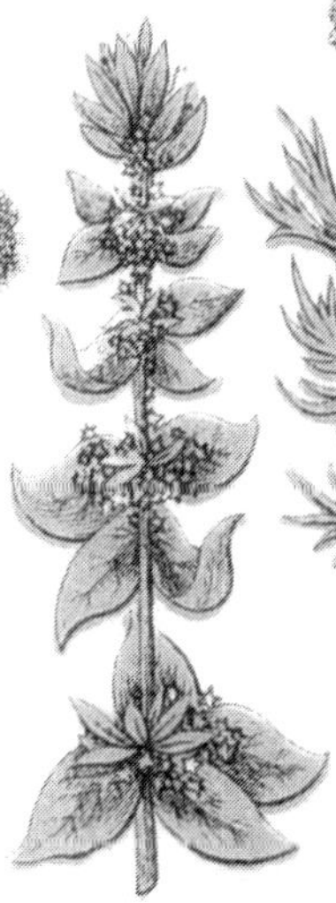

Cross Wort

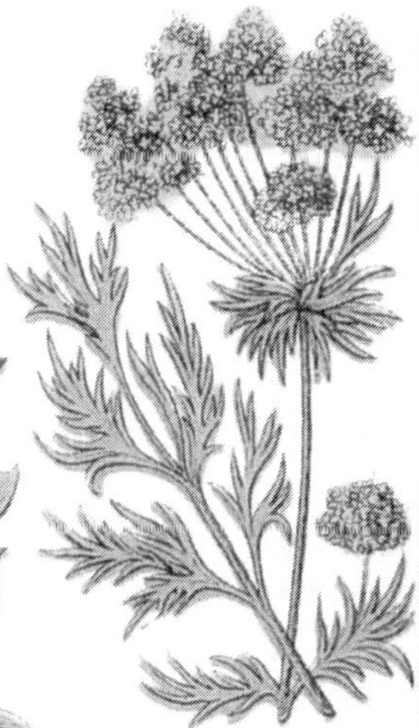

Wild Carrots

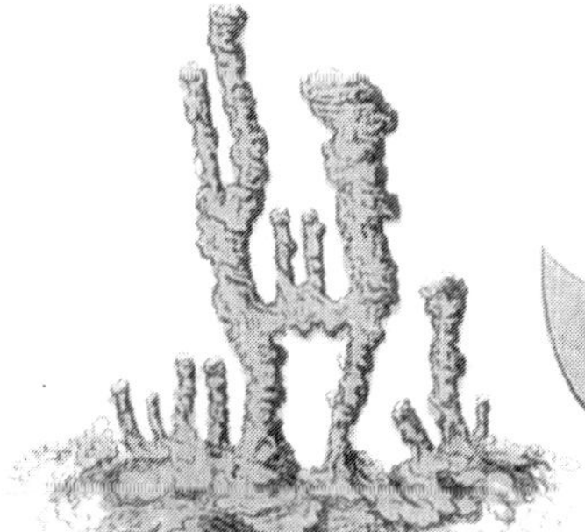

Cup Moss

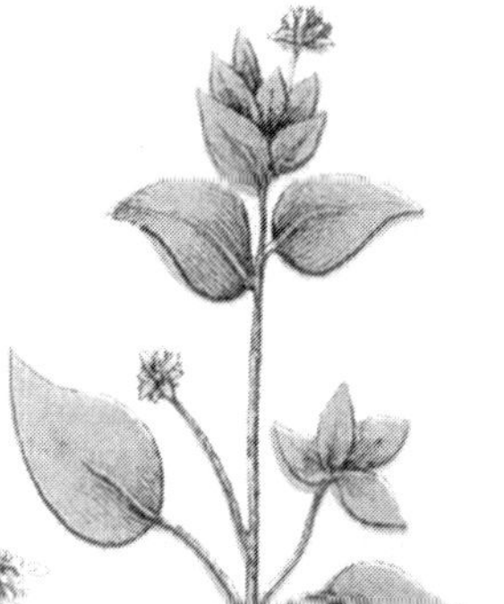

Chickweed

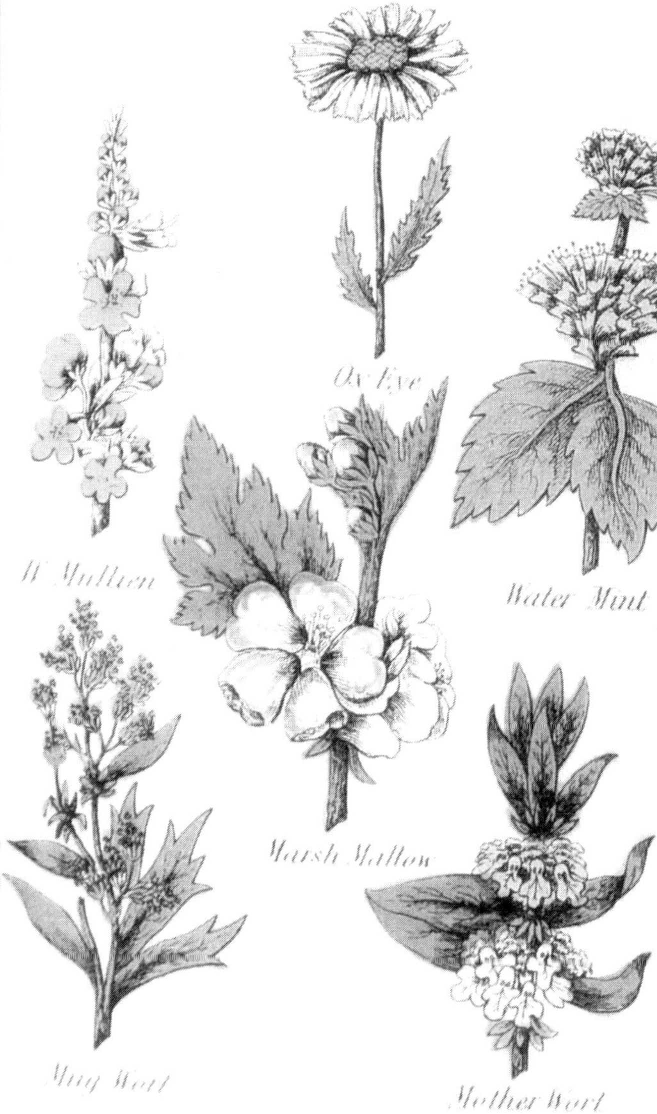
Ox Eye
W. Mullien
Water Mint
Marsh Mallow
Mug Wort
Mother Wort

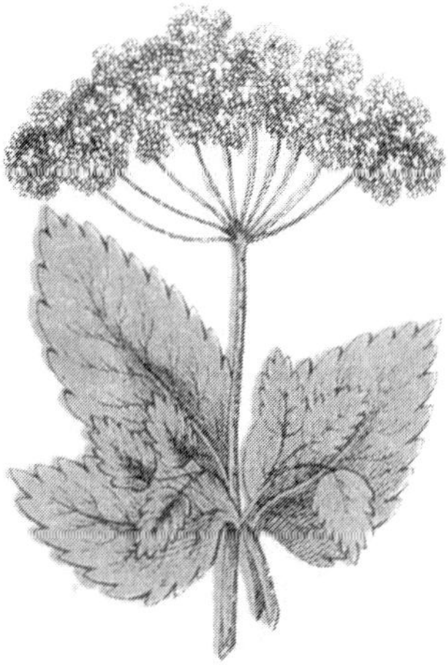

Goutwort

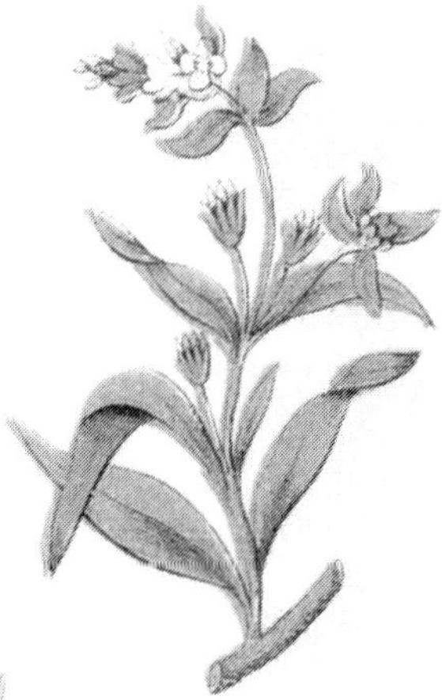

Gromwell.

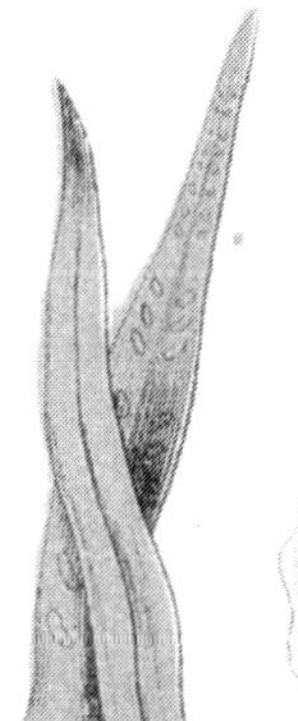

Hartstongue

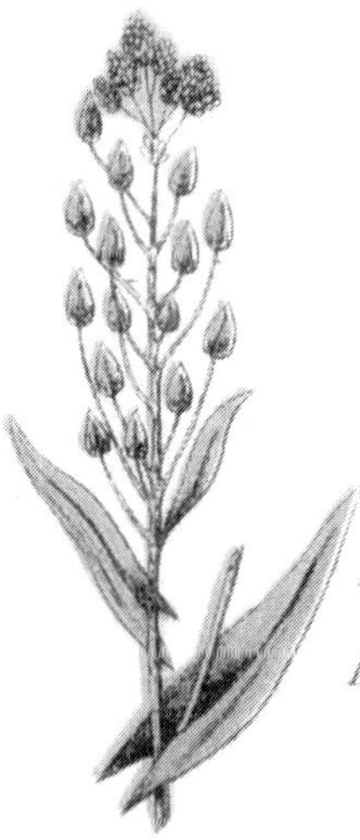

Gold of Pleasure

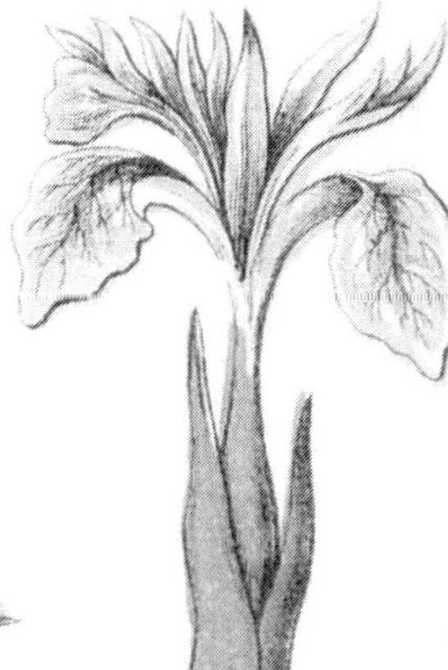

Gladwyn.

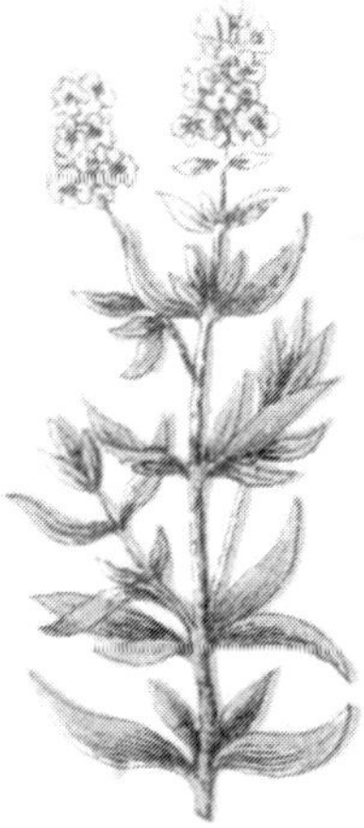

Hyssop

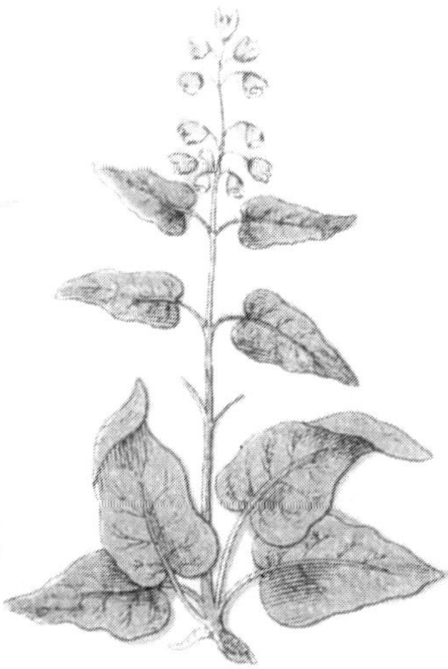

Betoney

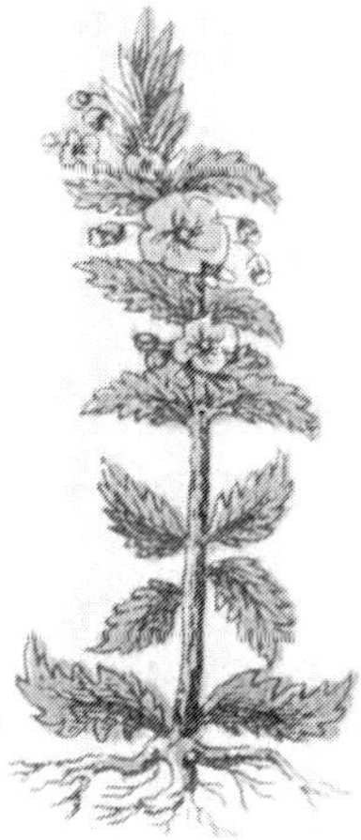

Self Heal

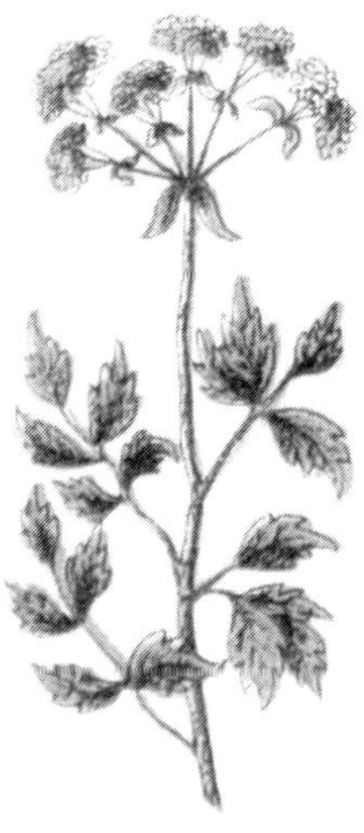

Lovage

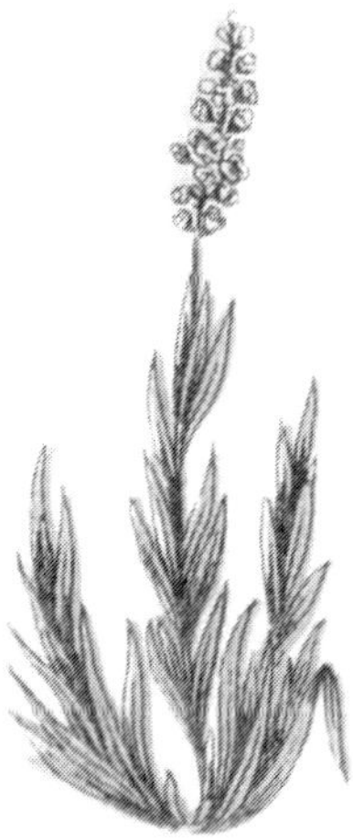

Lavender

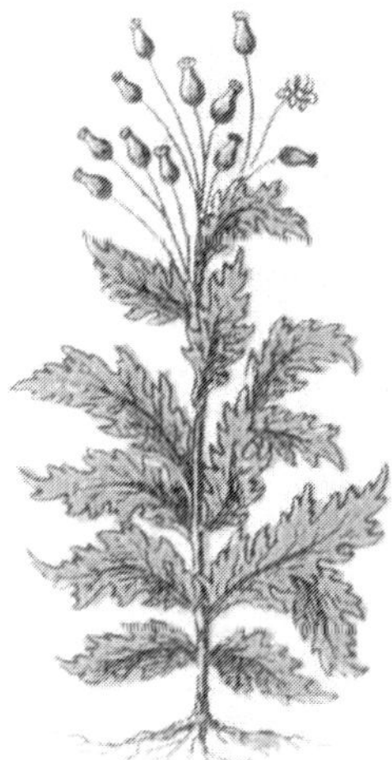

Groundsell

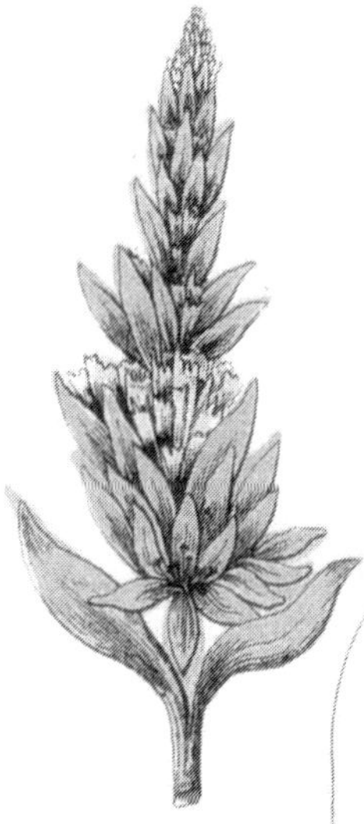

Purple Loosestrife

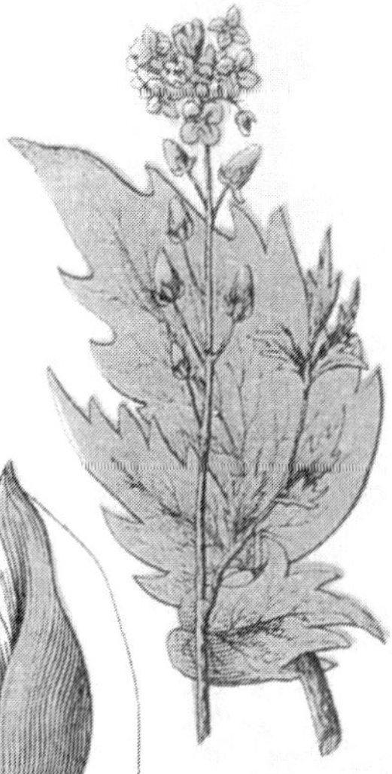

Scurvy Grass

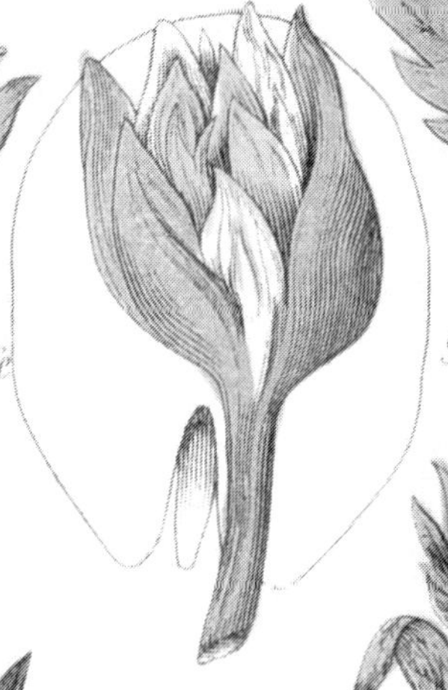

Water Lily

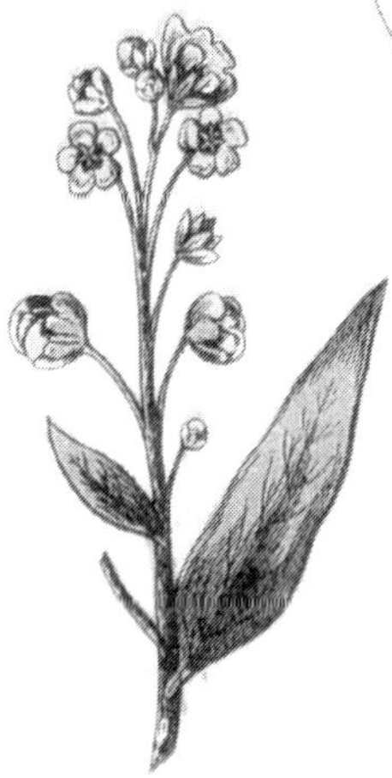

Houndstongue

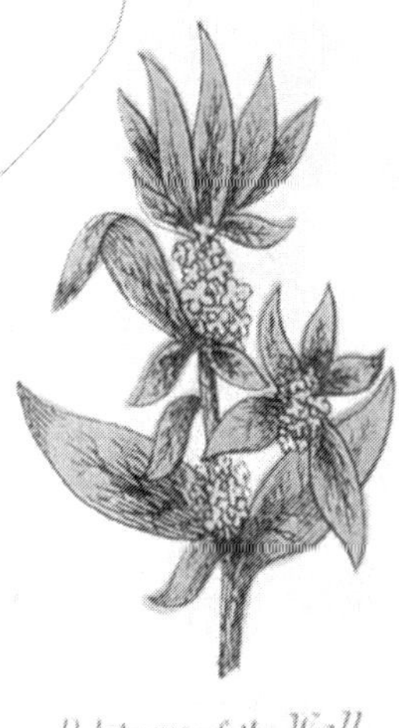

Pelitory of the Wall

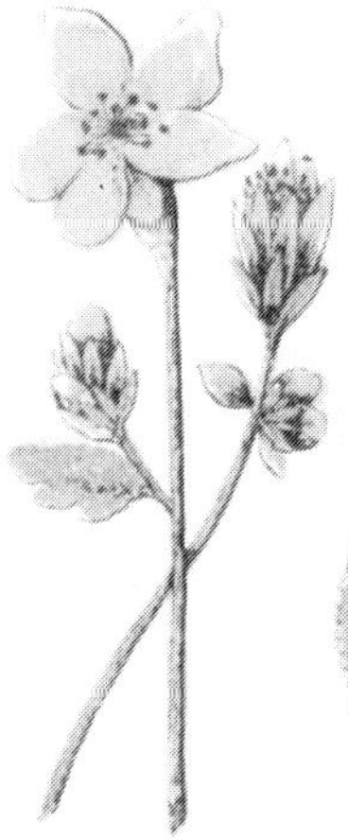

W. Saxifrage

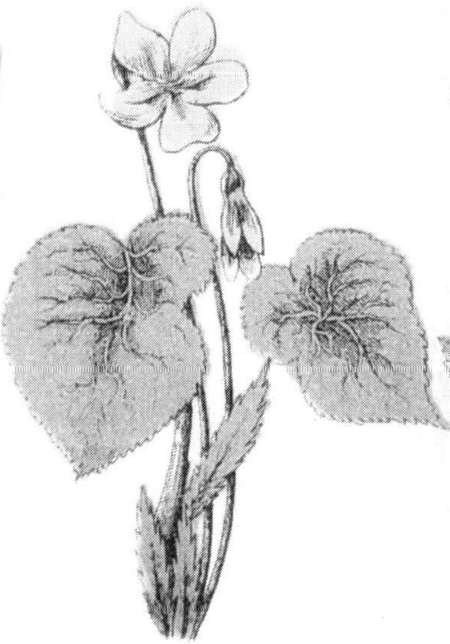

Violet

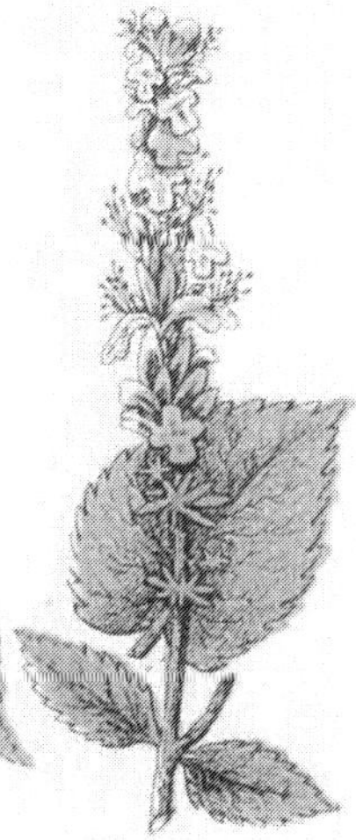

Wood Sage

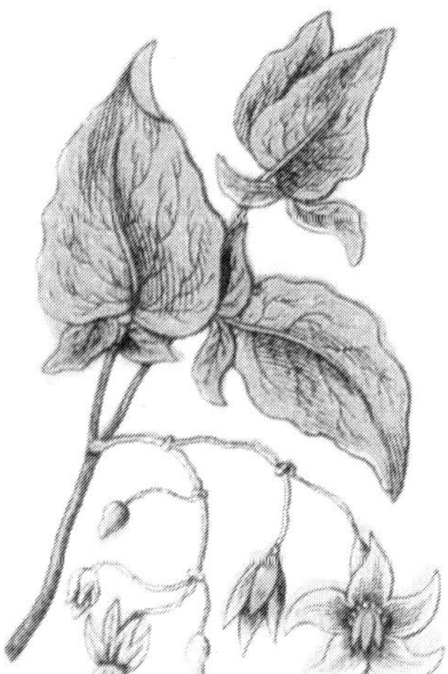

Bitter Sweet

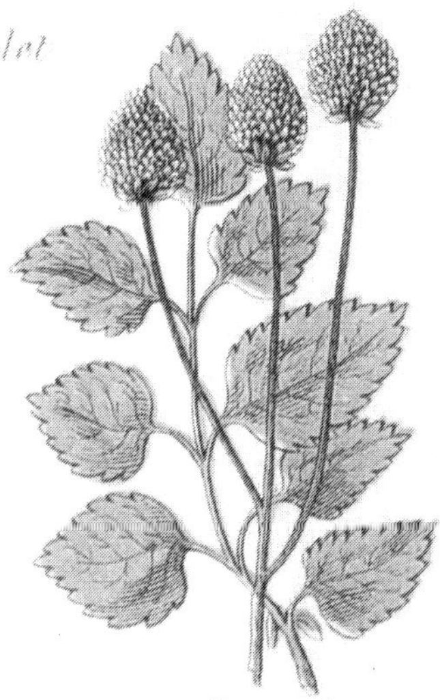

Burnel

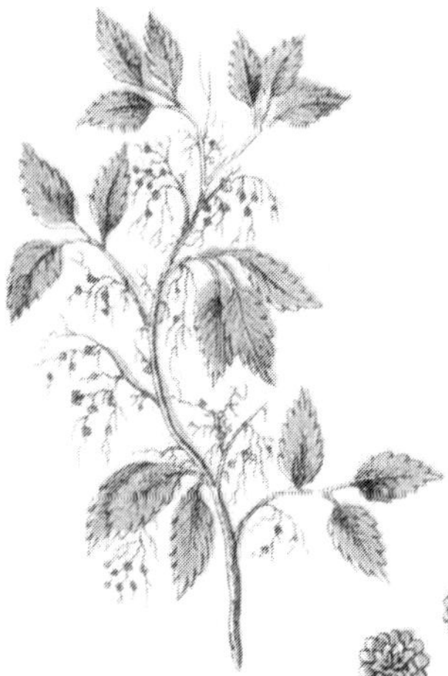

Dodder

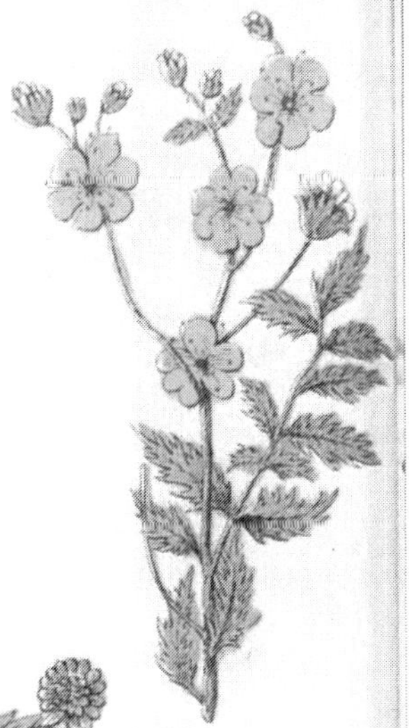

Dropwort

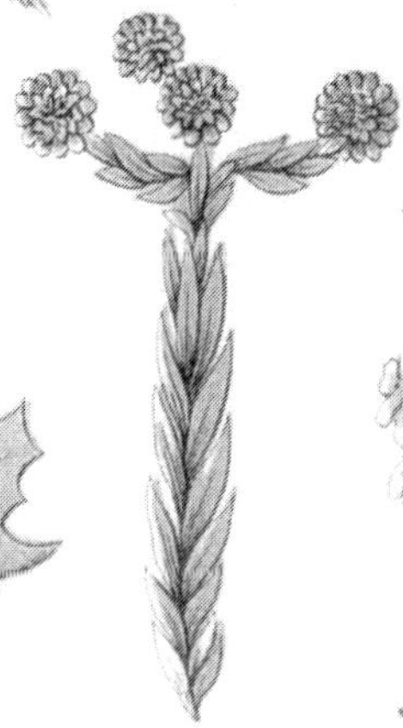

Cudweed

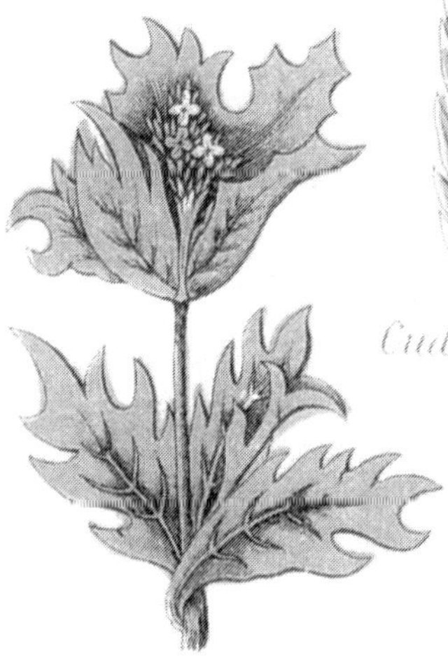

Eringo

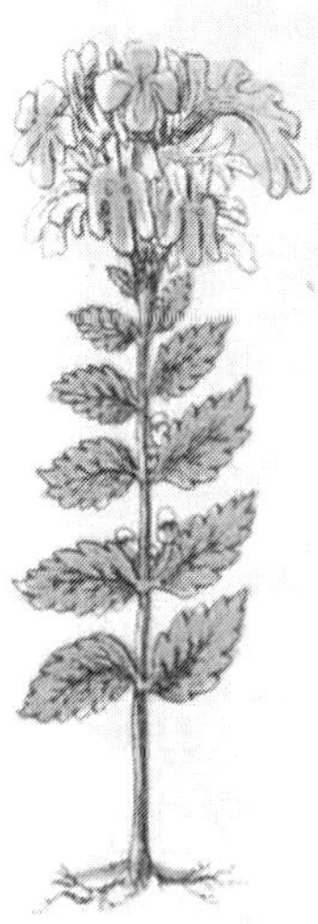

Eye Bright

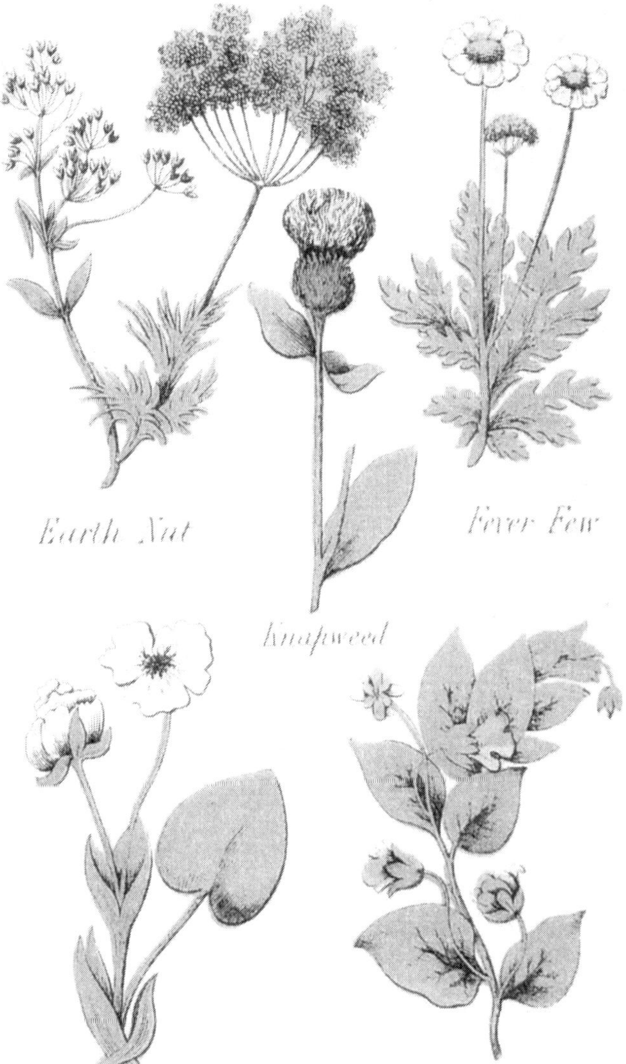
Earth Nut
Knapweed
Fever Few
Frogbit
Fluellin

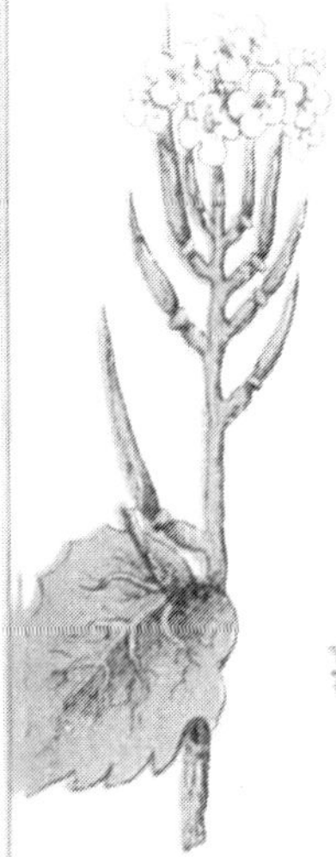

Jack by the Hedge
Or Sauce Alone

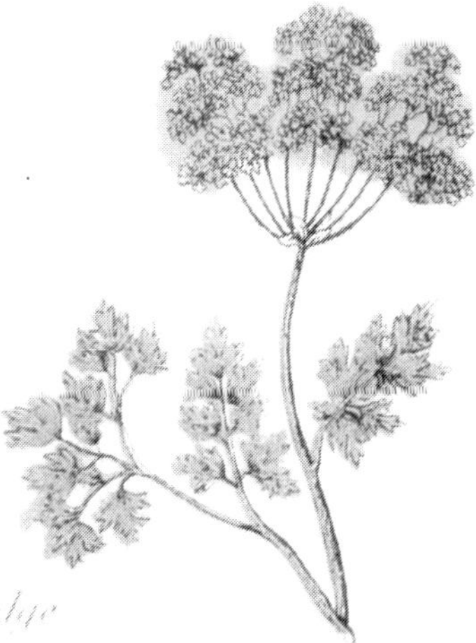

Hemlock

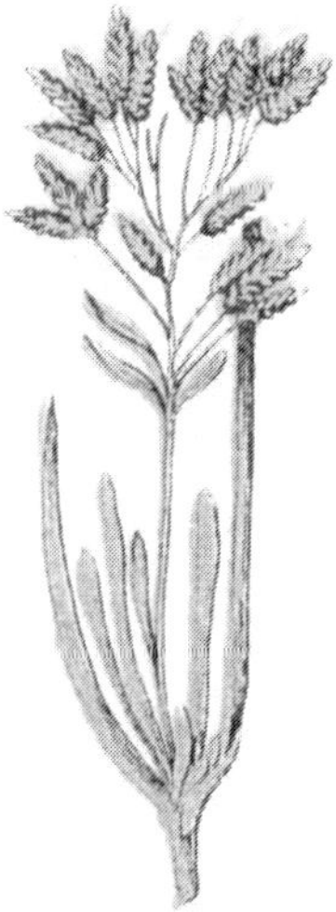

Long Cyperus

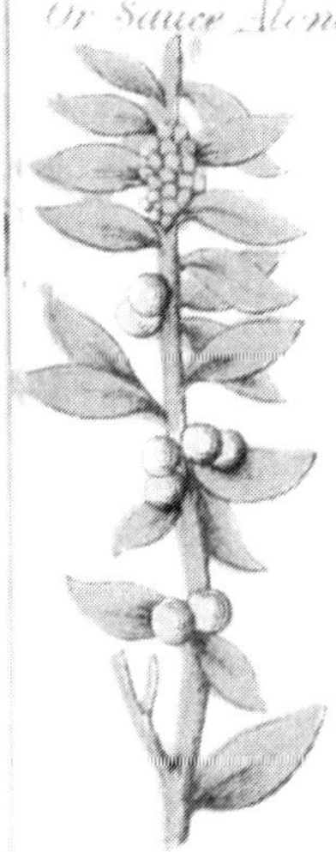

Juniper Shrub

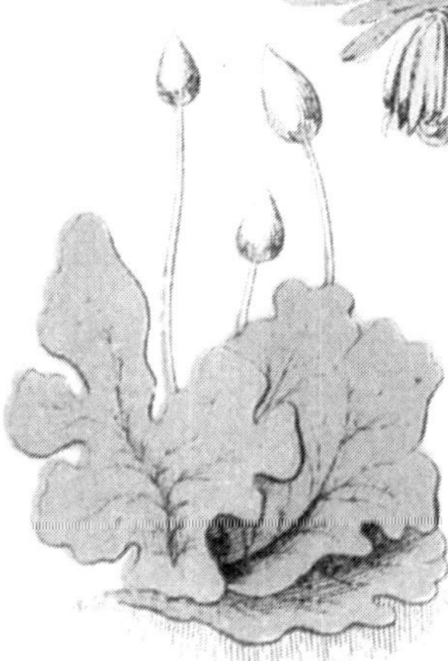

Liver Wort

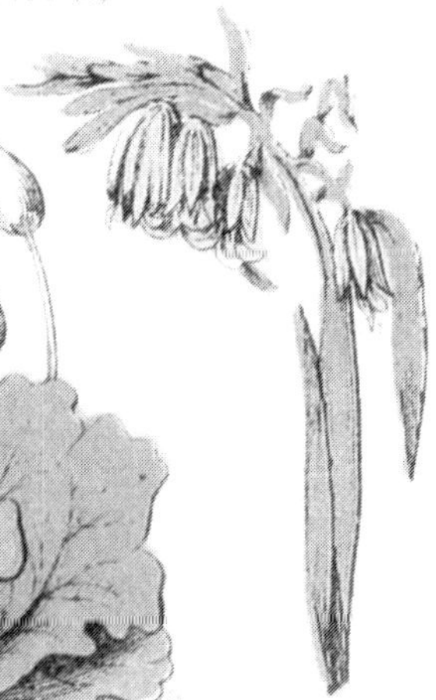

Hyacinth

THE DOCTORS WITHOUT A SYSTEM.

THAT the doctors have no system, is a fact pretty generally acknowledged by themselves: or at least they have none that has been fixed upon as a general rule for their practice. Almost every great man among them has had a system of his own, which has been followed by their adherents, till some other one is brought forth more fashionable. This is undoubtedly a great evil, for it makes every thing uncertain; where it is constantly changing, there can be no dependance on any thing, and the practice must always be experimental; no useful knowledge can be obtained by the young practitioners, as they will be constantly seeking after new theories. What should we say of a carpenter who should undertake to repair a building without having any rule to work by, and should, for the want of one, destroy the half of all he undertook to repair. The employers would soon lose all confidence in him, and dismiss him as an ignorant blockhead. And is it not of infinitely more importance for those who undertake to repair the human body, to have some correct rule to work by. Their practice is founded on visionary theories, which are so uncertain and contradictory that it is impossible to form any correct general rule as a guide to be depended upon. In order to show the opinions of others, as well as my own, I shall make a few extracts from late writers on the subject, —Speaking of the revolutions of medicines, one says:—

"We have now noticed the principle revolutions of medicine: and we plainly perceive that the theory of medicine, not only has been, but is yet in an unsettled state; that its practical application is wavering, fallacious and extremely pernicious: and taking a survey of the various fortunes of the art, we may well say with BACON, that medicine is a science that hath been more professed than laboured, and yet more laboured than advanced; the labour having been in a circle, but not in progression."

"Theories are but the butterflies of the day—they buz for a while and then expire. We can trace, for many centuries past, one theory overturning another, yet each, in its succession, promising itself immortality.

"The application of the rules which the practitioner lays down to himself, is direct, and in their choice, no one can err with impunity. The least erroneous view leads to some consequence. We must remember the lives of our fellow-creatures are at stake. For, how many cruel and premature deaths, how many impaired and debilitated constitutions have paid for the folly of theories? Follies which have proved almost always fascinating. The study of a system is more easy than an investigation of nature; and, in practice, it seems to smooth every difficulty."

"In my lectures on the art of physic, (says Dr. Ring,) both theoretical and practical, I have fully proved that there is no necessity for that bane of the profession, conjecture or hypothesis; and if I were asked whether, if I myself were dangerously ill, I would suffer any hypothetical, however plausible, physician, to prescribe for my malady, my answer would be NO, assuredly NO, unless I wished to risk the loss of my life. I could give a remarkable instance of this."

"*Speculation and hypothesis are* always at variance with *sound experience* and successful *practice.*"

The above extracts evince the pernicious effects of false theory and hypothesis, which, at the present day, constitute nearly the whole art of physic.

The following just remarks are copied from the writings of the Rev. JOHN WESLEY:

As theories increased, simple medicines were more and more disregarded and disused, till in a course of years, the greater part of them were forgotten, at least in the more polite nations. In the room of these, new ones were introduced, by reasoning, speculative men, and those more and most difficult to be applied, as being more remote from common observation. Hence, rules for the application of these, and medical books were immensely multiplied, till at length physic became an abstruce science, quite out of the reach of ordinary men.

Physicians now began to be held in admiration, as persons who were something more than human, and profit attended their employ, as well as honour, so that they had now two weighty reasons for keeping the bulk of mankind at a distance, that they might not pry into the mysteries of their profession. To this end they increased those difficulties by design, which were, in a manner, by accident. They filled their writings with abundance of technical terms, utterly unintelligible to plain men.

"Those who understood only how to restore the sick to health, they branded with the name *Empirics*. They introduced into practice abundance of compound medicines, consisting of so many ingredients, that it was scarce possible for common people to know which it was that wrought the cure—abundance of exotics, neither the nature nor names of which their own countrymen understood."

"The history of the art of medicine, in all ages, (says Dr. Blane,) so teems with the fanciful influences of superstitious observances, the imaginary virtues of medicines, with nugatory, delusive, inefficient, and capricious practices, fallacious and sophistical reasonings, as to render it little more than a chaos of error, a tissue of deceit, unworthy of admission among the useful arts and liberal pursuits of man."

GENERAL REMARKS ON BRITISH HERBS,

FOR DISEASES OF STOMACH AND BOWELS, AND ASSISTING DIGESTION.

Camomile, agrimony, betony, thistle (blessed,) caraway seeds, sweet flag, fennel, garlic, horehound, hyssop, lavender, masterwort (the root,) mint, mustard seed, pennyroyal, horse radish, rue, wormwood.

Decoctions of the above are made by pouring boiling water on them. A little should be taken in the morning fasting.

For purging the Bowels.—Class 1. The powerful are the following: common dock, hellebore (white,) in doses not exceeding four grains; black helebore, from two to five grains; marsh-mallow leaf decoction, and mountain flax.

Class 2. more moderate; buckthorn berry, broom, and dandelion.

For Worms.—Bear's-foot, cowhage, camomile, garlic, fern root, savin, and wormwood.

Astringents, which serve to correct excessive discharges, logwood, red roses, sage, and tormentil root.

Carminatives, or those herbs which allay pain, or dispel wind from the stomach; aniseed, caraway seed, peppermint, spearmint, ginger, and dill root.

Demulcents, or those which are useful in diarrhœa, dysentery, gravel, gonorrhœa, &c.; colt's-foot, liverwort, mallows, liquorice root, wheat, &c.

Diaphoretics, or those which promote perspiration; burdock, centaury, bay tree, betony, balm, germander, lovage, and rue.

Tonics, or those which give strength and vigour to the body; bistort, balm, bog-bean, camomile, centaury (lesser,) logwood, gentian, southernwood, tansy, tormentil, valerian, and wormwood.

To heal Ulcers.—Adder's tongue, agrimony, archangel, arse-smart, cuckow-point, blue bottle, burdock, bryony, soapwort, celandine, centaury, chickweed, cinquefoil, comfrey root, mugwort, cudweed, dog grass, water dock, figwort, flaxweed, foxglove, glasswort, ground ivy, ground pine, tormentil, tansy, bugle, scurvy grass, and nightshade.

Either made into ointments, with hog's-lard, or washes made of them, and daily applied to the parts.

To purify the Blood.—Agrimony, borage, burdock (sea,) chickweed, chervil, fennel, fir tree, fumitory, garden cresses, wild water cresses, ground pine, hops, maiden hair, sorrel, and tansy.

Made into decoctions with hot water, and taken every morning.

NEW BRITISH HERBAL.

ACACIA TREE.

Foreign. Grows in Egypt. We have from it two drugs; the Acacia juice, like liquorice juice, hard and black. Also the Gum Arabic; both astringent, useful in stranguries, and in coughs, hoarseness, &c. Given in solution. An ounce boiled in a quart of barley water, or in powder as an electuary. In diseases of the lungs, kidneys, or intestines, on account of its demulcent properties, it neutralises irritation. Gum Arabic powdered, or in thick solution, is a good application for burns and excoriations, forming a crust over, and protecting the parts from the atmosphere. Combined with powdered resin, it is a good styptic. As diet it is nutricious. The wandering Arabs, sometimes subsist wholly upon it.

ACANTHUS.

It is also called Brank Ursine and Bear's Breech. *Acanthus*, Greek, a thorn; and Latin, *mollis*, soft.

Description. This thistle has many large thick, green leaves upon the ground, with a thick and juicy middle rib. The leaves are parted with deep gashes on the edges; and remain a long time before a stalk appears, three or four feet high, bearing white flowers hooded and gaping, and standing with brownish husks, and a small long undivided leaf under each leaf, It has many thick roots, blackish without, and whitish within, and full of clammy sap. It is a Garden Plant, and flowers in June and July; and it ought to be in every garden.

Medicinal Virtues.—The leaves boiled, and the liquor used as a clyster, beneficially cleanse the bowels, and strengthen the rectum. The decoction is good for the bloody flux. The leaves boiled and applied as a poultice serve to unite broken bones, and strengthen joints that have been dislocated! As a decoction, or as a poultice, the leaves or roots are beneficial in scrofula or king's evil, when the sore is broken. It is a first-rate remedy for burns, drawing out the fire, and heals it without a scar. It is a valuable remedy in hectic fevers, as it restores radical moisture to the consumptive. It has been much used as a diuretic. It is excellent in diseases of the urinary organs, given in the form of powder—that is, from the leaves—from 12 to 40 grains three or our times a day. It is a powerful dissolvent of stones in the kidneys.

ACONITE.

DESCRIPTION.—*Aconitum Napellus.*—There are many poisonous Aconites not used. It is also called *Wolf's Bane*, or *Monk's Hood.* The Purple Monk's hood, formerly called the Purple Helmet-flower, is the most common. It is well known by its purple flowers resembling a Monk's hood. Children and delicate persons should not approach too near it, as even inhaling the scent has sometimes produced sickness and fainting.

MEDICINAL VIRTUES.—The leaves and roots are medicinal. In proper doses they are anodyne, sedative, diuretic, and diaphoretic; and very useful in dropsy, consumption, and enlargement of the heart. The Tincture of Aconite may be procured at the shops, and is a valuable external application for Rheumatism, Lumbago, Neuralgia, &c. *Liniment* as follows; Extract of Aconite, 1 scruple; Soap Liniment, and Compound Camphor Liniment, of each 1 ounce, rubbed into the affected part night and morning, or oftener.

☞ No one should take it inwardly except under the direction of a skilful physician.

ADDER'S TONGUE.

Ophiglossum Vulgatum. It is also called Serpent's Tongue.

DESCRIPTION.—It is a small plant, common in moist meadows, buried among the grass. It has but one leaf, oval, on a stalk a finger's length above the ground, flat, and of a fresh green colour; broad like Water Plantane, but less, without any rib in it. The stalk rises from a root composed of small fibres, about four or five inches high. The spike rises to the same height above it, and the tongue, or seed vessel is notched on each side. The root is perennial. It is to be found only in April or May.

MEDICINAL VIRTUES.—The juice of the leaves drank with distilled water of Horse-tail is good for wounds, and for vomiting, or bleeding at the mouth or nose. It is good for sore eyes. The leaves make an excellent balsam for green and fresh wounds, for old and inveterate ulcers, and for inflammations. It is a fine cooling herb, which gives it rare adaptation as a curative of wounds, &c. Make the ointment as follows;—Two pounds of leaves chopped very fine, put into half a pint of oil and one and a half pound of suit melted together. Boil the whole, (but do not burn it) till the herb is rather crisp; strain off from the leaves, and the liquid will be, when cool, a beautiful and efficacious Ointment. Some Surgeons add a little fine clear turpentine.

AGRIMONY.

Agrimonia Eupatoria.—A plant of the natural order *rosaceæ*, common over all England in the hedge-rows, pastures, and woodsides.

DESCRIPTION.—It has long leaves, dented at edges, green above, and grayish underneath, and a little hairy. The stalk which is strong, round, hairy, and brown, is two or three feet high, with smaller leaves upon it. At the top grow small yellow flowers, one above another, in long spikes, after which come rough heads of seeds, pendant, and which adhere to garments, like burs. The root is black, long, and perennial. It flowers in July and August.

MEDICINAL VIRTUES.—This herb ought to have high reputation on account of its great medicinal qualities. The leaves may be used fresh or dried. It is a famous *vilnerary* herb. The leaves are astringent and aromatic, and therefore very useful in jaundice, diabetes, and incontinence in urine. It is given for a lax tone of the bowels, on account of its astringency, and combined with raspberry leaves, would arrest diarrhœa.

Few herbs have been so efficacious in spitting of blood, bloody urine, and disorders of the liver.

The best method of using it is by infusion, sweetened with a little sugar. It should be taken in the morning fasting, and repeated two or three times during the day. It has been found useful in colic, and in coughs. It cleanses the chest and the lungs. In Ague, the decoction of it taken hot before the fit in time cures the disease. The leaves and seeds infused in wine cure the bloody flux. Made into an ointment, (with Hog's Lard) it cures wounds, sores, ulcers, &c. In liver affections it is very serviceable. By it some very obstinate cases have been cured. It is a most effectual cleanser of the skin, and purifier of the blood, and it is an excellent gargle for sore throats. For diabetes and incontinence of urine, boil in milk. Agrimony tea, with alum and honey is a remedy for tape worms.

Take equal quantities of Agrimony, St. John's Wort, and Camomile flowers, and Wormwood, make into a decoction, and you have a good fomentation, for violent pains, cramps, &c. The plant should be gathered when in bloom, and carefully dried, and hung up in a warm place. *How few know the value of this plant!*

AGRIMONY.—WATER AGRIMONY.

Eupatorium Canabinum. In some countries it is called Water Hemp, Bastard Hemp, and Bastard Agrimony.

DESCRIPTION.—The stalks grow several feet high, of a dark purple colour; the branches are numerous, growing distant from one another. The leaves are winged, and indented. The flowers grow at the top of the branches, of a brown yellow colour, black spotted, having a centre like a daisy. The seeds are long, and adhere to any woollen substance. It is principally found in the north of England, in cold grounds, by ponds and ditches, by running waters, sometimes in the midst of waters. It flowers in July and August, and the seed is soon ripe.

MEDICINAL VIRTUES.—It heals and cleanses cancer, and relieves tough humours of the breast, taken as a decoction. It relieves the dropsy and yellow jaundice, and removes obstructions of the liver, and applied outwardly, mollifies the hardness of the spleen. It is a good remedy for the ague, provokes urine and the terms. As a purge it operates powerfully, yet safely, and dropsies are said to have been cured by it. It strengthens the lungs, and is an excellent vermifuge. Farmers give it to cattle troubled with cough, or broken winded.

ALDER TREE ;—COMMON

DESCRIPTION.—*Alnus Glutinosa Vulgatus.* The common Alder-tree is well known. Its stem is tree-like and full of branches ; the bark is rough, of a dark brown colour, and irregularly blotched with white, having large round leaves irregularly notched on the edges and clammy to the touch, especially while young. Its flowers are white, and the berries are black. It grows in hedges, moist woods, and watery places. It flowers in April or May and the seed is ripe in September.

MEDICINAL VIRTUES.—The decoction, or distilled water of the leaves, is good for burns and inflammations. And especially for inflammation in the breast. An infusion of the inner green bark of the trunk in wine, or of the expressed juice of the berries in the dose of half an ounce, is said to purge moderately, and in small doses prove an efficacious deobstruent, promoting all the fluid secretions. The decoction, as thick as treacle nearly, makes a good pill for indigestion, impetigo, or pustular eruption. A strong decoction is recommended. The fresh leaves laid upon swellings dissolve them, and stay the inflammation. The leaves put under the bare feet galled with travelling, greatly refresh them. The leaves with morning dew on them, and brought into a chamber troubled with fleas, will gather them, which being suddenly cast out, will rid the chamber of them.

ALDER TREE ;—BLACK.

Alnus Glutinosa. It is also called the berry-bearing Alder.

DESCRIPTION. The Alder is often confounded with the Elder. The Alder is more like a shrub than a tree, and it seldom grows to a great size. The branches are smooth, slender, numerous, of a dark brown or purple colour. The inner bark next the wood is yellow, which when infused, produces a saffron colour. The leaves resemble those of the ordinary Alder-tree, or the Female Cornet, or Dog-berry-tree. The flowers are white, with leaves at the joints, which produce small round berries, first green, and blackish when ripe. It grows plentifully in some woods. It flowers in May, and the fruit is ripe in September.

MEDICINAL VIRTUES.—The inner yellow bark decocted is useful in billious affections, and the dropsy. The bark boiled with Agrimony, Wormwood, and Fennel, and taken every morning, is very effectual against jaundice and dropsy, a decoction of the dried bark removes obstruction of the liver and spleen, and removes the hardness of the former. The outward bark is astringent, and is useful in Fluxes. The outward bark boiled in vinegar kills lice, cures the itch, and removes scabs. It is a good wash for the teeth, easing tooth-ache and fastening loose teeth. As a decoction it is an excellent drink in the beginning of spring. On account of its purifying and exhilarating qualities, it ought to be esteemed as a jewel.

ALKANET.

Anchusa Officinalis. It is also called Orchanet, and Spanish Bugloss.

DESCRIPTION.—It has a large thick root, of a reddish colour, long, narrow, hairy leaves, green like the leaves of Bugloss, which lie very thick upon the ground. The stalks are thick with leaves. The flowers are small, hollow, and of a reddish colour. The plant grows in Kent, Devonshire and Cornwall.

MEDICINAL VIRTUES.—It is serviceable in old ulcers, inflammations, burns, and St. Anthony's fire. The best way is to make it into an ointment; or make a vinegar of it, as you make a vinegar of roses. It is useful in the yellow jaundice, spleen, and gravel. Dioscorides saith, it cures venomous bites, whether it be taken inwardly, or applied to the wound. It stays the flux, and kills worms. Its decoction made in wine, strengthens the back, and removes its pains. It is good for bruises and falls, and to drive out the small pox and measles. Made into an ointment, it is excellent for green wounds, punctures, &c.

ALL-HEAL

It is also called Wound Wort, Panay, Opopane Wort, Latin, *Stachys Sylvatica.*

DESCRIPTION. – It grows in wet grounds, has long hairy leaves, each leaf has five or six pairs of winged leaves, almost like ash-tree leaves set one against the other upon foot stalks, broad at the base, and narrow at the end. The leaves have a strong smell and a bitterish taste. The flowers, which are yellow, stand in clusters round the stalks at the joints, and they bear light yellow flat seeds, bitter in taste. The root is perennial, long, thick, of a hot biting taste. It flowers in Autumn, and soon sheds its seeds.

MEDICINAL VIRTUES.—As its name imports, it is a good wound herb; the leaves being bruised and applied to a new wound; they stop the bleeding and cure the wound. It relieves gout, cramp, and pains in the joints, vertigo, falling sickness. Made into an ointment it cures the itch.

ALMONDS.

Foreign.—The Essential Oil of *Bitter Almonds* is used for flavouring Custards; but on account of its poisonous nature great care ought to be exercised. *Sweet Almonds* are emollient and demulcent; and an emulsion of them is useful in bronchial diseases, in tickling coughs, hoarseness, dysentery, and affections of the urinary organs, often decreasing the acrimony of the secretions in a remarkable manner.

ALOE.

Foreign.—The juice which resolves itself into a very bitter resin is used in medicine as a stimulant cathartic, acting chiefly on the lower bowels; it is a tonic when taken in small doses. —There are three kinds of Aloes, Socotrine, or Cape, Barbadoes, and Hepatic. The former is the best, being the mildest in its effects. For indigestion, lowness of spirits, and jaundice, aloes are serviceable, as they stimulate action on the rectum; and also on the uterus; therefore must not be prescribed in piles, nor in pregnancy. Pills are the best form for taking it. It is best to combine them with other purgatives to prevent after constipation. As they act on the colon and rectum, they expel ascarides, or seat worms. Dose from 3 to 10 grains, if taken alone.

AMARANTHUS.

Amaranthus Blitum. It is also called Flower Gentle, Flower Velure, Floramor and Velvet Flower.

DESCRIPTION.—It is a garden flower, well known. It grows from one to two feet high, streaked, and red towards the root, but very smooth, divided towards the top with small branches, among which stand long broad leaves of a reddish green colour, slippery; the flowers are not properly flowers, but tufts, very beautiful, but of no smell, of a reddish colour; if bruised they yield juice of the same colour; being gathered they keep their beauty a long time; the seed is of a shining black colour. They flower from August till the frost nips them.

MEDICINAL VIRTUES.—There are several kinds of the Amaranthus; but that used in medicine is the large one with the drooping purple spike. The flowers dried and powdered are used as a styptic, arresting the profusion of Menses, diarrhoea, bleeding at the nose. &c. One species bears a white flower, which stops the whites and cleanses and strengthens the kidneys.

ANEMONE.

Called also Wind Flower, because, they say the flowers never open but when the wind bloweth. The seed also flies away with the wind.

DESCRIPTION.—It has a perennial thick root, full of knobs, very acrid to the taste. Its leaves are supported on long leaf stalks, which are divided into three parts, each of which support a number of pointed and jagged segments, having a round slender and purple stem, six or eight inches high, with three leaves surrounding it near the top. The flowers are large and white, with more or less of a purple tinge, which stand on tender foot stalks, which rise from the centre of the leaves, surrounding the stem. It is found in woods, and by hedges; but it is mostly cultivated in gardens where its colours are more beautiful and various. It flowers early in the spring.

Medicinal Virtues.—The leaves provoke the terms, when taken as a decoction. Bathing the body with it cures leprosy. The leaves being stamped, and the juice snuffed up the nose, purge the head. Being made into an ointment, and the eye-lids anointed with it, it is good for inflammations of the eyes, and other diseases peculiar to them. amaurosis, cataract, and opacity of the cornea.

ANGELICA.

Description.—*Angelica Archangelica*, a plant of the natural order *Umbelliferæ* or *Apiaceræ*. It is a large beautiful plant cultivated in gardens, and it grows wild in some parts. It grows eight feet high, the stalks are strong, and divided into branches. The leaves are large, each of which is composed of many smaller, set upon a divided pedicle. They are notched at the edges, and of a bright green. The flowers are small and white, but in large tufts of a globose form. Two seeds follow each flower, which seeds are flat on one side, on the other convex, and marked with three furrows. It flowers in July, and the seeds are ripe in September.

Medicinal Virtues.—The stalks, leaves, and seeds possess stimulant, carminative, and tonic properties, which are strongest in the latter. It has a pungent taste, and an agreeable aromatic odour. The whole plant has the same virtues. It is cordial and sudorific, and has always been reckoned good against pestilential and contagious diseases. The root is valuable; but the best roots come from Spain. Water distilled from the root removes flatulent pains, and pains arising from cold. This water with some of the powdered root is good in the pleurisy, diseases of the lungs and breast, as coughs, shortness of breath, and a syrup of the stalks has the same effects. It is good in the colic, stranguary, and stoppage of urine, and removes obstructions of the liver and spleen. The juice dropped into the eyes removes dimness of sight; and into the ears, deafness. Also some have found relief in tooth-ache by applying the juice. The juice or the root powdered, cleanses sores and ulcers, and the distilled water eases gout, sciatica, rheumatism.

Dose, of the *powdered root* from 10 to 20 grains.—*Distilled water*, 1 ounce.—*Extract* from 5 to 15 grains.—*Infusion*, a tablespoonful or more.—*Tincture*, a drachm.—*Spirits*, from half a drachm to 3 drachms.

Angelica Cordial.—A small handful of the Angelica stems, from which strip the leaves, and pick out the threads; then cut them into little pieces. To a pound put 12 pints of brandy, or more, two drachms of cinnamon, and one of mace, with 12 cloves; dissolve 4 pounds of sugar in 6 pints of water, and mix the whole in a jar that must be well corked, to stand for about 6 weeks; then filter it, and bottle for use. It is most serviceable in windy complaints.

ANISEEDS.

Foreign.—Aniseeds are produced by a small plant growing on the island of Malta and elsewhere. They possess stimulant and carminative properties, useful in indigestion, flatulency, and colic. Dose of bruised or powdered seeds 10 to 30 grains, infused in distilled water, a wine-glassful;—compound spirit 1 to 4 drachms, essential oil 4 to 20 drops, on sugar.

ARCHANGEL, RED, WHITE, AND YELLOW.

Description. *Lamium, Album, Flavus, Rubeus.* Called also Dead Nettle, and Bee Nettle. It grows about hedges, about a foot high, and its leaves are shaped like those of the nettle, but they do not sting. The stalk is square, and the leaves are hairy. In the White Archangel, the flowers are white and large; they stand at the joints, where the leaves issue and are very pretty. The leaves are in pairs. The Red Archangel has, of course, flowers of a pale reddish colour, The Yellow plant is like the others in the stalks and leaves;

except the stalks are rather more straight and erect, and the joints with leaves are farther asunder and the flowers a little larger, of a good yellow colour in some, and rather paler in others. They flower from the beginning of the spring and throughout the summer.

Medicinal Virtues.—The Archangels are used with great success in removing the hardness of the spleen or milt, which is supposed to be the seat of melancholy, &c. A decoction is to be made with wine, and the herb applied hot to the region of the spleen, as a plaster; or foment with the decoction. The flowers of the White Archangel are preserved or conserved, and used to stay the whites, and the decoction is good for floodings, bleeding at the nose, and spitting of blood, or any kind of hæmorrhage. It is an exhilarating herb, driving away melancholy, and it makes the heart merry. Bruised and mixed with salt, vinegar, and lard, and applied to hard tumours, swellings, or king's evil, it is of great service, it also gives ease to the gout, sciatica, and other pains of the joints and sinews. It is very effectual in the healing of green wounds, bruises and burns. The Yellow Archangel is the most effectual for old sores and ulcers, though they have become hollow; and to dissolve tumours.

ARRACH, WILD AND STINKING.

Called also Dog's Arrach, Goat's Arrach, and stinking Motherwort.

Description.—It has small and roundish leaves, of a dusky mealy colour, growing on slender stalks that spread on the ground, with small flowers in clusters set with the leaves, which leave small seeds. It is an annual, and smells like rotten fish, or something worse. It usually grows upon dunghills, and flowers in June and July, and the seed is soon ripe afterwards.

Medicinal Virtues.—Stinking Arrach is a valuable medicine for diseases of the womb, especially those which produce hard labour in child-birth; for it cleanses and strengthens the womb, and cures barrenness. It promotes and moderates the menses. In these respects it is very valuable. The best way of using it is to make it into a syrup, by sugar or honey.

ARRACH, GARDEN.

It is also called Orach and Arage, and it is cultivated for domestic use.

Description.—It is well known to every housewife. It is an annual, and is grown in the garden as a vegetable. It flowers from June till August.

Medicinal Virtues.—Eaten as a vegetable, it is laxative and healing to the bowels. If bruised, and applied to the throat, is good for swellings in the throat. The best way is to boil it to drink the decoction and then apply the herb outwardly. It is also excellent for the jaundice.

ARSESMART.

Description.—*Polygonum Hydropiper.*—The hot Arsesmart is also called Water-pepper, or Culrage. The mild Arsesmart is called dead Arsesmart, Persicaria, or Peach-wort, because the leaves are like the leaves of a Peach-tree; it is also called Plumbago.

It has broad leaves set at the great red joint of the stalks, with semi-circular blackish marks on them, either bluish or whitish, with such like seed following. The root is long, with many strings. It has no sharp taste (as another sort hath, which is quick and biting) but rather sour like sorrel, or else a little drying, or without taste. It groweth in watery places, ditches, and the like, which are for the most part dry in Summer. It flowereth in June, and the seed is ripe in August.

Medicinal Virtues.—It possesses great virtues. It is of a cooling nature, and effectually cures putrified ulcers, kills worms, and cleanses putrified places. The juice is good for cold swellings, and it softens and removes congealed blood of bruises, by strokes, falls, &c. A piece of the root, or some of the seeds bruised, and held to an aching tooth, takes away the pain. The leaves bruised cure the felon. It destroys worms in the ears. If the hot Arsesmart be strewed in a chamber, it will soon kill all the fleas; and the herb or juice of the cold Arsesmart, put to the sores of cattle, will drive away the fly in the hottest time of Summer. The mild Arsesmart is good against all imposthumes and inflammations at the beginning, and to heal green wounds.

The hot Arsesmart grows not so high or tall as the mild, but has many leaves like peach leaves, seldom spotted ; in other particulars it is like the former, but may easily be known from it by breaking a leaf of it across your tongue, for the hot will make your tongue smart, but the cold will not. If you see them both together you may easily distinguish them, because the mild hath broader leaves. It effectually cures obstructions of urine, in gravel and stone, and in the jaundice and dropsy it has wrought great cures. Dr. Eberle considers this plant one of the best promoter of menses we have. Use the cold watery infusion. Never boil or scald it.

ARTICHOKE.

This requires no description.—*Cynaria.* It has good medicinal qualities. The leaves yield a bitter juice, which is diuretic, and useful in dropsy. The fresh root sliced and boiled in water, six ounces to a quart of water, makes a decoction, has been known to cure the jaundice. The following decoction which was long kept a secret by a person at Andover, is said to have carried off the water from several persons in the dropsy. Take off Artichoke leaves and stalks, three handfulls, bruised juniper berries, one quart, a handful of scraped Horse-radish, bruised white mustard-seeds two table-spoonfuls ; boil the whole in two gallons of water to one and strain the liquor through a cloth. Half a pint for an adult, morning and evening. Add sugar if required.

ASARABACCA.

Description.—*Asarum, Europæum.* It is an evergreen, putting forth new leaves in spring. It is wild in many parts of Europe, and in Berkshire, and the Southern counties, and is common in gardens. The roots creep about the surface of the ground, the leaves grow singly from them, without stem or stalk ; the leaves are grassy green and kidney-shaped ; the blossom greenish, with purple-brown streaks on a short stem ;

these flowers are near the ground. The roots are small and whitish; sweet in their smell, but more so when they are dry, and of a sharp, but not unpleasant taste.

Medicinal Virtues.—It is acrid, emetic, purgative, and sternutatory, or provocative of sneezing. The powdered root in the form of snuff is an effectual remedy for removing obstructions in the head, removing headaches, giddiness, drowsiness, and colds in the head. It has been useful in deafness arising from catarrhs. Two or three grains snuffed up the nose going to bed, will cause a copious discharge of offensive mucous from the head the following morning, and be of service all the day following. A decoction of it proves an emetic, and it purges downwards, and by urine also, and removes phlegm, and relieves colic. As a fomentation it relieves pains. Boiled in whey it removes obstruction of the liver and spleen, and is therefore good for dropsy and jaundice. Steeped in wine and drank, it is good for the ague. The oil of it with a little laudanum, promotes perspiration, the ridge of the back being anointed therewith. The roots have the same effect, but not so forcibly. Let it be used with caution; for I am opposed to much vomiting and purging medicines; they weaken nature. A physician should strengthen as much as he can, and debilitate or weaken as little as possible. To make the *snuff*—take three parts of Asarabacca, one part of Marjoram, and one part of Lavender flowers. Reduce to a powder, and cork in bottles.

The Cephalic and Eye snuffs are composed of Asarabacca, root of White Hellebore, Lily of the Valley, and Betony.

ASH.

Description.—*Fraxinus Excelsior*. It is a tree common in hedges and woods. The bark of the branches is gray, and the leaves are winged. The flowers are of a whitish green, and come before the leaves. More description is useless, as the tree is so well known.

Medicinal Virtues.—The distilled water taken every morning is very good for the dropsy and obesity. The decoction in white wine helps to dissolve the stone and expel, and to cure the dropsy. The ashes of the bark made into ley to wash with, cure scabby and leprous heads. The bark, as a decoction removes obstructions of the liver and spleen. The bark of the common Ash has been used as a substitute for Cinchona in larger doses. By some medical men the leaves have been recommended as a substitute for Senna, having a less griping effect, and they answer well. They are useful in rheumatic affections. They should be gathered in June, well dried, powdered, and kept in well corked bottles. For use, infuse 1 drachm in a pint of boiling water until cold, then strain. Take a teacupful twice a day. As a purgative, half an ounce of the Powder is required.

From the *Fraxinus Ornus*, or flowering Ash, is derived the concrete juice, called Manna, a very useful purgative for children and weakly persons. It is a pleasant and mild laxative.

ASPARAGUS.

Description.—*Asparagus Officinalis*. This vegetable requires but little description, as it is well known, and often seen in markets, tied in bundles of a hundred for sale. It is cultivated in gardens; but in the south of England, near the sea coasts, it grows wild; and the roots of the wild are medicinally better than those in gardens.

Medicinal Virtues.—The roots generally used, which are very diuretic, aperient, and alterative, or deobstruent; their action being caused by the presence of an alkaloid, called *Asparagin*, given chiefly for dropsy, consumption, and undue action of the heart. It has been known singly to cure the jaundice and dropsy. It is best given in decoction. The dose is a teacupful three times a day. Of the extract from 20 to 60 grains. Of the Syrup from 1 to 4 ounces a day. The latter is most useful in *Phthisis*. The roots decocted in white wine, is a good external remedy for pains in the kidneys, bladder, cramp, and benumbed limbs!

This is the French method of making *Asparagin*, which is so effectual:—Wrap the stalks of Asparagus in moistened linen for a few days in a warm place, till decomposed, which may be known by their unpleasant smell. Beat in a mortar with water sufficient to dilute the viscid juice, press the juice strongly through a cloth, and heat in order to coagulate the albumen and chlorophylle. Then filter, and concentrate in a marine bath; do it a second time, and then boil down to the consistence of syrup, and put it in a cool place. The vessel containing the liquid will be lined with crystals of asparagine, covered with extractive matter; purify them by washing in cold water, or diluted spirit.

ASSAFŒTIDA.

This stinking drug is the concrete juice of the *Ferula Assafœtida*. It is antispasmodic, expectorant, stimulant and gently aperient. It is a valuable remedy for all nervous disorders; for spasmodic cough, asthma, and other disorders of the chest. The pills may be made thus:—Assafœtida, galbanum, myrrh, each 1 ounce; rectified oil of amber, half a drachm; beat them into a mass with simple syrup The dose is ten grains twice a day in hysteria and asthma.

AVENS

Description.—It is also called Colewort, and Herb Bennet. It is a wild plant, and grows about hedges, rising about fourteen inches high; the stalk is firm and slender, and divided into several branches. It has long, rough, dark green winged leaves; the stalks are hairy. The leaves growing up from the root are winged; they consist of three pair of small ones, and one much larger at the end. Those on the stalk are smaller, and have fewer parts, otherwise they are the same. On the tops of the branches stand small yellow flowers, consisting of five leaves, in the middle of which stands a small green head, which, when the flower is fallen becomes round, consisting of many long greenish purple seeds, which will adhere to clothes. The roots consist of many brownish strings or fibres, smelling like cloves.

Medicinal Virtues.—This plant is invaluable, and is much superior to most of the drugs kept in the shops. It possesses astringent, antiseptic, and tonic properties. The root powdered is equal to the Cinchona, or Peruvian Bark, in agues, a drachm of the powder being given every two hours. For diarrhœas, dysenteries, and the latter stages of continued fevers, a wine glass full of the infusion may be taken two or three times a day with good effect. It is made by pouring a pint of boiling water on a half ounce of the root. It is good for diseases of the chest or breast, for pains or stitches in the side. It expels crude humours from the bowels and stomach and revives the system by its warming qualities. It dissolves inward congealed blood, caused by falls &c., and spitting of blood, if the roots be boiled in wine and drank. In spring it is excellent, taken as a decoction, as a purifier; it removes obstructions of the liver. It removes the windy colic, and relieves those who suffer from rupture. It promotes digestion. As a wash, it removes spots or eruptions from the face.

A little of the root of Avens put in Ale gives it a fine flavour and makes it very wholesome. Hence the Augsburgh Ale which is so much prized on the Continent is said to owe its peculiar excellence to the custom which prevails of putting a small bag of Avens into each Cask.

Compound Tincture of Avens.

Avens Root bruised, 2 ounces
Tormentil Root, bruised, ½ ounce
Angelica Root, bruised, ½ ounce
Raisins, Muscatel, 2, or 3 ounces
French Brandy, 1 quart

Macerate for a month, in a warm place, then filter.—*Dose*, half an ounce.

BALM.

Melissa Officinalis. This plant is so well known, that it needs no describing.

Medicinal Virtues.—In some form or other this valuable medicine should always be kept in the house. It is a plant of balsamic odour, the leaves of which are used as a diluent in fever. It possesses high stimulant and carminative properties, which render it valuable as a remedial agent. Balm is a good tonic, which strengthens the stomach, braces the nerves and elevates the mind by its exhilarating virtues. It is really excellent in colds, attended with fever, as it is sure to promote a copious perspiration, after repeated draughts of the tea or decoction. It makes a good wash for aching teeth, and a suitable drink for those who have the bloody flux, or dysentery. The leaves with a little nitre, decocted, will relieve griping pains, and shortness of breath. It is good for inflamed liver. Used with salt, it removes wens, kernels, or hard swellings in the flesh or throat.

Dr. Copeland recommends Balm to be infused with Liquorice-root, Anise seeds, Fennel seeds, and Coriander seeds; 2½ drachms each of the Balm of Liquorice, and ½ drachm each of the seeds to two pints of water. Dose from 1 to 2 ounces.

Compound Spirit of Balm.

Fresh leaves of Balm, 8 ounces;
Lemon Peel bruised, 4 ounces;
Nutmegs and Carraway seeds, each 2 ounces;
Anise seeds, 1 ounce;
Cloves, Cinnamon, Angelica root, of each 1 ounce.

Infuse for 3 weeks in a quart or more of Brandy, and well cork in bottles.

Some make tea of it combined with Hyssop, and Blackberry-leaves, which very much resembles that from China.

BARBERRY.

Description.—*Berberis Vulgaris*, natural order, *Berberidacæa.* It is a well-known plant, the berries having come much into use lately for making tarts and pies. They are a pleasant acidulous fruit, and may be eaten with safety. The Barberry is found wild in hedges in some parts of England; but it is common everywhere in gardens; it grows eight or ten feet high. The bark is whitish, with abundance of prickles about the branches. The leaves are oval, indented about the hedges, and of strong green colour. The flowers are small, of a pale yellow colour;—the stamens have a remarkable sensibility, when touched by anything, towards the pistillum. The leaves are tender, and very subject to the *rubigo*, which will infest the corn in its neighbourhood. The berries are oblong, red, and acid in taste.

MEDICINAL VIRTUES.—The inner rind of the Barberry tree boiled in white wine cleanses the body from choleric humours, from scabs, itch, ringworms, inflammation of the liver, and dysentery. The bark of the stem infused in beer, has the reputation of curing the jaundice, for it is tonic, and deobstruent. The dose of the infusion is from 1 to 2 ounces twice a day. The berries are cooling, antiscorbutic, and deobstruent, containing *malic and citric acid.* They are very useful in all inflammatory fevers, especially typhus fever, and bilious disorders, and scurvy. The fruit in the form of jam is very refreshing in acute diseases. The active principle of the bark, called *Berberine*, is tonic, and in large doses, laxative. It is an excellent remedy for dyspepsia, with functional derangement of the liver. The dose is from 4 to 10 grains; if more is given, it acts as a purgative. It is an excellent gargle for sore mouth from any cause. The bark dyes a beautiful yellow.

BARK,—PERUVIAN.

Foreign.—The Bark most generally used is the Peruvian, or Jesuits' Bark, *Cinchona.* It is a powerful tonic, febrifuge, and antiseptic, very useful in intermittent fevers and in general and nervous debility, typhus fever especially when tending to gangrene. In confluent small-pox, it promotes languid eruption, and suppuration, diminishes the fever, and prevents putrescence and gangrene; the same in gangrenous sore throats. In contagious dysentery after due evacuation, it has been used, taken internally and by injection, with and without opium.

Many eminent physicians have great confidence in it, joined with sulphuric acid, and the tincture of cayenne pepper, in cases of phthisis, scrofula, ill-conditioned ulcers, rickets, scurvy, and in states of convalescence. In dropsy it is often alternated or conjoined with diuretics or other evacuants, and by its early exhibition after the water is once drawn off, or even begins to be freely discharged, a fresh accumulation is prevented, and a radical cure obtained. In ague and typhus fever the bark is one of the most valuable remedies. The powder is more powerful when taken as an infusion in Port Wine, or mixed with strong brandy and water. Externally, Cinchona Bark is used as an application to bad carious, or gangrenous ulcers. The powder is an excellent dentrifice for spongy and bleeding gums and the decoction is an excellent gargle or wash.

It is given in the form of powder, infusion, decoction, or tincture. Dose of powder, 10 grains to 2 drachms. In agues, begin with 15 grains, and repeat in 3 or 4 hours.

Huxham's Compound Tincture of Bark.—Peruvian Bark in powder 2 ounces; exterior peel of Seville oranges, dried 1½ ounce. Virginia Snake-root, bruised, 3 drachms; saffron, 1 drachm; cochineal powder, 2 scruples; proof spirit, 20 ounces; digest for 14 days and strain. In taking, begin with 2 or 3 drachms. See *Quinine.*

BARLEY.

Hordeum Pretense, or Districhum, or Perlatum. It is so well known as a cereal, or in its prepared state, Pearl Barley, as to require no description. Barley in all its compositions (except malt) is more cooling than wheat, and a little cleansing. Barley-water, and all other preparations of Barley, give nourishment in fevers, agues, and heats in the stomach. A poultice made of barley-meal or flour boiled in vinegar and honey, and a few dry figs put in them, dissolves hard imposthumes, and reduces inflammations. Combined with mellilot, camomile-flowers, linseed, fenugreek, and rue in powder, and applied warm it eases pains in the side and stomach, and flatulence. The meal of barley and fleaworts boiled in water, and made a poultice with honey and oil of lilies, applied warm, cures swellings under the ears, throat, neck, &c., and a plaister made thereof with tar, wax, and oil, is good for the king's evil; boiled with vinegar and quince, it removes the pains of gout; barley flour, salt, honey, and vinegar mingled together, cure the itch. The water distilled from the green barley in the end of May, is very good for humours in the eyes, and dropped into them allays pain. To make Barley Water:—Take 2 or 3 ounces of Pearl, or French Barley, wash it first in cold water, then in hot water; then boil in 2 quarts of water till reduced to 1 quart, and strain. It is an excellent diluent drink in fevers; it is very soothing for inflamed mucous surfaces, especially those of the urinary organs; it may be improved by a few slices of lemon. It may be made into a laxative by adding chopped figs and stoned raisins and liquorice-root. The demulcent properties may be increased by the addition of an ounce of Gum Arabic.

BARRENWORT.

Description.—*Epimedium Alpinum.*—It is a curious, but very pretty plant. It is not so common in England. It is a wood plant, with beautiful purple and yellow flowers. It grows a foot high. The leaves are oval and formed like a heart, indented at the edges, and of a dusky green. The flower stalks are weak, brittle, and often crooked; the flowers stand in a very loose spike, ten, or more, on the top; they are purple on the back with a red edge. It is called Barrenwort because it only flowers in the shade, and not in the sun.

Medicinal Virtues.—The roots boiled in milk are given by some to domestic female animals to arrest the natural emotions for the males. It has been successfully administered to females subject to hysterics. It must not be given in large doses, as it might produce stupor.

BAY TREE.

This Plant is the laurel of antiquity, and the *Laurus nobilis* of Linnæus. It needs no description; it is so well known.

Medicinal Virtues.—The leaves and bark heal very much, and the berries more than the leaves; the bark of the root is less sharp and hot, but more bitter, and astringent and effectual in dissolving stone, and removing obstructions of the liver, spleen, and other inward parts, which bring the jaundice, dropsy, &c. The berries are very effectual against the sting of wasps and bees; and against infectious diseases. They are good for cold and rheumatic distillations from the brain to the eyes, lungs, or other parts; and made into an electuary with honey, they are good in consumption, old coughs, shortness of breath, &c. They expel wind, and provoke urine, and kill worms. The leaves have the same effects. A bath of the decoction of the leaves and berries, is good for female stoppages, for diseases of the bladder, pains in the bowels by wind and stopping of urine. A decoction of equal parts of Bay berries, cummin seed, hyssop, with honey, and the head bathed therewith removes distillations and rheums. The oil made of the berries is useful in affections of the joints, nerves, arteries, stomach, belly, or womb, palsies, convulsions, cramp, and tremblings, by anointing the affected parts. It is excellent for the earache being dropped into the ears. The oil also removes marks on the skin, caused by bruises, falls, &c.

BAZIL,—Garden or Sweet Bazil.

Description.—*Clinopodion hortus.* The greater or ordinary Bazil is cultivated in gardens, on account of its fragrant scent. It rises up with one upright stalk, branching forth on all sides, with two leaves at every joint, broad and round, yet pointed, of a pale green colour, a little snipped about the edges, and of a strong healthy scent. The flowers are small and white, of the same shape as those of the dead nettle; they stand on the upper parts of the branches in loose spikes. The *Wild Bazil* is similar, but not so fine as that which is cultivated.

Medicinal Virtues.—This plant is but little used, but it deserves to be. A decoction of the leaves is a good remedy for all obstructions. No plant has such efficacy in gently promoting menses, and the disorders caused by their obstruction. It may be used in infusion. It arrests vomiting, and allays nausea. The infusion of the seed is a remedy in gonorrhœa and nephritic affections.

BEANS.

Faba. Both the garden and field Beans are well-known.

Medicinal Virtues.—The distilled water of the flower of Garden Beans, is good to clear the face and skin from spots and wrinkles. The water distilled from the green husks, is very effectual against the stone, and it provokes urine. Bean flower is used in poultices to reduce inflammations in wounds, and the swelling of women's breasts. Flour of beans and fenugreek mixed with honey, and applied to felons, boils, bruises, or blue marks by blows, or the imposthumes in the kernels of the ears, is an excellent remedy, and with rose leaves, frankincense, and the white of an egg, it may be beneficially applied to eyes that are swollen or water, or have received any blow upon them. Bean flower boiled to a poultice with wine and vinegar, and a little oil, is good for swelled testicles.

BEANS,—FRENCH.

Phaseolus. Called also Kidney Beans, and it is cultivated for domestic use. It needs no description.

MEDICINAL VIRTUES.—The ordinary French Beans are of easy digestion, and make an excellent vegetable for the table. Dried and powdered they greatly strengthen the kidneys. A dram taken in wine occasionally, prevents stone, and removes obstructions in the kidneys and bladder. Shortness of breath is much relieved by their use.

THE BEECH TREE.

Fagus. It is needless to describe it, it is so well known. It grows in woods, and forests, and in other places. It blooms in the beginning of May, and the fruit is ripe in September.

MEDICINAL VIRTUES. The leaves of the Beach-tree are cooling and binding, and therefore good to be applied to hot swellings. A decoction of the bark is used in diabetes. A decoction of the leaves is excellent for obstinate ulcers, various cutaneous diseases, and dyspeptic affections, accompanied with great weakness, headache, and lowness of spirits. The nuts contain much nutriment for some animals, as deer, pigs &c. The water that is found in the hollow places of decaying Beeches will cure both man and beast of any scurf, scab, or running tetters, if they be washed therewith ; you may boil the leaves into a poultice, or make an ointment of them when the time of year serves.

The Beech-Tree is said to be a non-conductor of lightning. Dr. Beeton, of America, says that the Beech-Tree is never known to be struck by atmospheric electricity, whilst others are often shattered into splinters.

BEETS

DESCRIPTION.—*Beta Vulgaris.* There are two sorts, the white and red Beets. The common white Beet has many leaves next the ground, somewhat large, and of a whitish green colour. The stalk is great, strong, and ribbed, bearing many leaves, almost to the very top of it. The flowers grow in very long tufts, small at the end, and turning down their heads, which are small greenish yellow buds, giving cornered prickly seeds. The root is great, long and hard. The common red Beet differs not from the white, only it is less. The leaves are differently red, some only with red stalks or veins ; some of a fresh red, and others of a dark red. The root is a deep red, spongy, and eaten when boiled either alone or mixed with sallad.

MEDICINAL VIRTUES.—The juice of the root is a remedy for the headache, and toothache, when the jaw is affected, snuffed up the nose to promote sneezing. The white Beet opens and cleanses the bowels, and promotes digestion, and it is a good diuretic. The juice removes obstructions of the liver and spleen, and is good for affections of the brain. Being applied to the temples, it stops inflammations in the eyes. Mixed with oil and a little alum, it is good for burns, and St. Anthony's fire. It is good for all weals, blisters, and blains in the skin ; and made into a poultice, it is good for chilblains. The decoction with some vinegar, heals the itch, if bathed therewith, and cleanseth the head from dandriff, scurf, and dry scabs, and is excellent for running sores, ulcers, and cankers in the head, legs, or other parts, and for baldness.

The red Beet root stays the bloody flux, women's courses, and the whites, and is a remedy for the yellow jaundice.

WATER BETONY.

DESCRIPTION.—*Betonica Aquatica.*—It is also called Brownwort, and Bishops-leaves. Water Betony rises up with square, hard, greenish stalks, set with brown dark green leaves dented about the edges, somewhat resembling the leaves of the Woody Betony, but much larger. The flowers are many, set at the tops of the stalks and branches, being round; opened at the brims, and divided into two parts, the upper one is like a hood, and the lower like a lip hanging down, of a dark red colour, and succeeded by small round pointed heads, wherein lie small brownish seeds. The root is a thick bush of strings and shreds growing from the head. It grows by the ditch-side, brooks, and other water-courses, and is seldom found far from the water-side. It flowereth about July, and the seed is ripe in August.

MEDICINAL VIRTUES.—It is appropriated more to wounds and hurts in the breasts than Wood Betony; it is a good remedy for sick hogs, it is of a cleansing quality. The leaves bruised and applied are effectual for old filthy ulcers; and especially if the juice of the leaves be boiled with a little honey, and the sores dressed therewith; as also for bruises or hurts, inward or outward. The distilled water of the leaves is used for the same purpose, as also to bathe the face and hands spotted or blemished, or discoloured by sun burning.

WOOD BETONY

DESCRIPTION.—*Betonica Offianalis.*—This is one of the herbs that ought to be kept in every family.

It has many leaves rising from the root, which are rather broad and round at the end, roundly dented about the edges, standing upon long foot stalks, from which rise up small, square, slender, upright hairy stalks, with some leaves thereon to a piece at the joints, smaller than the lower, whereon are set several spiked heads of flowers like lavender, and of a purple colour, the seeds are in the husks that hold the flowers, and are blackish, The roots are many white thready strings; the stalk perisheth, but the roots, with some leaves thereon, abide all the Winter. It grows in woods, and in shady places. It flowers in July, after which the seed is quickly ripe, yet it is in its prime in May.

MEDICINAL VIRTUES.—Antonius, physician to the Emperor Augustus Cæsar, wrote a book on the virtues of this herb, in which he says, that it preserves the liver, and the body from epidemical diseases, and promotes digestion, cures belching of the stomach. It is good for disorders of the head, and for all nervous complaints. The herb or root, or the flowers in broth, drunk, or made into conserve, syrup, water, electuary or powder, is a good remedy for the jaundice, falling-sickness, the palsy, convulsions, or shrinking of the sinews, the gout, and for dropsy, and continual pains in the head. The powder with honey, is most excellent for all coughs or colds, shortness of breath, distillations of thin rheum upon the lungs, which cause consumptions. The decoction made with mead, and penny royal, is good for putrid agues, and to draw down and evacuate the blood and humours, that by falling into the eyes, hinder the sight. The decoction thereof made in wine, and taken, destroys worms, and removes obstructions of the spleen and liver. It cures stitches, pains in the back or sides, and griping pains of the bowels, and the flatulent colic. Mixed with honey it purges. It is of great service in the falling down of the womb, obstruction of the menses, and stone in the bladder. The decoction with wine gargled in the mouth, easeth the tooth-ache. A dram of the powder of Betony, taken with a little honey in some vinegar, is very refreshing for those that are wearied by travel. It stays bleeding at the mouth or nose, and helps those that spit blood, or make bloody urine, and is good for those that have a rupture and are bruised. The green herb bruised, or the juice applied to any outward green wound in the head or body, will quickly heal it, and any veins or sinews that are cut. It is a curative of old sores and ulcers, though they be fistulous and hollow. The fume of the decoction while it is warm, received by a funnel into the ears, eases pain, destroys worms, and cures the running sores in them. The juice dropped into them does the same. On the whole, Wood Betony is one of the most valuable herbs we have in Great Britain.

Betony must be gathered when about to flower. Some persons mix it with tobacco and smoke it. With the Eye-bright, and Coltsfoot, it has been made into tobacco, and it relieves difficult breathing. For a snuff, take Betony, Marjarom, a little of the root of Florentine Iris, and Eye-bright, powder when dry, and you have a remedy for the head-ache, sore eyes, and obstructions in the head.

BENZOIN.

Foreign.—Styrax Benzoin.—Commonly called Gum Benjamin. It is a good stimulant and expectorant. When burned, its vapour is deodorant and antiseptic, and therefore useful for sick rooms. Benzoin mixed with ointment prevents it from becoming rancid; its vapour is supposed to be good for hooping cough. In Cosmetic washes it is an ingredient, and also in *Friar's Balsam*, a most useful Styptic and healing application, as well as an inward Medicine.

Friar's Balsam to be made thus:—Gum Benzoin, 3½ ounces; Strained Storax, 2½ ounces; Balsam of Tolu, 10 drachms; Aloes, 5 drachms; rectified spirit, 2 pints; let it stand 14 days, shaking frequently, and before use. This preparation is stimulant, expectorant, and antispasmodic, and is beneficial in old Asthmatic cases, chronic catarrh, and phthisis with a feeble circulation. The dose is about ½ a drachm in mucilage, or dropped upon Lump Sugar. Applied to wounds it stimulates gently, and protects from the action of the air. A piece of lint, or soft rag dipped into it, and wrapped round a cut finger, will produce smarting at first, yet it will commonly stay hæmorrhage, and effect a cure without the necessity for another dressing, unless the wound be extremely severe. Probably *Friar's Balsam* was used by the monks of old time to dress the wounds of travellers, and others, who called and rested in their convents.

BILBERRIES,

CALLED BY SOME WORTS, THE WORTLE-BERRIES.

Vaccinium Myrtillus. Two sorts are common in England, viz, the black and red berries. And first of the black.

Description. The small bush lies upon the ground, nearly a foot high, with small dark green leaves a little dented above the edges; at the foot of the leaves come forth small, hollow, bluish coloured flowers, the brims ending with five points, with reddish threads in the middle, which pass into small round berries, about the size of juniper berries, but purple colour, and of a sweetish sharp taste; the juice gives a purplish colour to the hands and lips of those who eat and handle them.

The Red Bilberry or Wortle-bush, rises up like the former, having sundry hard leaves, like the Box-tree leaves, green and round pointed, standing on the several branches, at the top of which, and not from the sides as in the former, come forth round, reddish, sappy berries, when they are ripe, of a sharp taste.

The first grows in forests, on moors, and in woods. They flower in March and April, and the fruit of the black is ripe in July and August.

Medicinal Virtues.—It is a pity they are used no more in physic than they are. The Black Bilberries are good in hot agues, and to cool the heat of the liver and stomach ; they are astringent, and stay purgings, vomitings, and loathings. The juice of the berries made into syrup, or the pulp made into a conserve with sugar, is good for the purposes aforesaid, as also for an old cough, or for an ulcer, or other diseases in the lungs. The red Worts are more binding, and stop women's courses, spitting of blood, or any other flux of blood or humours, being used as well outwardly as inwardly.

BILFOIL, or TWABLADE.

Description.—*Listera Ovata.* From a root somewhat sweet, shooting downwards many long strings, rises up a round green stalk, bare or naked, next the ground for an inch, two or three in the middle thereof, as it is in age or growth ; as also from the middle upward to the flowers, having only two broad plaintain-like leaves (but whiter) set at the middle of the stalk, one against another, compassing it round at the bottom of them. It is an inhabitant of woods, copses, and many other places.

Another sort grows in wet grounds and marshes. It is a smaller plant, and greener, having sometimes three leaves ; the spike of the flowers is less than the former, and the roots of this, run or creep in the ground.

They are often used by many to good purpose for wounds, both green and old, and to consolidate or knit ruptures. A decoction of Twablade is good for the piles, and also the external application of its fresh juice.

BIND WEED.

Description.—*Convolvulus Sepium.*—A common wild plant climbing about hedges, and bears large white flowers, the form of the Garden Convolvulus. It is well known.

Medicinal Virtues. The root is used as a purge, boiled in ale. It answers well, though on account of the nausea which it tends to produce, it is not fit for the delicate. For people of a strong constitution, there is not a better purge.

THE BIRCH TREE

Description.—*Betula Alba.*—Its appearance in summer is elegant, and in winter the bark is frequently variegated with red and white streaks.

It is a tall straight tree, with many boughs, and slender branches bending downward; the old being covered with a discoloured chapped bark, and the younger being much browner. The leaves are dented about the edges. It bears small short catskins, somewhat like those of the hazlenut-tree, which growing ripe, fall on the ground, and their seed with them. It usually grows in woods.

Medicinal Virtues.—The juice of the leaves, while young, or the distilled water of them, or the juice from the tree bored with an augur, and distilled afterwards, any of these being drunk for some days together, tends to break the stone in the kidneys and bladder, and is good also to wash sore mouths. The leaves have been used in the itch, dropsy, &c., either externally applied, or taken in decoction. Birch-wine made from the juice of the tree, is an excellent remedy for consumptions, and scurvy; and the fungus which grows on the tree, is a good styptic.

BIRD'S FOOT.

Description.—*Avis Pes.*—This herb groweth not above a span high, with many branches spread upon the ground, set with wings of small leaves. The flowers are small, and of a pale yellow colour, being set a head together, which turneth into small jointed cods, resembling the claws of small birds, whence its name.

There is another sort of Bird's foot like the former, but a little larger; the flower of a pale whitish red colour, and the cods distinct by joints like the other, but a little more crooked. They grow on heaths, and in open untilled places. They flower and seed in the end of Summer.

MEDICINAL VIRTUES.—They are of a drying, binding quality, and very good to be used in wound drinks; as also to apply outwardly for the same purpose. But the latter Bird's-foot is found by experience to break the stone, and drive them forth, if the decoction be taken; and it is very serviceable in ruptures, taken inwardly, and outwardly applied to the place.

BISTORT, OR SNAKEWEED.

DESCRIPTION.—*Polyginum Bistorta*, natural order, *Polygonaceæ*. It is also called Sapentary Dragonwort, Osterick, and Passions. It is a beautiful wild plant, growing in shadowy moist woods, at the foot of hills, and in some meadows. It flowers about the end of May, and the seed is ripe in July. It grows about a foot and a half high. The leaves are broad and pretty, and long like a dock leaf, a little pointed at the ends, of a bluish green colour on the upper side, of an ash-coloured grey, and rather purplish underneath. The flowers grow in a thick spike or ear, at the top of the stalks, and are of a bright red colour. The stalks on which the flowers stand have a rim of the leaf running down them; the stalks are round, firm, and erect, of a pale green, almost without leaves, or with very few and narrow, placed at distances. The spike of the flowers is as long and as thick as a man's thumb. It has a thick short knobbed root, crooked, with black threads, and it has an astringent taste. March is the best time for gathering it, when the leaves begin to shoot.

MEDICINAL VIRTUES.—Both the leaves and the roots have a powerful faculty to resist poison. The root is one of the *best astringents in the world*, and is used in mucous discharges, passive hæmorrhages, and fluxes. Combined with the bitter

Flagroot (*Calamus*) it has been effectual in the cure of intermittent fever and ague. Its active principles are *Tannin and Gallic Acid.* The powder or decoction of the roots is a most effectual remedy for profuse menstruation, and also for diabetes, and for fluor albus. The decoction is an excellent gargle for scurvy in the gums, and ulcerated sore throat, and for washing. The leaves kill the worms in children. A dram of the powder of the root taken in water, in which red hot iron has been quenched, is a powerful remedy. The dose of the powdered root is from 1 scruple to a drachm; of the decoction, from 1 to 2 ounces. It makes also an excellent injection when an astringent is required. The herb is invaluable; therefore no family should be without it.

BISHOP'S WEED.

DESCRIPTION.—*Episcopi Herba ignobilis.*—Some persons call it Ethiopian Cummin-seed, and others Cummin royal, as also Herb-William and Bull-wort.

Common Bishop's weed rises up with a round straight stalk, usually three or four feet high, beset with small, long, and broad leaves, cut in some places, and dented at the edges, growing one against another, of a dark green colour, having various branches, and at the top small umbels of white flowers which turn into small round seeds, like parsley seeds, of a quick hot scent and taste. It grows wild in many places in England and Wales, as between Greenhithe and Gravesend.

MEDICINAL VIRTUES.—It is hot and dry in the third degree, of a sharp bitter taste. It dispels humours, provokes urine and women's courses, dispels wind, and taken in wine it eases pain and griping in the bowels. It is used with good effect in medicines given to counteract the poisonous operation of Cantharides upon the passage of the urine. Mixed with honey, and applied to black and blue marks, produced by blows or bruises, it takes them away.

BLITES.

DESCRIPTION.—*Blitum.* A kind of spinach or beet, having no taste. Of these there are two sorts known, viz., White and

Red. The White has leaves like beets, but smaller, rounder, and of a whitish green colour, each standing upon a small long foot-stalk; the stalk rises up two or three feet high, the flowers grow at the top in long round clusters, containing small round seeds; the root is very full of threads or strings.

The Red Blite is like the white, except its leaves and tufted heads are very red at first, and afterwards turn purplish.

They grow in gardens, and wild in many places. They seed in August and September.

Medicinal Virtues. They are cooling, astringent, and useful in fluxes of blood, especially the red; which restrain the overflowing of the courses, as the white Blites stay the whites. It is an excellent secret, you cannot well fail in the use.

BLOOD WORT.

Description.—*Lapathum Sanguineum.*—A beautiful kind of dock kept in gardens, and wild in some places. It grows to four feet high; the stalks are firm, stiff, upright, branched, and striated. The leaves are very long and narrow, broadest at the base, and smaller all the way to the end. They are not at all indented at the edges, and they stand upon long foot-stalks: their colour is a deep green, but they are in different degrees stained with a beautiful blood red; sometimes the ribs only are red, sometimes there are long veins of red irregularly spread over the whole leaf; sometimes they are very broad, and in some plants the whole leaves and the stalks also are of a blood colour; the flowers are very numerous and little. They in all respects resemble those of the common wild docks. The root is long and thick, and of a deep blood red colour.

Medicinal Virtues.—The roots are used: they are best dry, and they may be given in decoction, or in powder. They are a powerful astringent: they stop bloody fluxes, spitting of blood, and the overflowings of the menses. It is also good against violent purgings and against the whites.

BLUE BOTTLE

Description.—*Centaurea Cyanus.* It is called Cyanus from the colour of it; Hurt-sickle, because it turns the edge of the sickles that reap the corn; Blue-blow, Corn-flower, and Blue-bottle.

Its narrow leaves spread on the ground, being of a whitish green colour, amongst which rises a stalk divided into divers branches, with long leaves of a greenish colour, a little indented; the flowers are of a blue colour, consisting of many small flowers set in a scaly head, like those of knapweed. The seed is smooth, bright and shining, wrapped up in a woolly mantle.

They grow in corn-fields generally; towards the full of the moon, they will grow more double than they are, and many times change colour. They flower from the beginning of May to the end of harvest.

MEDICINAL VIRTUES.—The powder or dried leaves of the Blue-bottle are given with good success to those that are bruised by a fall, or have broken a vein inwardly, and void much blood at the mouth. The herb is a valuable styptic, and exceeds all other things, and may save a life when surgical aid is not available. The leaves fresh gathered and bruised will stop the bleeding of a fresh wound, even if a large vessel be cut. An infusion of them works gently by urine. The leaves or seed taken in wine, is very good against all infectious diseases, and pestilential fevers. The juice put into fresh or green wounds, rapidly heals them, and it is very effectual to heal all ulcers and sores in the mouth, the juice dropped into the eyes takes away inflammation, and the distilled water of this herb has the same virtues.

BORAGE AND BUGLOSS.

DESCRIPTION.—*Borago Officinalis, et Sycopsis.* These are rough plants, common in gardens, with great leaves and beautiful blue flowers. They are so well known, as to need little description. There is a third kind called *Languae de beœuf.* The leaves are smaller than those of bugloss, but much rougher; the stalk rises about a foot and a half high, and is mostly of a red colour; the flowers stand in scaly rough heads, being composed of many small yellow flowers, not unlike those of the dandelions, and the seed flies away in down; the flowers are very bitter. The virtues of this plant are the same as those of

Borage and Bugloss. They flower in June and July, and the seed is ripe shortly after.

MEDICINAL VIRTUES.—All three are great cordials, and strengtheners of nature. The leaves and roots are very useful in putrid fevers, to defend the heart, and to expel the venom of other creatures. The seed and leaves are good to increase milk in women's breasts, and to drive away melancholy; to clarify the blood, and mitigate heat in fevers. The juice made into a syrup has the same effect, and is a valuable remedy for the yellow jaundice, the itch, ringworm, &c. The flowers candied or made into a conserve, are useful for persons weakened by long sickness, and for those who are subject to swoonings. The distilled water is as effectual, and cures inflammation of the eyes. The roots of Bugloss made into an electuary, promote expectoration, and remove a cough. They are excellent for affections of the lungs. A good way of taking it is to infuse it in wine, which partly neutralizes its nauseousness.

BOX TREE.

Busus.—It is well known.

MEDICINAL VIRTUES.—The wood and the root make a good purifier of the blood. It has greater virtues than the Guiacum. Leprosies have been cured by a decoction of the wood and root. The decoction of the bark, or powdered, successfully cures intermittent fevers, and is a good tonic for debility, for billious disorders, jaundice, and low spirits.

THE BRAMBLE, OR BLACK-BERRY BUSH.

Rubus Fruticosus.—This needs no description.

MEDICINAL VIRTUES.—The buds and leaves while they are green, are of good use in ulcers and putrid sores of the mouth and throat, and in quinsy, and to heal fresh wounds and sores; but the flowers and unripe fruit are very binding, and very useful for the bloody flux, and for spitting of blood. The decoction of powder of the root being taken, is good to break gravel and the stone. The leaves and brambles, green and dry, make a good lotion for sores in the mouth, or secret parts. It is a powerful astringent, and restrains laxity of the bowels, and the undue flow of the menses. The decoction is good for the piles, fevers, and the distilled water of the branches, leaves, and flowers, or of the fruit, is effectual in fevers, and hot distempers of the body, head, eyes, and other parts. The leaves boiled in ley, and the head washed therewith, heal the itch, and tend to turn the hair black.

BROOK LIME, or WATER PIMPERNEL.

Description.—*Veronica Beccabunga.* This is one of those neglected vegetables which might occasionally be used for culinary purposes, particularly as a sallad.

It has a creeping white root, shooting forth strings at every joint, as it runs, divers and sundry green stalks, round and sappy, with some branches on them, somewhat broad, round, deep green and thick leaves, set by couples thereon; from the bottom whereof shoot forth long footstalks, with small beautiful sky-blue flowers on them, consisting of five small round pointed leaves a-piece.

It grows in small standing waters, and usually near water cresses. It flowers in June and July.

Medicinal Virtues. It is a hot and biting plant. Brook-lime and water cresses are generally used together in diet-drink, with other things serving to purge the blood and body from all humours destructive to health, and are good for diseases of the bladder, and help to break the stone, and pass it away. The plant is useful in removing female obstructions. It is of itself a good scorbutic medicine. Dioscorides states that its leaves drunk in wine relieve the strangury, and diseases of the bladder. It operates gently by urine, and is a great purifier of the blood.

BROOM, AND BROOM-RAPE.

Description.—This is the *Spartium Scoparium* of botanists, a plant very common in England; for with it floors are swept; it therefore needs no description.

The Broom-rape springs up on many places from the roots of the broom. The stalk is about the size of a finger or thumb, above two feet high, having a show of leaves on them, and many flowers at the top, of a beautiful bright yellow. It grows on waste grounds. It flowers in the Summer months, and seeds before winter. The flowers are shaped like a pea blossom, and are of a bright yellow.

Medicinal Virtues.—The tops of the Broom have a bitter disagreeable taste. The plant possesses cathartic and diuretic properties, which render it very useful in some cases of dropsy. The tops and seeds are the parts used, chiefly the former in the form of decoction—*one ounce to a quart of water*. Boil down to a pint, and take half a wine-glassful, or a wine-glassful two or three times a day. Dr. Cullen says, "It seldom fails to operate both by stool and urine, and by repeating every day, or every second day, some dropsies have been effectually cured." The green stalks infused in ale or beer operate by urine, and remove obstructions of the liver and other parts, they are very useful in jaundice. Some of the old physicians burned the tops to ashes, and infused them in wine; thus the salt was extracted and the wine turned into a ley. It works powerfully by urine; but the above-mentioned decoction is the best.—Bruised Broom-seed, infused in rectified spirit—let it infuse for two weeks. Strain. A table-spoonful in a glass of peppermint water to be taken daily.—A strong decoction has been recommended in cases of hydrophobia. The dose of the powder either of tops or seeds is from 1 scruple to 1 drachm. In liver complaints, the above decoction, with that of Dandelion, is very efficacious. Also in the ague, producing profuse perspiration, taken before the fit, the person lying in bed.

The decoction of Broom-rape has the same effect as the Broom.

BRYONY.

Description.—There are two kinds of Bryony; the *White Bryonia Alba;* (called by some persons the *Red Bryonia Dioica;*) and the Black, *Bryonia Nigra, vel Tamus Communis.*

The WHITE BRYONIA is a tall, climbing wild plant, growing in hedges. The leaves are somewhat like those of the vine; the flowers are white, but inconsiderable, the berries are red, and are very showy. The root is very large, rough, and whitish; the stalks are tough, ten or twelve feet long; but weak and unable to support themselves; by tendrils at the joints they fix themselves to bushes. The leaves are broad and divided deeply at the edge, of a hoary green colour. The whitish flowers are on a long tuft, consisting of five small leaves each open like a star. The berries hang like a cluster of grapes, very red when ripe, having a loathsome taste, producing nausea.

Medicinal Virtues.—The root powdered, or decocted, is a very strong purgative, even if a small dose be taken. Great caution ought therefore to be exercised in taking it. It is a capital remedy for dropsies, hysterics, given in minute doses. For dropsies, two drachms of the root to six ounces of water, sweetened to the taste—take a spoonful every two hours. Many cases of dropsies it has cured. Very weak people should begin with a less dose. The same will apply to hysteric complaints. Dr. Sydenham recommended for maniacal disorders—a drachm of the powder in a gill of milk—or an infusion of the leaves, say about half an ounce in a gill of white wine; begin with a tea-spoonful at a time. The infusion is milder than the root in substance; and Dr. Lewis says, that an extract prepared by water acts more mildly, and with greater safety, than the root itself; given from half a drachm to a drachm, it proves a gentle purgative; it operates powerfully by urine. It is good for diseases of the head by drawing away rheumatic humours. An electuary made of the root with honey proves a powerful expectorant. The root, leaves, and fruit boiled, are good to cleanse old sores, cankers, and gangrene; and the decoction frees the face from freckles, black and blue spots, &c.

The BLACK BRYONY, Bryonia Nigra, *vel Tanus Communis*. The plant climbs upon bushes and hedges like the former; but this by twisting its stalk about the branches of trees and shrubs, for it has no tendrils. It runs to fifteen feet in height; the stalk is tough and angular; the leaves are broad, and of a heart-like shape, perfectly smooth and shining, and of a glossy and deep blackish green. The flowers are very small, and of a greenish white; the berries are red; the root black without, white within, and full of a slimy juice.

MEDICINAL VIRTUES.—This herb ought not to be neglected, as its medicinal qualities are great, equal to any, and surpassing most herbs. It is very efficacious in epilepsy, and rheumatism. Dr. Thornton has witnessed its efficacy in cases of gout, rheumatism, and paralytic affections. The root is scraped with a knife, and the scrapings which feel like soap, are to be rubbed over the affected parts once a day. Immediately a momentary sense of tingling is felt, like that produced by nettles; and this mild rubefacient he has found also to do good in cases of Asthma, when rubbed over the chest.

The root of Black Bryony is one of the best diuretics known in medicine. It is a good remedy for gravel, obstruction of urine, and other disorders of the kidneys. The root has been thought to be the celebrated mandrake, and I believe that in some parts they call it by that name; but Mandrake is a different plant, though it possesses some of its properties.

Dr. Tissot says, a poultice made of the leaves of Bryony is an excellent remedy for painful tumours, rheumatism, and lumbago. The juice of Bryony, turpentine, and a small portion of wax, is a grand remedy for old sores, scrofulas, swellings, &c.

BUCKBEAN, OR WATER TREFOIL.

DESCRIPTION.—*Meyanthus Trifoliata.*—This perennial plant is very common in marshy places, and is one of the most beautiful of our native flowers. It grows a foot high, the leaves stand three upon each stalk, and these stalks rise immediately from the roots. They are thick, round, smooth, and fleshy; and the leaves themselves are large, oblong, and have some resemblance to those of garden beans. The flowers stand upon naked stalks, which are also thick, round, fleshy, and whitish: they are small, but they grow together in a kind of thick short spike, so that in the cluster they make a conspicuous appearance; they are white with a very faint tinge of purple, and are hairy within; the root is whitish, long, and thick.

The leaves of buck-bean are to be gathered before the stalks appear for flowering, and are to be dried.

Medicinal Virtues.—It is very tonic and astringent; in large doses purgative. Very useful in scurvy, scrofula, gouty affections, and fevers. A drachm of the leaves in powder, purges and vomits. In infusion, or extract, they are useful in intermittents, in several cachectic and cutaneous diseases. The dose of the extract is from ten to twenty grains.

It is surely Providential that this plant grows in places where agues prevail most. The remedy is near at hand. Boerhave says, "It overcomes the *tertian* and *quartan* ague." Haller says "that intermittents yield to it;" and the German soldiers made us of it in one of the wars, with almost unvaried success. They used it instead of bark. In cachectic disease, that is, disease and emaciation, and debility of the primæ vitæ, it is known to be of great service. It is applicable to arrest *consumption* in its incipient stages, especially if combined with a little Cayenne Pepper, to produce heat, and a decoction of Logwood, which is a most powerful antiseptic, or arrester of decay.

In scorbutic affections, and scrofula, it has often proved beneficial. Inveterate cutaneous diseases have been removed by an infusion of the leaves drunk freely every day for some weeks. Dr. Lewis says, "The leaves of the buck-bean have a bitter penetrating taste, which they impart both to watery and spirituous menstrua. They have come into use lately as an alterative and aperient, in impurities of the humours, and in dropsical and rheumatic cases. They are usually taken in the form of infusion, with the addition of some acrid anti-scorbutic herbs, which, in most cases, improve their virtue; also add orange-peel, or some other grateful aromatic, to alleviate their ill taste. The leaves have been used in brewing ale. One ounce, it is said, will go as far as half a pound of hops. Boerhave was himself cured of gout by taking it mixed with whey. He recommends it also as an external application for dissolving glandular swellings. Its seeds are said to be good for coughs of long standing, and for diseases of the chest.

BUCK'SHORN PLANTAIN.

Description.—*Plantago Coronopus.*—It is a very pretty plant, which grows in our sandy and barren places, with the leaves spread out in manner of a star, all the way round from the root; and in the heads like other plantains, although so very unlike them in its leaves. The root is long and slender; the leaves which lie thus flat upon the ground are narrow and long, very beautifully notched, and divided so as to resemble a buck's horn, whence the name, and of a pale whitish green, and a little hairy. The stalks are slender, six inches long, but seldom quite erect: they are round, hairy, and whitish, and have at the top a spike of flowers of an inch or two in length, altogether like that of the other plantains, only more slender.

This plant has obtained the name of star of the earth, from the way of the leaves spreading themselves. These leaves bruised, and applied to a fresh wound, stop the bleeding, and effect a cure. It is said also to be a remedy against the bite of a mad dog; but this is idle and groundless.

It is a good remedy for stone, and inflammation of the kidneys, as it cools and strengthens the parts affected. The herb boiled in ale or wine, and taken night and morning for some time is serviceable in inflammation of the eyes.

BUCK'S HORN, CALLED BUCKTHORN.

Description. *Rhamnus Catharticus.*—A Prickly shrub, common in our hedges, with pale green leaves, and black berries. It grows to eight or ten feet high. The bark is dark coloured and glossy, and the twigs are tough. The leaves are oval, of a very regular and pretty figure, and elegantly dented round the edges. The flowers are little and inconsiderable; they are of a greenish yellow, and grow in little clusters. The berries, which are ripe in September, are round, glossy, black, as big as the largest pepper-corns, and contain each three or four seeds.

Medicinal Virtues.—Some persons call it the purging Buckthorn, on account of the cathartic properties of its berries, which must be used fresh or made into a syrup. It has been found useful in dropsies, rheumatisms and the gout. It has been found efficacious in the expulsion of worms, made into a syrup—begin with a table-spoonful. Of the fresh berries 20 may be taken, or from 1 to 2 drachms of the dried ones. It is a rough purge, but a very good one.

Syrup of Buckthorn.—Take the juice of the berries fresh gotten, one quart; bruised ginger two drachms; pimento powdered, half an ounce; refined sugar, two pounds. Set aside the juice for three days, that the fæces may subside, and then strain. Macerate the ginger and pimento in half a pint of the strained juice for four hours, and filter. Boil the rest of the juice to one pint; then add that part of the juice in which the ginger and pimento have been macerated, and form a syrup of it with the sugar.

Three or four spoonfuls of this Syrup acts as a brisk purge; but it is a very useful one.

BUGLE.

It is also called Middle Confound, and Middle Comfrey, Brown Bugle, Sicklewort, and Herb-Carpenter.

Description.—*Bugula Reptans.*—The flower-stalks grow eight or ten inches high, square, of a pale green, sometimes purplish, and have two leaves at every joint, the joints being a little distant. These leaves are similar in form as those which rise immediately, oblong, broad, blunt at the point, and of a deep green colour, slightly indented at the edges. The flowers are small, of a pretty blue colour, which produce small, round blackish seeds.

The white-flowered Bugle differs not in form or size from the former, saving that the leaves and stalks are always green, and never brown, like the other, and the flowers thereof are white.

They grow in woods, copses, and fields, throughout England, but the white-flowered Bugle is rather scarce. They flower from May until July.

Medicinal Virtues.—The decoction of the leaves and flowers made in wine, dissolves congealed blood in those that are bruised inwardly by a fall, and is very effectual for any inward wounds, thrusts or stabs in the body or bowels; and for obstructions in the liver. It cures ulcers and sores, gangrenes and fistulas, if the leaves be bruised and applied, or their juice be used to wash and bathe the place. By infusion, it is very useful in coughs, spitting of blood, and in incipient consumption. In its action it rather resembles digitalis, lowering the pulse, and lessening its frequency; it allays irritation, cough, and equalises the circulation, and is considered by Rafinesque, "as one of the mildest and best narcotics in the world." A lotion made of it and some honey cures sores in the mouth and gums, and other parts of the body. An ointment made with the leaves of Bugle, Scabious, and Sanicle bruised and boiled in hog's grease, until the herbs be dry, and then strained into a pot, is very good for all sorts of hurts in the body. It is good for the bad effects of excessive drinking, as sickness, headache, delirium tremens, &c.

BURDOCK.

DESCRIPTION.—*Aretium Lappa*, or *Bardanus.*—It is so well known, even by little boys, who pull off the bur to throw and stick upon one another that it needs no description. They grow plentifully by ditches, watersides, highways, and on waste grounds.

MEDICINAL VIRTUES.—It is a most excellent herb. It has been successfully used in many chronic diseases, as scurvy, rheumatism, gout, lues venerea, and affections of the lungs. It is a powerful diuretic, and it has been known to succeed in dropsical cases where other powerful medicines had been ineffectually used. As it neither excites nausea, nor increases irritation, it is worthy of a trial where more active remedies are improper. The seeds also possess a diuretic quality, and are very advantageous in stone or gravel, and in the form of an emulsion for coughs. A decoction may be made by boiling two ounces of the fresh root in two pints of water. This is excellent for provoking urine. It should be taken in one or two days. The leaves bruised and mixed with the white of an egg, is excellent for burns, scalds, &c. The decoction applied to sores stops gangrene; but the ointment of Burdock must also be applied. Powder the root and mix with hog's lard, and a little vinegar. In short, it is aperient, diuretic, and sudorific. It has cured *dropsies alone*, and has arrested the progress of fevers. In fact it is a most valuable herb; but its commonness is against it. *Remember*, that Providence has made some of the most useful plants the most common. The leaves bruised and moistened with Spirits of Hartshorn and Laudanum, form an excellent application for sprains, bruises, and other external injuries, it is good for old ulcers and sores.

BURNET.

Description.—*Pimpinella Sanguisorba.*—The great wild Burnet hath winged leaves rising from the roots like the garden Burnet, but not so many; yet they are twice as large, and notched in the same manner about the edges, of a greyish colour on the under side; the stalks are greater, and rise higher, with similar leaves, and greater heads at the top, of a brownish colour, and out of them come small dark purple flowers like the former, but larger. The root is black and long like the other. It has very little scent or taste.

The first grows in gardens. The wild grows by waysides, and in dry places. They flower in June and July.

Medicinal Virtues. It is a most precious herb, little inferior to Betony. The continual use of it preserves the body in health, and the mind in vigour. It is a friend to the heart, liver, and other principal parts of a man's body. Two or three of the stalks, with leaves put into a cup of wine, especially claret, are known to quicken the spirits, and drive away melancholy. It is a special herb against infection, the juice being taken in some drink, and the party laid to sweat. It has also an astringent quality, and will stop fluxes of blood or humours, staunch bleedings inward or outward, women's too-abundant courses, the whites, and the choleric belchings of the stomach. It is a good herb for all sorts of wounds, both of the head and body, either inward or outward, used either in juice or decoction, or by powder of the root, or distilled, or made into an ointment.

BUR-REED

Description.—*Sparganium Ramosum.*—A common water plant, with leaves like flags, and rough heads of seeds: it is two or three feet high. The stalks are round, green, thick, and upright. The leaves are very long and narrow, sharp at the edges, and with a sharp ridge on the back along the middle;

they are of a pale green, and look fresh and beautiful. The flowers are inconsiderable and yellowish: they stand in a kind of circular tufts about the upper parts of the stalk: lower down stand the rough fruits called burs, from whence the plant obtained its name; they are of the size of a large nutmeg, green and rough. The root is composed of a quantity of white fibres.

MEDICINAL VIRTUES.—The unripe fruit is used: they are astringent, and good against fluxes of the belly, and bleedings of all kinds: the best way of giving them is infused in a rough red wine, with a little cinnamon. They use them in some parts of England externally for wounds. A strong decoction of them is made to wash old ulcers, and the juice is applied to fresh hurts, and they say with great success.

BUTCHER'S BROOM.

DESCRIPTION.—*Ruscus Aculeatus.* It is sometimes called Kneeholm, Kneeholy, and Pettigree.

The stalks are thick, whitish, and short, somewhat like those of Asparagus, but a foot and a half high, spread into divers branches, green, round, tough, flexible and crossed, having broad and almost round hard leaves and prickly, pointed at the end, of a dark green colour, two at a place close together. The flowers are small, and whitish green, and grow in a singular manner upon the backs of the leaves; they are succeeded by a small round berry, red when it is ripe, about the size of a pea. The root is thick, white, and great. It grows in copses, and upon heaths and waste grounds, and under or near the holly bushes. It shoots forth its buds in the Spring, and the berries are ripe in September, the leaves are green all the winter.

MEDICINAL VIRTUES.—The root is the part used, and it is an excellent deobstruent. It works powerfully by urine, and is good in the jaundice, in gravel, and female obstructions. As such it was recommended by Dioscorides and other ancient physicians. In scrofulous tumours, great advantage has been realized by administering the root in doses of a drachm, every morning. The decoction sweetened with honey, clears the chest of phlegm, and relieves difficult breathing. A conserve made of the berries is a remedy for gonorrhœa and scalding urine.

BUTTER-BUR.

DESCRIPTION.—*Tussilago Petasites.*—Some Herbals denominate this herb *Colt's Foot.* But it is a very different plant. It springs up in February, with a thick stalk a foot high. The flowers appear before the leaves. The stalks are round thick and spongy, of a whiteish colour, and have a few imperfect leaves upon them. On the top of each is a spike of flowers, of a pale reddish colour, and before it has been a month above ground, it withers, and the leaves begin to spring, which being full grown, are very large and broad, being rather thin and almost round, whose thick red sour-stalks above a foot long, stand towards the middle of the leaves; the lower part being divided into two round parts, close almost one to another, and are of a pale green colour, and hairy underneath. They grow in low and wet grounds by rivers and water-sides; their flowers rising and decaying in February and March, before the leaves which appear in April.

MEDICINAL VIRTUES. It is a great strengthener of the heart, and cheerer of the vital spirits. The roots are, by long experience, found to be very good against pestilential fevers, by provoking sweat, to be taken in wine. The decoction of the root in wine, is good for those that wheeze much, or are short winded. It provokes urine and is good for gravel, and kills flat and broad worms. The powder of the root is a remedy for sores hard to be cured, and it takes away spots and blemishes of the skin.

CABBAGES AND COLEWORTS.

Description is useless here. They belong to the genus *Brassicae.* As an article of diet they are wholesome and nutritious; but not very suitable for persons who have weak digestion.

MEDICINAL VIRTUES.—Cabbages or Coleworts boiled in broth open the body. The juice mixed with honey is good for hoarseness, or loss of the voice, and for those troubled with Asthma. The often eating of them well boiled is good for those that are entering into a consumption. The juice boiled with honey, and dropped into the corners of the eyes, clears the sight, by consuming any film beginning to dim it The decoction of Coleworts allays the swellings of sore and gouty legs and knees, wherein many gross and watery humours are fallen, the place being bathed therewith warm. Colewort stalks mixed with old hog's grease, are very effectual to anoint the sides of those who have had pains long therein. Cabbages are very windy: but Colewort flowers are more tolerable, and the more wholesome food of the two. A red Cabbage leaf placed on the side is effectual in removing pains, stitches, &c.

CALAMINT.

Description.—*Thymum Calamintha.*—It is also called Mountain-mint, it is a useful herb, but requires caution in some cases.

It seldom rises above a foot high, with square hairy, and woody stalks, and two small hoary leaves set at a joint, about the size of marjoram, a little dented about the edges, and of a very strong scent. The flowers stand at several spaces of the stalks, from the middle almost upwards, which are small and gaping like those of Mints, and of a pale bluish colour; after which follow small, round blackish seed. The root is small and woody, with fibres spreading the ground. It grows on heaths, and uplands, and dry grounds. It flowers in July, and the seed is ripe soon after.

Medicinal Virtues.—As a decoction, it is very useful in affections of the brain; for cramps, shortness of breath, colic pains in the stomach, yellow jaundice; and taken in wine, it arrests vomiting. The juice dropped into the ears relieves deafness. It is good for sciatica. A decoction of the leaves and wine, promotes perspiration, and removes obstructions of the liver and spleen. It regulates the flow of the gall, and is serviceable in old coughs.

WATER CALTROPS.

Description. *Tribulus Aquaticus, Tribulus Marinus.* Called Water Nuts, and Water Chesnuts.

There are two Caltrops; the first has a creeping and jointed root, sending forth tufts at each joint, from which joints arise long, flat, slender-knotted stalks, to the top of the water, divided into many branches, each having two leaves on both sides, two inches long, and half an inch broad, almost transparent, they look as if they were torn; the flowers are long, thick and whitish, set like a bunch of grapes, succeeded for the most part by sharp-pointed grains altogether, containing a small white kernel in them.

The second differs little except it delights in clearer water. Its stalks are round; its leaves are more pointed. They grow in the water, as their name implies.

MEDICINAL VIRTUES. Made into a poultice, they are good for inflammations, swellings, cankers, sore mouths and throats, being washed with the decoction. They cleanse and strengthen the neck and throat, and reduce the swellings of the same. It is a good remedy for the king's evil; for the stone and gravel, especially the nuts, being dried.

CAMOMILE.

Anthemis Nobilis. It is too well known to need description.

A decoction made of Camomile, removes pains and stitches in the side.

MEDICINAL VIRTUES.—The dried flowers have stomachic and tonic properties, which renders them very useful in dyspepsia and general debility. The flowers are an excellent remedy in spasmodic diseases, flatulent colics, in suppression of the menstrual discharge, in the vomiting of puerperal women, in the after pains, in agues, and in typhus fever. No bitter is so common as the Camomile. Light watery infusions of the flowers are much used to promote, and to assist the operation of other emetics, and strong infusions of it in small doses, from two to four ounces, twice or three times in the day, have been found, when used moderately to be good stomachics, and to assist digestion; and with the addition of a few drops of diluted vitriolic acid, have been effectual in removing feverish complaints, and in intermittent fevers. Dr. Morton says that he has cured intermittents which resisted Peruvian Bark by giving frequently in the day a scruple of flowers of Camomile in powder, with ten grains of wormwood, and as much diaphoretic antimony. It is good for Liver complaints. The flowers steeped in boiling water make an excellent fomentation for abscesses and inflamed parts, to promote suppuration and relieve pain. Flannels dipped in the hot decoction do as well.

Of the powdered flowers, 5 to 10 grains may be taken; of the Infusion from 1 to 3 ounces; of the Extract, from 5 to 20 grains; distilled water, 1 to 8 drachms; volatile oil, 1 to 4 drops. Syrup made of the juice of Camomile, with the flowers in white wine, is a remedy against the jaundice and dropsy.

CAMPHOR.

Foreign.—Arabic, *Camfur.*—The concrete juice of the *Camphora Officinarum.* As a medicine, it is diaphoretic, antiseptic, stimulant, antispasmodic, narcotic, and externally, anodyne. It is good in typhus, confluent small-pox, and all fevers and eruptions, of the typhoid class; also in measles, febrile delirium, hiccup, asthma, hysteria, epilepsy, gout, melancholy, and acute rheumatism. But it must never be taken in large doses. It exhilarates and raises the pulse with producing fever, it promotes perspiration, and promotes sleep, even where opium has failed. It corrects the effects of strong purges, diuretics, and narcotics. Dose, from 5 to 20 grains, in pills, powder, or emulsions. *Camphor Mixture*, dose from 1 to 2 ounces, made by simply putting a lump of the gum in cold water, and let it stand for a few hours; or previously dissolve the camphor in spirits of wine.

Camphor, Tincture of—Camphor ½ ounce, or 1 ounce; spirits of wine, half-pint, mix till the Camphor is dissolved. An external application of great value in rheumatism, paralytic numbness, inflammations, for dispersing tumours, preventing or restraining gangrenes.—Not to be taken internally.—The Camphor may also be dissolved in a little spirit of wine, and then mixed with oil—this is called, *Camphorated Oil.*

CAMPION WILD.

DESCRIPTION.—*Lychnis flore albo.* There are forty-five kinds of Campion:

The common English Campion is the only kind used in medicine. The Wild White Campion has many long and rather broad dark green leaves lying upon the ground, somewhat like plaintain, and hairy ; broader, and not so long ; the hairy stalks rise up in the middle two or three feet high, with great white joints, all which bear on several footstalks white flowers at the top, consisting of five broad-pointed leaves, each cut in on the end unto the middle, making them seem to be two a-piece, and each of them standing in a large green striped hairy bush, large and round below next the stalk. The seed is small and greyish in the hard heads that come up afterwards.

The Red Wild Campion differs in its leaves which are not so plainly ribbed, but shorter, rounder, and more woolly in handling. The flowers are of the same form and size, in some of a pale, in others of a bright red colour. They flower in summer, some earlier than others.

Medicinal Virtues. The decoction of the herb, either in white or red wine stops inward bleedings ; applied outwardly, it has the same effect. It is an excellent diuretic, removing stone, and obstructions in the kidneys. Two drachms of the seed drunk in wine, purges the body of coleric humours. It is good for old sores, ulcers, fistulas, to cleanse and heal them, and preventing putrefaction.

CAPSICUMS.

Foreign.—The pungent berries of the *Capsicum fustigratum.* They are very stimulant, useful in debilitated stomachs, dyspepsia, or indigestion. Used with vegetables to render them non-flatulent. They make an excellent gargle in malignant sore throats, and relaxed state of the uvula; and other organs of that part, as well as chronic hoarseness. Cayenne Pepper, which is Capsicum powdered, is taken from 2 to 8 grains. Taken moderately it is a superior medicine, Two parts Cayenne, three of compound rhubarb pill, and one of quinine form an excellent dinner pill.—See *Cayenne Pepper at the end of the book.*

CARAWAY.

Description.—*Carum Carui.*—The Caraway is propogated chiefly for the seeds. It bears divers stalks of fine cut leaves a little like the leaves of carrots, from among which rise a square stalk, at whose joints are set leaves a little like those of the carrot, but smaller, and at the top small umbels of white flowers, which turn into small blackish seed, which are well known. The root is whitish, small and long, like a parsnip, but with more wrinkled bark, and much less. It is usually sown in gardens. It flowers in July and seeds quickly after.

Medicinal Virtues, It is a good remedy for expelling wind, and for colic. The young root is better food than parsnips; it is comfortable to the stomach, and promotes digestion. The powder of the seed made into a poultice, takes away black and blue spots produced by blows and bruises. The herb itself, or with some of the seed bruised, laid hot in a bag or double cloth to the lower part of the belly, removes wind and colic. Combined with senna, these seeds correct its griping effects. The oil of Caraway, given in six or eight drops on a lump of sugar, is good for pains of the stomach, heart-burn, &c.

CARDAMOM.

Description.—*Elettaria Cardamomum*, a plant of the natural order *Zingiberacæa.*—This is an Indian plant, rather resembling our reeds. It produces a triangular fruit, about the size of a horsebean. These fruits or pods are an elegant and useful aromatic, of a grateful smell and flavour, very warm, yet not fiery like pepper. They strengthen the stomach and promote digestion. They are good for the headache, arising from a billious affection, and they also relieve the colic. Some dyspeptics regularly chew them, and they are not disagreeable. The large Cardamom, or Grain of Paradise is an excellent tonic.

Tincture of Cardamom.—Three ounces of the seeds, proof spirit, two pints. Bruise the seeds, and digest for 8 days.

Compound Tincture of Cardamoms.—Lesser Cardamom seeds powdered, Caraway seeds powdered, Cochineal powdered, two drachms of each, Cinnamon bruised, half an ounce; raisins stoned, four ounces, proof spirit, two pints. Digest for 14 days, and strain. Dose of the *Tincture*, two to three drachms, and of the *Compound Tincture* from three drachms to half an ounce. In dyspeptic habits, half a glass taken before dinner serves to rouse the nerves of the stomach, and to aid digestion.

WILD CARROTS.

DESCRIPTION.—*Daucus Sylvestus.*—Garden Carrots need no description ; but in medicine they are not so efficacious as the wild.

The Wild Carrot grows altogether like the garden but the leaves and stalks are whiter and rougher. The stalks bear large tufts of white flowers, with a deep purple spot in the middle, which are contracted together when the seed begins to ripen, and the middle part being hollow and the outward stalk rising high, make the whole umbel appear like a bird's nest. The roots small, long, and hard, and unfit for meat, being sharp and strong.

The wild kind grows by the field sides, and untilled places. They flower and seed in the end of Summer.

MEDICINAL VIRTUES. Wild Carrots expel wind, and remove stitches in the sides, promote urine and women's courses, and expel the stone. The seed also has the same effect, and is good for the dropsy, and for expelling wind. The leaves applied with honey cleanse running sores and ulcers. The seeds are antiflatulent, and an excellent diuretic.

CASTOR OIL.

Foreign.—This valuable oil is obtained from the seeds of a tree called *Palma Christi—Ricini Communis.* It is the mildest, safest, and most certain purgative known, seldom griping, or causing flatulency. In most persons it acts quickly, without pain, clears the bowels, leaves them with a greater tendency to relaxation than before, and does not require the dose to be increased in consequence of repetition. With most purgatives, the immediate effect is followed by constipation ; it is not so with Castor Oil. The usual dose for children is 1 to 2 drachms ; for adults from ½ ounce to 2 ounces.

The great objection to Castor Oil, its sickly nauseousness has produced many modes of taking it:—floated in brandy and water, barley-water, &c. &c. But perhaps the simplest way is to take it in a small quantity of Oat-meal and water—the meal neutralizes the taste.

CATECHU.

Foreign. A substance obtained from the wood of the *Acacia Catechu.* As a tonic it is most valuable in diarrhœa, chronic dysentery; it makes an excellent gargle for sore throats, or elongated uvula. It is good for sponginess of the gums, being allowed to dissolve in the mouth; it makes an excellent dentrifice. It is serviceable in gleet, Cucorrhœa, in passive hæmorrhages, especially those of the bowels and uterus, and for ulcerated mouth, chapped nipples, used as a tincture.

CATMINT.

Description.—*Nepeta Cataria.*—It grows a yard high, and has broad whitish leaves, and white flowers like mint. The stalks are square, whitish, hairy, and erect; the leaves stand two at a joint; they are broadest at the base, and terminate in an obtuse end; they are a little indented at the edges, and of a whitish green on the upper side, and very white underneath. The flowers are small and white; and they grow in spiked clusters, surrounding the stalks at certain distances. The plant has a strong and not very pleasant smell.

Medicinal Virtues.—Its virtues are considerable. It is a good female medicine; an infusion of it prevents hysteric complaints, vapours, and fits; it is also good to promote the evacuations after child delivery. It is good for pains in the head produced by colds, catarrh, &c. A decoction sweetened with sugar, or honey relieves an obstinate cough. The green leaves bruised, and applied to the anus, relieves the piles; the juice made into an ointment has the same effect. The decoction is good for cleansing the head.

CELANDINE,—LITTLE.

The greater and the Lesser Celandine are two different plants. They agree in nothing, except they have yellow flowers. The Great Celandine is much like the Poppy; and the Lesser Celandine resembles the Crow-foot. Their virtues also differ. It is surprising the old Herbalists did not make a distinction.

Description.—*Chelidonium Minus.* It is also known by the name of *Pilewort and Fogwort.* Celandine, or Pilewort spreads many round pale green leaves, set on weak and trailing branches, which lie upon the ground, and are flat, smooth and somewhat shining, and in some places marked with black spots, each standing on a long footstalk. The flowers, which are yellow, rise singly from the root, on long, slender, and naked stalks, consisting of nine or ten small narrow leaves, very like Crowsfoot. The seed also is not unlike, being many small kernels like a grain of corn, of a whitish colour, with fibres at the end of them. It grows mostly in moist corners of fields, and near water sides; yet it will grow in drier ground if it is a little shady. It flowers about March or April, is quite gone by May.

Medicinal Virtues.—If you dig up the root of it, you will perceive the perfect image of the disease commonly called the piles. Experience proves that the decoction of the leaves and roots is a wonderful remedy for the piles and hemorrhoids, the king's evil, or any other hard wens or tumours.

Pilewort made into an oil, ointment or plaister, has the same effect in curing the piles, or hemorrhoids, and the king's evil. The herb borne about one's body next the skin, helps in such liseases, though it never touches the affected place. With his I cured my own daughter of the king's evil, broke the sore, lrew out a quarter of a pint of corruption, and cured without ıny scar at all in one week's time.

CELANDINE,—GREAT.

Description.—*Chelidonium Majus.*—A common wild ılant having large leaves, and yellow flowers. It grows nearly hree feet high. The stalks are tender, round, green and naked, with thick joints. This plant, when broken in any part, emits a yellow juice, bitter in taste, and strong in scent. The leaves stand two at each joint; they are large, long, and deeply divided at the edges, and are of a yellowish green. The flowers produce small long pods, with blackish seed.

They grow by old walls, hedges and way-sides, in untilled places, and in gardens. They flower all the Summer.

MEDICINAL VIRTUES. It is a most valuable remedy for diseases of the eye, used as a decoction, or made into an ointment. The juice is the best way of adminstering it, it is an efficacious remedy for the jaundice, scurvy, and all obstructions of the liver and other viscera. The addition of a few aniseeds in making a decoction of it with wine, increases its efficacy in removing obstructions of the liver and gall. The juice applied to warts soon removes them, also ring-worms. The juice mixed with sulphur is a remedy for the itch. It has been given with great effect in scrofula. An ointment made of the roots and hogslard is a good remedy for the piles. Boil them together.

LITTLE CENTAURY.

DESCRIPTION.—*Centaurium Minus.*—There are two kinds of this plant, one bearing pale red flowers, the other white; but their virtues are the same. It usually grows with one round and somewhat crusted stalk, about a foot high or better, branching forth at the top into many sprigs, and some also from the joints of the stalks below; the flowers stand at the tops in one cluster. They are of a pale red, tending to carnation colour, consisting of five or six small leaves, very like those of St. John's wort. The root is small and hard, perishing every year. The plant is very bitter in taste.

It grows in fields, pastures, and woods. It flowers in July, and seeds a month after.

MEDICINAL VIRTUES. Centaury is justly esteemed as one of the most efficacious bitters in this island. It is often substituted for Gentian, which it much resembles. It is milder than Wormwood, or Holy Thistle. It is an excellent stomachic, both in substance and infusion and celebrated for the cure of intermittent fevers. It is a good remedy for worms; and like camomile, is made into tea for assisting the operation of emetics. As a bitter it is often taken to create an appetite. It removes obstructions of the liver and spleen; and is most useful in the jaundice, dropsy, green sickness, colic. It is very serviceable in obstructed menstruation, in connection with some mild purgative. The green herb bruised is very good for wounds, sores, &c. An ounce of Centaury, with two drachms each of Avens, and Angelica, infused in one quart of boiling water, and then add two ounces of Cardamoms—these make an excellent stomachic. Take a wine-glassful two or three times a day. *Remember* that the long continued use of any bitter impairs the coats of the stomach, and produces an incurable debility of that organ.

There is, besides these, another small Centaury, which bears a yellow flower, like the former, save that the leaves are larger, and of a darker green. In diseases of the blood, use the red Centaury; if of choler, use the yellow; but if phlegm or water, you will find the white best.

CHERRY-TREE.

DESCRIPTION.—*Cerasum Durasinum.*—This tree is well known.

MEDICINAL VIRTUES.—Cherries, as they are of different tastes, so they are of different qualities; the sweet digest more speedily, but have little nourishment. The acid are more pleasing to a hot stomach, procure appetite to meat, and help to cut tough phlegm, and gross humours; but when they are dried they are more constipating than when they are fresh, being cooling in hot diseases, and grateful to the stomach, they provoke urine. The gum of the Cherry-tree, dissolved in wine, is good for a cold, cough, and hoarseness of the throat; it improves the complexion, and the eye-sight. Cherries improve the appetite, black Cherries bruised with the stones, and dissolved, the water thereof is used to expel wind and the gravel.

CHERRIES,—WINTER.

DESCRIPTION.—*Alkekengi.* A very singular and pretty plant cultivated in gardens.

The Winter Cherry has a running root in the ground, shooting forth at several joints in several places. The stalk rises about a yard high, whereon are set many broad and long green leaves, somewhat like Night shade, but larger: at the joints come forth whitish flowers, composed of five leaves each, which produce green berries inclosed with thin skins, which are reddish when ripe, and as large as a cherry. The pulp encloses flat yellowish seeds, which being gathered and strung up, are kept all the year for use.

They flower in July; and the fruit is ripe about August, or the beginning of September.

MEDICINAL VIRTUES. The leaves being cooling, may be used in inflammations, but they are not so purgative as the berries and fruit. They promote a copious and an easy discharge of urine, and are excellent for the gravel. The berries and leaves distilled, or made into a decoction, with milk and a little sugar, must be drunk morning and evening. Or, take three or four good handfulls of the berries, either green or dried, and having bruised them, put them in so many gallons of beer or ale when it is new and tunned up. This drink, taken daily, has been very useful in urinary diseases, &c. It prevents the accumulation of stone. The decoction of the berries in wine and water is the most usual way, but the powder of them taken in drink is more effectual.

CHERVIL, *Sweet*, or SWEET CICELY.

DESCRIPTION.—*Myrrhis Odorata.*—It grows much like the great Hemlock, with large spreading leaves, cut into divers parts, yet of a fresher green than the Hemlock. The stalks grow a yard high, are creased hollow, and having smaller leaves at the joints. The stalks are crowned with tufts of white flowers, which produce long black shining seeds, pointed at each end, of a sharp, sweet, and pleasant taste. The root is large and white, deep in the ground, and its smell is stronger than that of the plant.

Medicinal Virtues.—The plant is a wholesome addition to salad. The root boiled, and eaten with vinegar, warms and stimulates cold stomachs; it is beneficial in complaints of the chest and lungs. It relieves flatulency, and promotes appetite, and removes female obstructions. The juice is good to heal old ulcers.—It is so harmless that it cannot do any harm.—Pulverize the root, and take half a spoonful in brandy for flatulency, colic, &c.

CHERVIL.

Description.—*Scandix Odorata.*—As a salad herb it is cultivated in gardens. It is like Parsley in its manner of growth; but after it is grown, the leaves rather resemble those of Hemlock, hairy, and sometimes rather red. The stalks are round, striated, hollow, and of a light green; they divide into several branches, and they grow two feet high. They bear white flowers in large tufts, which produce blackish seeds, of a sweet taste. It sometimes grows wild, two or three feet high, in meadows, by the hedge sides, and on heaths. It flowers and seeds early.

Medicinal Virtues.—As a garden vegetable, it ought to be generally cultivated. The roots decocted work moderately by urine. As a vegetable they warm the stomach, and purify the blood. The leaves, combined with a few Hemlock leaves, made into a poultice, relieve the sore breasts of women giving suck; by removing the knotty pants, it causes the milk to flow freely. It should be applied warm. Applied to the belly it gives relief in gravel. It is an expectorant, and relieves Asthma, if boiled in whey. Bruised and applied, it removes swellings, and marks occasioned by blows or bruises.

CHESTNUT TREE.

Alsculus Hippocastanum.—It is needless to describe a tree so commonly known.

MEDICINAL VIRTUES.—It is a powerful astringent, and it has been used as a substitute for Cinchona, in cases of Ague, intermittent fevers, &c. The inner skin of the nut is so binding, that a scruple taken by a man, or ten grains by a child, instantly stops fluxes. The dried nut powdered, and a drachm taken is good for the overflowing of the menses. The powder made into an electuary relieves coughs and spitting of blood.

CHESTNUTS.—EARTH CHESTNUTS.

DESCRIPTION.—*Bunium Fexuosum.*—They are called Earth Nuts, Earth Chestnuts, Ground Nuts, Pig Nuts. The root is the size of a Chestnut, brown outside, and white within, and sweet in taste. The plant grows a foot high; the leaves are divided into fine and numerous partitions; the stalk is firm, upright, round, and green; the flowers are small, white, and grow in tufts.

MEDICINAL VIRTUES. They are rather hot and dry in quality; the seed is good to provoke urine; and also the root, but it is not so efficacious as the seed. The root dried and beaten into a powder, and made into an electuary, is a singular remedy for spitting of blood, and for bloody urine.

CHICKWEED.

Alsine Media. It is well known. It is very common in gardens.

MEDICINAL VIRTUES.—The plant chopped and boiled in lard makes a fine green cooling ointment, and is good for piles, ulcers, sores, &c. The juice taken inwards, is good for scurvy. A cloth saturated with the juice, and applied to opposite the liver, reduces inflammation; the juice is good for inflammations of the eyes, when dropped into them. The leaves boiled with Marshmallows, and made into a poultice with fenugreek and linseed, applied to swellings and imposthumes, break them, reduce the swelling, and ease the pain. A poultice made of the leaves is a great cooler for inflammations.

"Some German physicians affirm that this plant, combined with Elecampane, is a specific in Hydrophobia, I administered it in a case, and the patient recovered."—DR. BEACH, *America.*

CHICK PEAS, or CICERS.

The garden sorts, whether red, black, or white, are so well known as to require no description.

MEDICINAL VIRTUES.—They are less windy than beans, but nourish more; they provoke urine, have a cleansing faculty, and break the stone in the kidneys. To drink the cream of them, being boiled in water is the best way. It purges, and promotes menstruation. One ounce of Cicers, two ounces of French barley, and a small handful of marsh-mallow roots, washed and cut, and boiled with a chicken, and four ounces taken in the morning, and fasting two hours after, is a good medicine for pains in the side. The white Cicers are used more for meat than medicine, yet have the same effects. The wild Cicers are much more powerful than the garden kind.

CHOCOLATE AND COCOA.

Foreign.—Both are prepared from the seeds of the *Theobroma Cacao,* a tree growing in the West Indies, and other places. Cocoa when genuine and properly prepared, is wholesome and nutritious, containing a large quantity of oily or fatty matter, starch, &c. Cocoa does not affect the nervous system in the same manner as tea and coffee, and therefore it may be used where they are not proper. Cocoa can seldom be obtained in a perfectly pure state; the only way is to purchase the nibs and crush and boil them.

Chocolate is of the same nature, but very liable to be adulterated. That of French make is generally to be preferred. Chocolate when pure is exceedingly nutritious.

CINQUEFOIL.

DESCRIPTION.—*Pentaphyllon.*—In some countries it is called five-fingered grass. It spreads and creeps far upon the ground, with long slender strings like strawberries, which take root again, and shoot forth many leaves made of five parts, and sometimes of seven, dented about the edges and somewhat hard. The stalks are slender, leaning downwards, and bear many small beautiful yellow flowers, with yellow threads in the middle. The root is of a blackish brown colour, growing long, with small strings, by which it soon spreads over the ground. It grows by wood sides, hedge sides, the pathway in fields, and in the borders and corners of them.

MEDICINAL VIRTUES.—The root is to be used, which must be dug up in April, and the outer bark taken off and dried; the rest is not used. Few drugs have power equal to this root for all kinds of fluxes. As an astringent, it stops purgings, and profuse menstruation. A scruple of the powder in wine will cure the ague. It may be repeated once or twice when the complaint is obstinate. It stops bleeding of the lungs, or bronchial tubes, bleeding at the nose, and is useful in coughs, jaundice, and ulcers in the kidneys. By washing the eyes in a decoction of the root inflammations are removed. The juice of the root is very efficacious. The juice and wheat bread boiled first is a good styptic. For the decoction, boil $1\frac{1}{2}$ ounce of the root in a quart of water down to a pint. The juice mixed with honey, relieves coughs, and hoarseness.

GARDEN CLARY

DESCRIPTION.—*Salvia Verbeneca.*—Some know it by the name of Clear-eye. Garden Clary has four square stalks, with broad, rough, wrinkled, whitish, or hairy green leaves, evenly indented on the edges, and of a strong sweet scent. The flowers grow at certain distances, with two small leaves at the joints under them, somewhat like the flowers of sage, but smaller and of a whitish blue colour. The seed is brownish, and somewhat flat. It is propagated by seed annually.

MEDICINAL VIRTUES.—The whole of this herb is used fresh or dry. It is cordial and rather astringent. It strengthens the stomach, relieves headaches, and cures the whites. A decoction is good for inflamed eyes. The mucilage of the seed diluted with water, and applied to tumours, or swellings, takes them away ; the leaves used with vinegar, or with a little honey, cures boils, felons, and inflammations caused by the same. The powder of the dried root provokes sneezing, and purges the head of much rheum. It is of much use both for men and women who have weak backs ; and it strengthens the reins.

WILD CLARY grows on the banks of ditches, and in dry ground. It is less than Garden Clary. Its medicinal virtues are rather more powerful. It is a capital remedy for dimness of sight. The plan is to put the seed into the eyes. They immediately collect a coat of mucilage about them, and this catches hold of any little thing it meets with in the eye—the seeds drop out of themselves, and cause little pain.

CLEAVERS.

DESCRIPTION.—*Aparine.*—It is also called Goose-share, and Goose-grass. The common cleavers has divers very rough square stalks, rising two or three yards sometimes, if it meets with any tall bushes or trees, whereon it climbs without claspers, or it creeps on the ground, full of joints, each of which shoots out a branch, and leaves usually six, set in a round compass, like a star, or rowel of a spur: From between the leaves or the joints at the top of the branches come forth very small white flowers. The seeds grow two together; they are rough. The stalks, leaves, and especially the seeds are so rough that they will stick to any thing they touch.

It grows in hedges, and by ditch-sides, and it is injurious to whatever grows near it. It flowers in June or July, and the seed is ripe in August.

MEDICINAL VIRTUES.—The juice of the herb is a good styptic for bleeding wounds. It is taken in broth, to keep those lean who are apt to grow fat. The distilled water drank twice a day is good for the yellow jaundice ; and the decoction also has the same effect, and stayeth lasks, both are useful in the bloody flux. The juice is also very good to close up the lips of green wounds, and the powder of the dried herb cures old ulcers. Boiled in hog's lard, it relieves hard swellings, or kernels in the throat. The juice is good for ear-ache. It is a renowned diuretic, most appropriate to remove speedily suppression of urine, gravelly complaints, removing slimy matter and obstructions from the kidneys and bladder. It has been found useful in the cure of scurvy. The infusion should always be made in cold water; say 4 ounces to 2 pints.

CLOVE.—SPICE.

Foreign.—Cloves are excellent against disorders of the head, and the stomach; they are warm, cordial and strengthening; they expel wind, and are a good remedy for the colic. Dose of Powder 2 to 3 grains. Infusion, 1 to 2 ounces. Tincture 20 to 30 minims. The Oil of Cloves is excellent for the toothache, and better still combined with Cajeput oil, opium, and Camphor.

CLOWN'S WOUND WORT.

DESCRIPTION—*Rusticum Vulna Herba.* It grows usually about two feet high, with square, green, rough stalks, but slender, joined far asunder, and two of them are very long, narrow dark green leaves, bluntly dented at the edges, ending in a long point. The flowers stand towards the tops, compassing the stalks at the joints with the leaves, and end in a spiked top, having long and and gaping hoods of a purplish red colour, with whitish spots in them, and standing in somewhat round husks. The root is composed of many long fibres, with tuberous long knobs of a pale yellowish or whitish colour. The plant has a strong smell.

It grows frequently by path-sides in fields, and in or near ditches. It flowers in June or July, and the seed is ripe soon after.

MEDICINAL VIRTUES. It is very effectual in fresh and green wounds, and therefore beareth not its name for nought. And it is very available in staunching of blood, and to dry up the humours in old ulcers, cankers, &c. that hinder the healing of them.

A syrup made of the juice of it is inferior to none for inward wounds, ruptures of veins, bloody flux, vessels broken, spitting, or vomiting blood. Ruptures are wonderfully cured by taking now and then a little of the syrup, and applying an ointment or plaister of this herb to the place. Also, if any vein, or muscle be swelled, apply a plaister of this herb to it—the addition of a little Comfrey to it, renders it more effectual. This Herb is very valuable, and should not be overlooked.

COCK'S HEAD.

Description.—*Galli Caput.*—It is also called Red Fitching, and Medœ Fitch. It has various weak, rough stalks, drooping, set winged leaves, longer and more pointed than those of lintels, and whitish underneath ; from the tops of these stalks arise other slender stalks naked unto the tops, where there grow many small flowers like a spike, of a pale reddish colour, with some blueness among them ; after which rise up in their places, round, and somewhat flat heads. It grows under hedges, and in the open fields.

Medicinal Virtues.—It has power to rarify and digest ; and therefore the green leaves bruised and used as a plaister, disperse knots, or kernels in the flesh ; and if when dry it be taken in wine, it relieves the stranguary ; and being anointed with oil, it provoketh sweat. It is a singular food for cattle, to cause them to give much milk, and boiled in ordinary drink it must be useful for nurses !

COFFEE.

Foreign.—The berries of the *Coffea Arabicus.* It is a tonic and stimulant, and possesses exhilarant and antisoporific properties. It is good in cases of poisoning by opium and laudanum. It is good for hooping-cough and asthma. It is not suitable where there is a profuse secretion of bile, as it stimulates the system too much. It is far more nutritious than tea. Coffee should be used freshly ground, infused in boiling, and never boiled. It assists digestion, expels wind, and gently promotes urine. It suspends the inclination to sleep, especially when taken at night. It is a first-rate *disinfectant.* Even the smell of musk and castor, which cannot be overpowered by any other substance, is completely dispelled by the fumes of Coffee —the same remark applies to the odour of asafœtida.

CASCARILLA.

Croton Eleuteria—The Bark is imported from the Bahama islands, in curled pieces. It has a light agreeable smell, and a moderately bitter taste with some aromatic warmth. When burning, it has a very fragrant smell, like that of musk. It produces a sense of heat, and excites the action of the stomach. It may be advantageously employed in flatulent colics, internal hæmorrhages, dysenteries, diarrhœa, &c. It is much used among the Germans, as a febrifuge, for stopping agues. In the year 1719, it was of great service in an epidemic dyssentery which raged at Paris, and had not yielded to ipecacuanha. Dr. Lewes, in his New Dispensatory, says that it deserves to be more regarded than it is at present.——*Dose*, from ten grains to half a drachm, or more.——*Tincture* :—Four ounces of the bark powdered; two pints proof spirits; digest with gentle heat seven days, and strain. It is a fine stimulating medicine, and excellent in the gout, or after that disease, to give to the stomach tone and system. *Dose*, two drachms four times a day in cinnamon water.

COLEWORTS.—SEA.

Description.—*Soldanella.*—This has rather long and broad, large, and thick wrinkled leaves, a little crumpled about the edges, and growing upon a thick footstalk, very brittle, of a greyish green colour, from which rises up a strong thick stalk, two feet high, with leaves thereon to the top, where it branches forth much; and on every branch standeth a large bush of pale whitish flowers, consisting of four leaves a piece. Some of these plants have red flowers, shaped like a bell. They grow on the sea-coasts.

Medicinal Virtues.—The whole plant is to be gathered

fresh when about flowering, and boiled in ale with nutmeg and cloves, and taken according to a person's strength. It is strongly purgative and sometimes promotes urine very beneficially. The bruised seed decocted, kills worms, and is very effectual in clap or gonorrhæa.

COLOCYNTH.

Foreign.—Bitter Apple, a plant of the natural order, *Cucurbitaceæ.* It is the fruit of a creeping plant, growing on the shores of the Mediterranean. An extract from the dried pulp is used in medicine. It is very useful in habitual constipation, in affections of the brain, as a revulsive. In small doses it is expectorant, diuretic, and alterative. Dose;—powder 2 to 8 grains; Extract, from 4 to 10 grains. It is best to take it with some aromatic, to neutralise its griping tendency. For Pills, combine with rhubarb, ginger, and extract of gentian. It is a most valuable aperient, tending to discharge watery humours.

COLT'S FOOT.

Description.—*Tussilago, Farfara.* Called also Coughwort, Foal's-foot, Horse-hoof, and Bull's foot. It shoots up a slender stalk, with small yellowish flowers as large as those of the Dandelion; these come before the leaves; they fall away quickly, and then come round leaves, sometimes dented about the edges, with a little down or frieze over the green leaf on the upper side, which may be rubbed away, and whitish or meally underneath. The root is small and white, spreading much under ground.

It grows in wet grounds and also in dry places. It flowers in February.

Medicinal Virtues.—It is a most valuable herb, and is not sufficiently appreciated. Its powerful expectorant qualities have rendered it celebrated as a remedy for coughs. It abounds with mucilage; it is slightly bitter; and possesses tonic and demulcent properties. A decoction is made by boiling a handful of the leaves in a quart of water till reduced to a pint, sweetened with Sugar Candy, and acidulated with a slice of Lemon. A wine-glassful may be taken three or four times a day. This is very useful in coughs and in all diseases of the lungs, shortness of breath, wheezing, &c. It thickens the expectoration when thin, and of course must allay inflammation. The Syrup of Colt's foot is much recommended by French physicians for chronic bronchitis. Boiled in milk it is excellent for consumptive patients with distressing coughs.

Dr. Cullen found this plant of great service in scrofulous diseases. He gave a decoction of the dried leaves, and found it succeed where other remedies had failed. Fuller relates that a girl with twelve scrofulous sores was cured by drinking daily as much as she could of a strong decoction. Dr. Percival found it useful in hectic diarrhœas. A decoction with wormwood has done wonders in calculous complaints. Sweetened with honey, it is good for colds and asthma.

The leaves are the basis of the British Herb Tobacco—to them are added the leaves of Eye-bright, Buckbean, Betony, Rosemary, Thyme, Lavender, and Camomile Flowers. This Tobacco is first-rate for Asthma. Let the Colt's foot preponderate.

COLUMBINES.

Aquilegia Vulgaris.—These are well known, growing almost in every garden.

Medicinal Virtues.—The leaves of Columbines are commonly used in lotions with good success for sore mouths and throats. Tragus says, that a drachm of the seed taken in wine, with a little saffron, opens obstructions of the liver, and is good for the yellow jaundice, if the party after taking it, sweat well in bed. The Spaniards used to eat the root in a morning fasting, many days together, to cure gravel, and other diseases of the kidneys.

COMFREY.

Description.—*Symphytum Officinal.*—The common great

Comfrey has large hairy green leaves lying on the ground, so hairy or prickly that if they touch any part of the body, they will cause it to itch. The stalk rises two or three feet high, hollow and cornered, and is very hairy. It has many such leaves as grow below, but decreasing in size to the top. At the joints of the stalks it is divided into many branches, with some leaves thereon, and at the ends stand many flowers in order one above another, which are long and hollow like the finger of a glove, of a pale whitish colour, after which come small black seeds. The roots are large and long, spreading large thick branches under ground, black on the outside, and whitish within.

There is another sort like this, but rather less, and which beareth flowers of a pale purple colour. They grow by ditches and water-sides, and in moist fields. They flower in June or July, and give their seed in August.

MEDICINAL VIRTUES. What was spoken of Clown's Woundwort, may be said of this. The Great Comfrey relieves spitting of blood, and bloody urine. The root boiled in water or wine, relieves inward hurts, bruises, wounds, and ulcers of the lungs, and loosens tough phlegm. It relieves those colds in the head which deposit rheum in the lungs; cures bloody flux, immoderate courses, the whites, and diseases of the kidneys. A syrup made thereof is effectual for all inward hurts, and for outward wounds and sores in the fleshy or sinewy part of the body. The roots are more effectual than the leaves. They are good for fresh wounds or cuts when bruised and laid thereon, and also for ruptures, and very powerful in knitting broken bones. It is an excellent remedy for sore nipples. The roots beaten small, and spread upon leather, and laid upon any place affected with the gout, immediately relieves the pains; also pained joints, and is very useful in moist ulcers, gangrenes, and mortifications.

COPAIBA, OR COPAIVA.

Foreign.—A resinous juice procured from the bark of the *Copaifera Multynga.* It is very diuretic, and stimulates the mucous membranes generally. In large doses it is purgative.

It is very useful in diseases of the urinary organs, especially gonorrhœa; in chronic affections of the chest, and piles, and externally for chilblains and indolent ulcers. Take 10 to 40 minims or drops in plain or aromatic water. Of oil of Copaiba, take 10 to 20 minims, or drops.

CORALWORT.

Description.—*Corallium Herba.* It is also called Toothwort, Tooth Violet, Dog Teeth Violet, and Dentaria. This plant shoots forth one or two winged leaves, upon long brownish footstalks, which are doubled down at their first coming out of the ground; when they are fully opened, they consist of seven leaves, of a sad green colour, dented about the edges, set on both sides the middle rib one against another, as the leaves of the ash-tree; the stalk has no leaves on the lower half, the upper half bears three or four, each consisting of five leaves, sometimes of three; on the top stand four or five flowers upon short stalks, with long husks; the flowers are very like the flowers of stock-gilliflowers, of a pale purplish colour, consisting of four leaves a piece. The root is smooth, white and shining, creeping, and has various small round knobs set together.

Medicinal Virtues. It cleanses the bladder, and provokes urine, expels gravel and the stone; it eases pains in the sides and bowels, and is very good for inward wounds, especially such as are made in the breast or lungs. A drachm of the root powdered must be taken every morning in wine. An ointment made of it is good for wounds and ulcers.

CORIANDER.

Foreign.—The seeds produced by the *Coriandrum Sativum.* They are cordial, aromatic, and chiefly used to correct the griping tendency of active purgatives, as Senna, &c. They are excellent to expel wind, warm, and strengthen the stomach, and aid digestion, are good for pains in the head, and arrest purgings.

CORN COCKLE.

Description.—*Agreste Gith.*—A tall and beautiful plant, wild in corn-fields, with red flowers. It grows two feet high; the stalk is single, slender, round, hairy, firm, and very erect. The leaves stand two at a joint, not numerous; they are long, narrow, hairy, and of a bright green colour, the flowers stand singly, one at the top of each branch,—large, and of a beautiful red. They have a beautiful cup, composed of five narrow hairy leaves much longer than the flower.

Medicinal Virtues.—The seeds are used; they promote urine, the menses, and all obstructions, and are good in dropsy and jaundice. The best way is to give them in powder, made into an electuary, to be taken for some time; for the medicines, whose virtues are against chronic disease, do not take effect at once.

COSTMARY or ALCOST, or BALSAM HERB.

This is known to be an inhabitant in almost every garden, so that it is needless to describe.

Medicinal Virtues.—Costmary gently purges choler and phlegm, extenuating that which is gross, and cutting that which is tough and glutinous, and hinders putrefaction and corruption. It is astringent to the stomach, and strengthens the liver, and the other inward parts; and taken in whey, it is more effectual. Taken fasting in the morning it relieves chronic pains in the head, and dries up, and consumes all thin rheums or distillations from the head into the stomach. It is very profitable for those that are fallen into a continual evil disposition of the body, called Cachexy, but especially in the beginning of the disease. It is an especial relief to weak and cold livers. The seed is given to children for worms, and so is the infusion of flowers in white wine, about two ounces at a time. It makes a valuable ointment for sores, being boiled with oil of olive, and adder's tongue; and after it is strained, put a little wax, resin, and turpentine. to bring it to a convenient body.

COWHAGE.

Foreign.—The stiff hairs which cover the pods, or seed vessels, are used. This hair or pile scraped off, and mixed in some viscid vehicle, is the part to be taken to dislodge intestinal worms, especially the lumbrici, resembling earth worms. It is a most effectual remedy. The dose is from 3 to 10 grains, or more, on going to bed, in treacle, honey, or syrup; repeated for 3 or 4 days, and then administer a brisk purgative, as infusion of Senna. Cowhage is quite harmless, in a vehicle as above.

COWSLIPS, OR PEAGLES.

Primula Veris. The wild and garden Cowslips, are so well known, that they need no description. They flower in April and May.

Medicinal Virtues. The flowers are held to be more effectual than the leaves. An ointment being made with them, taketh away spots and wrinkles of the skin, sun-burning and freckles, and increases personal beauty; they remedy diseases of the head arising from heat and wind, as vertigo, phrenzies, falling sickness, palsies, convulsions, cramp, and pains in the nerves. The roots allay pains in the back and bladder, and are a good diuretic. The leaves are good in wounds, and the flowers take away trembling.

Because they strengthen the brain and nerves, and remedy palsies, the Greeks gave them the name Paralysis. The flowers preserved or conserved, and the size of a nutmeg taken every morning, is a sufficient dose for inward diseases. The ointment is made of the leaves and hog's lard.

The flowers of the Cowslip make an excellent wine of a rather sedative nature, easing pain, and disposing to sleep. It may be made as follows:—

Allow 4 pounds of sugar to a gallon of water, and boil and skin it till it be quite clear. Add a gallon of the flowers, picked from the stalks, and the rind of a lemon; and let them boil three minutes. Put into a vessel to cool, and then into the cask; add the juice of the lemon, and a little brandy.

CRANESBILL.

DESCRIPTION.—*Geranium.*—It is sometimes called Stork-bill, Dove's-foot. There are many kinds of it. It is more generally known by its Botanical name than otherwise, *Geranium.* While some are tender and cultivated in the Greenhouse, others grow wild in many places by the path-sides. That known as *Dove's-foot* has small, round, pale-green leaves indented at the edges, resembling mallows, standing upon long hairy stalks, lying in a round compass upon the ground, from which rise two or more reddish jointed, slender, hairy stalks, having similar leaves, upon which grow many small bright red flowers, of five leaves each.

MEDICINAL VIRTUES.—It is good for the colic, and for the gravel. The decoction in wine cures inward wounds, hurts, or bruises, arrests the bleeding, and expels the congealed blood. The decoction is a good fomentation for gout, joint-aches, or pain of the sinews. The root is very astringent, subtonic, and antiseptic. It is one of the most pleasant and valuable astringents known. It gives tone to the stomach and bowels, restrains all immoderate discharges, and prevents inward mortification. It is excellent for all bowel complaints. The best is a decoction by boiling the root in milk. An infusion of the root immediately suppresses bleeding at the lungs.—The dose of the root from 12 to 25 grains.

CRANESBILL.—STINKING.

DESCRIPTION.—*Geranium Robertianum.*—It is often called *Herb Robert.* It very much resembles the Cranesbill previously described, except the five leaves at the top of the stalks are much larger, and of a redder colour. The flowers are moderately large, and of a bright red, conspicuous and pretty; the fruit that follows is long and slender, resembling the long beak of a bird; hence the name.

MEGICINAL VIRTUES.—It is in great repute among farmers, being a cure for black water, bloody flux, given in decoction, and repeated. The whole plant is to be gathered, even to the root, and dried for use. It is a rare astringent, scarcely any plant can equal it. It may be given dried and powdered, or in decoction. It restrains profuse menstruation, dysentery, and all other bleedings. The decoction gives great relief in stone or gravel. It is a first-rate vulnerary, or wound herb. An ointment made of the green leaves and lard reduces scrofulous and cancerous swellings, and heals sore nipples. Herb Robert, and Tutsan, or St. John's Wort, are two of the best remedies for outward and inward bleedings.

CRESS,—GARDEN.

Nasturtium Hortense.—Every one knows this plant. It warms and strengthens the stomach. It is good for the scurvy, being a great purifier of the blood. The seeds open obstructions.

CRESS,—BLACK.

Description.—*Nasturtium Niger.*—It has long leaves, deeply cut and jagged on both sides, not much unlike wild mustard; the stalks small, very limber, though very tough; you may twist them round as you may a willow before they break. The flowers are very small and yellow, after which come small pods, containing the seed.

It usually grows by the way sides, and sometimes upon mud walls, but most among stones and rubbish.

Medicinal Virtues. It is a plant of a hot and biting nature. The seed of Black Cress strengthens the brain, and in that respect is little inferior to mustard-seed. It is good to stay rheums, which fall from the head upon the lungs. Beat the seed into powder, and make it into an electuary with honey; and you will have an excellent remedy for coughs, yellow jaundice, and sciatica. The herb boiled into a poultice, is an excellent remedy for inflammations, both in women's breasts and men's testicles.

CRESS,—SCIATICA CRESS.

Description.—*Nasturtium Silvestre.*—These also are of two kinds. The first rises up with a round stalk, about two feet high, spread into several branches, whose lower leaves are larger than the upper, yet all indented on the edges, like garden cress, but smaller; the flowers are small and white, at the tops of branches, which produce small brownish seeds, very sharp in taste, more so than garden cress; the root is long, white, and woody.

The other hath the lower leaves whole, rather long and broad, deeply dented about the edges towards the ends; but those that grow up higher are less. The flowers and seeds are like the former, and so is the root, and both root and seed are as sharp as it.

They grow by the waysides in untilled places, and by the sides of old walls. They flower in the end of June, and their seed is ripe in July.

Medicinal Virtues.—The leaves, but especially the root taken fresh in Summer-time, and made into a poultice or salve with lard, and applied to the places pained with the sciatica, for four or five hours, the place afterwards to be bathed with wine and oil mixed, and then wrapped with wool or skins after they have sweat a little, will assuredly cure not only the same disease in the hips, or other joints, as gout in the hands or feet, but all other old diseases of the head, (as inveterate rheums,) and other parts of the body that are difficult to be cured. Repeat in five or six days. It is also effectual in diseases of the spleen; applied to the skin, it taketh away blemishes, whether they be scars, leprosy, or scabs. It may ulcerate the part, yet that is to be healed with a salve made of oil and wax.

THE CANDY-TUFT, *Iberis Amara*, is of the same nature. Flowers, different colours. The leaves are used, and give relief in sciatica, or hip-gout. The best way is to beat them with a little lard. It is a good remedy, and ought to be more in use.

CRESS,—WATER CRESS.

Nasturtium Aquaticum.—This is well-known.

Medicinal Virtues. They are more powerful against the scurvy, and to cleanse the blood and humours, than Brooklime, (which see.) It removes the stone, and is very diuretic. It removes female obstructions. The decoction cleanseth ulcers, by washing them therewith. The leaves bruised, or the juice, is good to be applied to the face, or other parts troubled with freckles, pimples, spots, or the like, at night, and washed away in the morning. The juice mixed with vinegar, and the fore part of the head bathed therewith, is very good for those that are dull and drowsy, or have the lethargy.

CROSSWORT.

Description.—*Cruciata.*—It is so called from the situation of its leaves.

Common Crosswort has square hairy brown stalks, a little above a foot high, having four small broad and pointed, hairy, green leaves growing at every joint, each against other crossway. Towards the tops of the stalks at the joints, with the leaves in three or four rows downwards, stand small, pale, yellow flowers. The root is very small and full of fibres. It grows in moist grounds, and meadows. It flowers from May all the Summer long.

Medicinal Virtues.—This is a very good wound herb, and is used inwardly, not only to stay bleeding of wounds, but to consolidate them, as it outwardly does any green wound, which it quickly healeth. The decoction of the herb in wine, raises phlegm from the chest, and is good for obstructions in the breast, stomach, or bowels, and it rectifies a decayed appetite. It is also good to wash any wound or sore with, to cleanse and heal it. The herb bruised and boiled, applied outwardly, and renewing it often; and in the mean time the decoction of the herb in wine taken inwardly every day, certainly cures rupture, if it be not too inveterate; but very speedily if it be fresh and of late occurence. It is a good remedy for fever, rheumatism and dropsy.

CROTON OIL.

Foreign.—An oil extracted from the seeds of the *Croton Tiglii.* It is the most powerful of all known purgatives. No one ought to venture on more than a drop at first. In obstinate costiveness, in dropsy, in apoplexy, and paralysis, this oil is generally used. In lock-jaw, and mania, it is of great advantage, a drop or two placed on the tongue will be sufficient. Externally applied it is a valuable counter-irritant; soon producing eruption, and therefore is a special remedy for inflammation of the chest.

CROWFOOT.

DESCRIPTION.—*Ranunculus Acris.*—It is also called Frogsfoot, Crowfoot, Gold Cups, King's Knob, Poults, Butter-flowers, and Butter-cups.

The most common Crowfoot hath many dark green leaves, cut into divers parts, in taste biting and sharp, biting and blistering the tongue; it bears many flowers, and those of a bright resplendent yellow colour. They grow very common every where, especially in fields.

MEDICINAL VIRTUES.—This fiery and hot-spirited herb is not fit to be given inwardly; but an ointment of the leaves or flowers will raise a blister, and may be applied to the nape of the neck to draw rheum from the eyes. The herb being bruised and mixed with a little mustard, raises a blister as perfectly as Cantharides, and with far less danger.

CUCKOW-POINT.

DESCRIPTION.—*Arum Maculatum.*—By some it is called Aron, Arum, Ramp, Starchwort, Cuckow-pint and Wake-Robin.

It sends forth three, four, or five leaves from one root, each large and long, broad at the bottom next the stalk, forked, ending in a point, of a full green colour, each standing upon a thick round stalk, 4 to 6 inches long, among which, after two or three months that they begin to wither, rises up a bare, round whitish green stalk, spotted and streaked with purple, higher than the leaves: at the top of which are long hollow husks close at the bottom. but open from the middle upwards, ending in a point; in the middle whereof stand the small long pestle or clapper, of a dark purple colour, as the husk is on the inside, though green without, which, after continuing for some time, the husk with the clapper decays, and the foot thereof groweth to be a small long bunch of berries, green at first, and of a red colour when ripe, of the size of a hazel-nut kernel. They look very tempting, but are highly poisonous, as indeed the whole plant is. The root is round and long, of the size and shape of a walnut, externally brown, and white internally, and of a sharp acrid taste, and so is the whole plant. The root was anciently used instead of starch.

There is another sort of Cuckow-point, with lesser leaves than the former, and sometimes harder, having blackish spots upon them, which for the most part abide longer green in Summer than the former, and both leaves and roots are more sharp and fierce than it: in all things else it is like the former.

These two sorts grow under our hedges.

Medicinal Virtues.—The root is the part used. It is a good medicine in palsies. Half of one of the roots, fresh gathered and bruised, will sometimes restore the speech at once; if not, repeat the medicine. It is also good in scorbutic cases, and in all inward obstructions. Half a pound of the roots, 1½lb. of Sugar, beaten together in a mortar, is the best way of taking it. Take a drachm at a time. This is good for the above diseases, for gout, and severe rheumatism. An electuary made of the root and sugar is good for difficult breathing, coughs, and affections of the chest. The juice of the leaves is good for Polypus in the nose. The water, in which the root has been boiled, dropped into the eyes, frees them from film or mist which hinder the sight, and also cures the eyes when inflamed. The root mixed with bean-flower, and applied to the throat or jaws that are inflamed, cures them. The juice of the berries diluted with a little water, and dropped into the ears, easeth pains in them.

CUCUMBER.

Medicinal Virtues.—The best of Galenists hold them to be cold and moist in the second degree, and then not so hot as either lettuces or purslain; they are good for a hot stomach, and hot liver; the immoderate use of them fills the body full of raw humours. The face being washed with their juice cleanses the skin, and is good for hot rheums in the eyes; the seed is good to provoke urine, and to cleanse the urinary passages when they are stopped. There is not a better remedy for ulcers in the bladder. The usual course is, to take the Cucumbers, bruise them well, and distil the water from them, and let such as are troubled with ulcers in the bladder drink no other drink. The face being washed with the same water, cures redness of the face; it is also good for sun-burns and freckles.

CUDWEED, OR COTTONWEED.

Description.—*Gnaphalium.*—It is also called Chaffweed, Dwarf Cotton, and Petty Cotton. The common Cudweed rises up with one stalk, and sometimes with two or three, thick set on all sides with small, long, whitish, and woody leaves, from the middle of the stalk almost to the top; with each leaf is a small flower of a brownish yellow colour; after the flowers are fallen, come small seed wrapped up, with the down therein, which is carried away with the wind; the root is small and thready.

There are smaller kinds of this plant, the flowers paler, and more open.

They grow in dry, barren, sandy, and gravelly grounds. They flower about July, and their seed is ripe in August.

Medicinal Virtues.—The plants are all astringent, binding or drying, and therefore profitable for defluxions of rheum from the head, and to stay the fluxes of blood. The decoction being made in red wine, or the powder may be taken. It is very useful in dysentery, and for the immoderate courses of women, and for inward or outward wounds, hurts, or bruises. It expels worms in children, and as a decoction or as an injection, it removes the disease called Tenesmus, or a feeling for evacuation without doing anything. The green leaves bruised, and laid to any green wound, stays the bleeding, and heals it quickly. The juice of the herb taken in wine and milk, is, as Pliny says, a sovereign remedy for the quinsy.

CUMMIN.

Foreign.—Cummin seeds are in tolerable repute; they are the produce of the *Cuminum Cyminum.* It is extensively cultivated in the East. The seeds are of a disagreeable flavour; but of excellent virtues. They remove flatulency, are good for the colic, and strengthen the stomach. The oil applied outwardly, in the form of plaster, will often remove local pains, especially those of the side.

CURRANTS,—RED AND BLACK.

These require no description. The former *Ribes Nigrum,* Black Currant, has a more astringent taste than the red or white, and is somewhat aromatic. The fruit in the form of preserve or jam, is very useful in colds, fevers, and coughs. The fruit is an expectorant, or having a tendency to loosen phlegm, and allay irritation in the mucous membrane. It is also useful in sore throats, and it gently acts upon the bowels. Black Currant leaves are used in infusion, as a domestic diuretic.—Boiling water is poured upon a quantity of the preserve, as a remedy for fevers, coughs, &c., forming one of the pleasantest and most useful of our fever beverages.

The Red Currant, *Ribes Alpinum;* its fruit is very wholesome, disagrees with few, and is particularly well adapted, either fresh or cooked, to form part of the cooling diet requisite for health in very hot weather. The mechanical action of its seed has a most beneficial effect in exciting the bowels. Some bilious persons say they find benefit from eating a few ripe red currants a short time before breakfast, and that the practice tends to prevent bilious attacks during the hot weather, when currants are in season.

DAFFODIL.

Pseudo Narcissus.—This is known by all. It grows in woods, and double in gardens

Medicinal Virtues.—The fresh root is to be used, which

has great virtues. It acts as a gentle emetic, and purgative. It is the best to give in the juice with wine; but its principal uses are external. The fresh root, bruised and applied to wounds, soon heals them. It takes away the swelling and pain of sprains and bruises.

DAISY.

Bellis Perenis.—It needs no description.

MEDICINAL VIRTUES.—It is good for wounds in the breast, and very fitting to be kept both in oils, ointments, and plaisters, as also in syrup. The greater wild Daisy, is a very good wound herb. The juice of the small Daisy reduces inflammation of the liver, and the other inward parts. A decoction cures ulcers and pustules in the mouth or tongue, or in the secret parts. The leaves bruised and applied, reduce swellings. A decoction made of Daisies, and Wallwort, and Agrimony, and places fomented therewith warm, gives ease to the palsy, sciatica, or gout. An ointment made thereof relieves inflamed wounds.

DANDELION.

Taraxacum dens Leonis.—No plant is better known than this. From its effects it has been called by country people, Piss-a-bed.

MEDICINAL VIRTUES.—The leaves and root are bitter, and contain a bitter milky juice. It is of an opening and cleansing quality, and therefore very effectual for obstructions of the liver, gall and spleen, and the diseases that arise from them, as the jaundice and hypochondriasis; it opens the passages of the urine both in young and old; powerfully cleanses imposthumes and inward ulcers in the urinary passage, and by its drying and temperate quality heals them; for which purpose the decoction of the roots or leaves in white wine, is very effectual. In progressing consumption, or in an evil disposition of the whole body, called Cachexy, by the use of Dandelion great relief will be obtained. It promotes rest and sleep to bodies distempered by the heat of ague fits or otherwise.

The Dandelion therefore is a most useful herb, and ought to be more extensively known, on account of its tonic, alterative, diaphoretic, and diuretic properties. It is as valuable as Sarsaparilla, and is often given in dyspepsia, dropsy, cutaneous eruptions, and chachectic disorders generally. A decoction is made of the fresh root sliced, 1 ounce to a pint of water, boil down to half a pint, and strain, adding 2 drachms of Cream of Tartar, and take a wine glassful twice or thrice a day. Physicians generally order the extract prepared thus :—obtain the juice from the root by pressure, and then evaporate till it is a little thicker than treacle—the dose is from 10 grains to half a drachm. The French use the leaves in Sallad, and the Germans roast the root for Coffee.

DARNEL.

Description.—*Lolium Rubrum.*—It is called Jum and Wray in Sussex, and some call it Crop; it is an enemy among corn.

All the Winter it has long, flat, and rough leaves, which when the stalk rises, which is slender and jointed, are narrower, but rough still; on the top grows a long spike, composed of many heads set one above another, containing two or three husks, with sharp short beards of awns at the end; the seed is easily shaken out of the ear, the husk itself being somewhat rough.

Medicinal Virtues.—It has many virtues. The meal of Darnel is very good to stay gangrenes and other eating cankers and putrid sores; it also cleanses the skin from ringworms and the like, if it be used with salt and Radish roots. And being used with brimstone and vinegar, it dissolves knots and kernels, and especially if boiled in wine with linseed. A decoction made with water and honey, and the places bathed therewith is good for sciatica. Darnel meal applied in a poultice draws forth splinters and broken bones in the flesh. The red Darnel boiled in red wine, restrains all fluxes, and the immoderate discharge of urine.

DEVIL'S BIT.

Description.—*Succisa Scabiosa.*—A wild plant in our meadows, with slender stalks, and globous flowers. It grows two feet high. The stalks are round, firm, and upright, and divided into several branches; they have two little leaves at each joint. The flowers are as big as a small walnut, and composed of many little ones; their colour is very strong and beautiful. The leaves which grow from the root are four inches long, an inch broad, obtuse, of a dark green, and a little hairy, not at all divided, or so much as indented, at the edges. The roots are white, and composed of a thick head, which terminates abruptly, as if it had been bitten or broken off, and of a multitude of fibres. The Devil, as old women say, bit it away, envying mankind its virtues.

Medicinal Virtues. The plant is venereal, pleasing, and harmless. The herb or the root, boiled in wine, is very powerful against fevers, poisons, and bites of venomous creatures: it relieves those inwardly bruised by any casualty, or outwardly by any falls and blows, dissolving the clotted blood; and the herb or root beaten and outwardly applied, takes away black and blue marks in the skin. The decoction of the herb, with honey of roses put therein, is very effectual in inveterate tumours and swellings of the throat, by often gargling the throat therewith: it is an expellant of wind. The powder of the root taken in drink expels worms. The juice of the herb is effectual for green wounds or old sores, and cleanseth the body inwardly, and outwardly from sores, itch, pimples, and freckles, especially if a little vitrol be dissolved therein.

DILL.

Description.—*Anethum Graveolens.*—It has seldom more than one stalk, neither so high nor so large as Fennel, being round, and having fewer joints thereon; its leaves are sadder and somewhat long, and is so like Fennel that it deceives many, but harder in handling, and somewhat thicker, and of a stronger unpleasant scent; the tops of the stalks have four branches, and smaller umbels of yellow flowers, which turn into small seed somewhat flatter than Fennel-seed. The root is long. It usually grows in gardens and grounds for the purpose, and is also found wild in some places.

MEDICINAL VIRTUES.—It is stimulant and Carminative, and much used in flatulency. The decoction of Dill is good to ease swellings and pains. The seed is of more use than the leaves, and more effectual to digest vicious humours, and is used in medicines that serve to expel wind, and the pains proceeding therefrom. An oil made of Dill is effectual to warm or dissolve humours and imposthumes, to ease pains and procure rest. The decoction of Dill, herb or seed, in white wine is a powerful expeller of wind. The Dill Water of the shops is made by rubbing down the oil of Dill with sugar or Magnesia, adding water; and straining—about one drop of oil to one ounce of water. Dose from half an ounce to two ounces for adults, and one or two tea-spoonfuls for children.

DOCK.

Lapathum.—This needs no description. All know it.

MEDICINAL VIRTUES. The red Dock is commonly called Bloodwort; it cleanses the blood, and strengthens the liver; but the yellow Dock root is best to be taken when either the blood or liver is affected by choler. It has a cooling drying quality. The seeds stay fluxes of all sorts, the loathing of the stomach through bile, and is good for those that spit blood. The roots boiled in vinegar remove itch, scabs, breaking out of the skin, if it be bathed therewith. The distilled water of the herb and roots have the same virtue. Blood-wort is very strengthening to the liver, and procures good blood, being as wholesome a pot-herb as any that grows in a garden.

DOCK.—GREAT WATER.

DESCRIPTION.—*Hydrolapathum maximum.*—This is the largest of all Docks. It is much like the Sharp-pointed Dock, but much larger. It grows about waters, five or six feet high. In all respect, it is the same as the former, except its great size.

MEDICINAL VIRTUES.—Like the rest it is renowned for the

cure of scurvy. So it was with the ancients; and it possesses great astringent qualities, and is good therefore for diarrhœa. In skin disorders it is a good remedy. In powder it is healing to old sores, ulcers, cleansing and healing them. The powdered root is a capital dentrifice for the teeth; removing scurvy from the gums As a tonic, to strengthen the stomach, ten or twelve grains will be sufficient. A decoction of it may be used for the same purpose. Take two ounces of the root sliced, to three pints of water, with a little cinnamon, or liquorice in powder, and boil down to a quart. A wine-glassful two or three times a day.

DOCK.—SHARP POINTED.

DESCRIPTION.—*Lapathum folio acuto.*—A common plant, like the ordinary Dock, but handsomer, and distinguished by its sharp-pointed leaves, being narrower and longer. It grows three feet high. The stalks are erect, round, striated, green and branched. The leaves are of a fine green, smooth, with large ribs. Flowers, small, at first greenish, and when ripe, brown.

MEDICINAL VIRTUES.—The root is the part to be used. It is excellent for scurvy, and is one of the best herbs for sweetening or purifying the blood. It is best given in diet-drinks, and decoctions. Used externally, it is good for cutaneous eruptions, and for this purpose it should be beaten up with lard.

DODDER.

DESCRIPTION.—*Epythymon.*—Dodder of Thyme, and other Dodders.

The first from seed gives roots in the ground which shoot forth threads of a purplish colour, grosser or finer according to the property of the plant besides which it grows, creeping and spreading on that plant whereon it fasteneth, be it high or low. The strings have no leaves at all upon them, but wind and interlace themselves so thick upon a small plant, that it takes away all comfort of the sun from it: and is ready to strangle it. After these strings are risen up to that height, that they may draw nourishment from the plant, they seem to be broken off from the ground, either by the strength of their rising or withered by the heat of the sun. Upon these strings are found small heads or husks, out of which shoot forth whitish flowers, which give small pale coloured seed, somewhat flat, and twice as big as Poppy-seed. It generally participates in the nature of the plant upon which it climbs. The Dodder of Thyme is accounted the best, and is the only true Epithymum.

Medicinal Virtues. Thyme is the hottest herb it usually grows upon: and therefore that which grows upon Thyme is hotter than that which grows upon colder herbs; for it draws nourishment from what it grows upon, as well as from the earth where its root is. It is accounted effectual for melancholy diseases, and to purge bad bile, which is the cause of many diseases of the head and brain, as also for trembling of the heart, faintings, swoonings; and all diseases of the spleen, that arise from the windiness of the hypochondria; it purges kidneys by urine; it opens obstructions of the gall, and relieves those who have the jaundice.

DOG'S GRASS, or COUCH GRASS.

Description.—*Canis Gramen.*—This is called Dog's Grass from its efficacy in relieving dogs when sick.

It is well known, that the grass creepeth far about under the ground, with long white jointed roots, and small fibers almost at every joint, very sweet in taste, as the rest of the herb is, and interlacing one another, from whence shoot many fair grassy leaves, small at the ends, and sharp on the edges. The stalks are jointed like corn, with similar leaves, and a spiked head, with a long husk in it, and hard rough seed. Watch the dogs when they are sick, and they will lead you to it. It grows almost everywhere.

Medicinal Virtues. It is the most medicinable of all the Quickgrasses. As a decoction it opens obstructions of the liver, gall, and urine; and eases the griping pains of the belly, and inflammation; and frets away stone in the bladder, and ulcers. The roots bruised and applied heal wounds. The seed is the most powerful. The distilled water with a little wormseed, kills worms in children.

The way is to bruise the roots, and having well boiled them, drink the decoction ; it is opening, but not purging, very safe ; a remedy against all diseases arising from obstructions ; and fully one half of diseases spring from this cause ; therefore this herb is invaluable.

DRAGONS.

They are well known to those who plant them in their gardens ; at the lower end of the stalks they look like a snake.

Medicinal Virtues.—In all herbs of this quality, the safest way is either to distil the herb in an alembick, or what vehicle you please, or else to press out the juice, and distil that in a glass still, in sand. It scoureth and cleanseth the internal parts of the body greatly, and externally applied, it removes freckles, itch, and sun-burning. The best way to use it externally is to mix it with vinegar ; an ointment of it is good in wounds and ulcers ; it consumes cankers, and Polypus in the nose. The distilled water dropped into the eyes, takes away spots, and removes dimness of sight.

DRAGON'S BLOOD.

Foreign.—Sanguis Draconis Arbor.—A beautiful tree of the Palm kind, native of the Canaries, &c. Dragon's Blood is kept by the Druggists ; it is a red friable resin. It is obtained by cutting the trunk of the tree in the great heats. It is a very good astringent ; and very useful in purgings, profuse menstruation, spitting of blood, &c. It may be given in powder.

DROPWORT.

Description—*Fillipendula Spiræa.*—It is called Dropwort, because it relieves those who may void urine by drops. It has many leaves, different sizes, dented at the edges, a little like Wild Tansy, or Agrimony. From them one or two stems arise two or three feet high, with leaves growing thereon, sometimes branching out and spreading at the top into white sweet-smelling flowers, having five leaves each, with threads in the middle of them standing together, in an umbel. The seeds are flattish, and grow several together. The root is composed of a great number of black tubers, united by filaments. It grows in the corners of dry fields, and hedge sides. It flowers at the end of June.

MEDICINAL VIRTUES.—The root is the part most used. It relieves fits of the gravel, for it is a powerful diuretic. For this purpose the juice must be given, or a strong decoction of the fresh root. It is a gentle and safe astringent, and is excellent for the whites or for purgings. All pains of the bladder and kidneys will be relieved by it. The root powdered, and made into an electuary with honey, reduces fulness of the stomach, arising from flatulency. It is beneficial in diseases of the lungs, shortness of breath, wheezing, hoarseness, and coughs. It is a capital expectorant.

DUCK WEED.

Lemna Trisulca.—This is so well known to swim on the top of standing water, as ponds, pools, &c., that it is needless to describe it.

MEDICINAL VIRTUES. It reduces inflammations, and St. Anthony's fire, and the gout, either applied by itself, or in a poultice with barley meal. The distilled water by some is highly esteemed against all inward inflammations and pestilent fevers; inflammation of the eyes and swellings of the private parts, and of the breasts. The fresh herb applied to the forehead, relieves head-ache arising from heat. It is a good remedy for the jaundice. Many have been cured by it alone. The juice is to be taken, and to be repeated for several days.

ELDER TREE.

Sambucus Nigra.—It is so common in hedges as to require no description.

MEDICINAL VIRTUES.—An infusion of the inner green bark in wine, or the expressed juice of the berries in the dose of half an ounce or an ounce, purges moderately, and in small doses it proves an efficacious deobstruent, promoting all the fluid secretions. The juice boiled in sugar till it is stiff, is a useful opening medicine; it promotes the natural evacuations; and, if continued for a sufficient length of time, is of considerable use in various chronical disorders. The young leaf-buds are strongly purgative, and require caution. The flowers are different in quality; have an agreeable aromatic flavour. They are made into an ointment, by boiling them in lard till they are almost crisp, and then pouring it off: this is very cooling. The juice of the berries boiled down with a little sugar to the consistence of honey is good for colds and sore throats. A decoction of the bark or berries, is successfully given in dropsy. A decoction of the middle or inward bark is more powerful. The juice of the leaves is good for inflammation of the eyes.

Elder Wine is an excellent beverage for sore throats, colds, &c., as it is a powerful promoter of perspiration.

ELDER,—DWARF ELDER.

DESCRIPTION.—*Ebulus.*—It is very much like the Elder-tree; but growing lower, and being more of a herbaceous nature. It is wild in England, but not so common.

MEDICINAL VIRTUES.—It is more powerful than the Common Elder, as a purgative, an expectorant, a diuretic, and sudorific. Dr. Butler states it to be an efficacious remedy for dropsy—made into a decoction by water or wine. This and the other Elder are said to turn the hair black.

ELECAMPANE.

DESCRIPTION.—*Inula Helenium.*—It is a large downy perennial plant, sometimes found wild in rich soils. It grows wild in some parts of England; but principally in gardens for the use of medicine; it grows five feet high, and the large flower is yellow. The stalk is round, thick and reddish. The leaves are long, large, rough, and pointed at the ends. The flowers grow at the top of the branches, and resemble a double sun-flower. They are two inches wide and very beautiful.

MEDICINAL VIRTUES.—The fresh roots of Elecampane preserved with sugar, or made into a syrup or conserve, are very effectual to warm a cold windy stomach, or the pricking therein, and stitches in the sides caused by the spleen; and to relieve cough, shortness of breath, and wheezing in the lungs. The dried root powdered and mixed with sugar, serves the same purpose The root is esteemed a good pectoral, and, like Angelica root, is candied, and sold as a sweetmeat. Dr. Hill says, he has found an infusion of the fresh root, sweetened with honey, to be very successful for the hooping-cough. It operates by urine powerfully, and by sweat; the juice will cure the itch, applied externally. The decoction of the root in wine, or the juice taken therein, expels worms; and gargled in the mouth, or the root chewed, fastens loose teeth, and keeps them from putrefaction. The decoction, or the juice in honey, is good for those who spit blood. The root boiled well in vinegar, beaten, and made into an ointment with hog's lard, is an excellent remedy for scabs or itch. In the roots of this herb lies the chief effect.

ELM.

Ulmus Campestris.– It requires no description.

MEDICINAL VIRTUES.—The leaves bruised and applied, heal green wounds. The leaves or the bark used with vinegar, cure scurvy. The decoction of the leaves, bark, or root, as a wash, heals broken bones. The water that is found in the bladder on the leaves, while it is fresh, is very effectual to cleanse the skin, and make it fair; and if cloths be often wet therein, and applied to the ruptures of children, it heals them, if they be well bound up with a truss. The decoction of the bark of the root as a fomentation, softens hard tumours, and the shrinking of the sinews. The roots of the Elm boiled for a long time in water, and the fat scummed off the top, and applied to the head is a cure for baldness. The said bark ground with brine and pickle, until it comes to the form of a poultice, and laid on the place pained with the gout, gives great ease. The decoction of the bark in water is excellent to bathe such places as have been burnt with fire. It is one of the best gargles for a sore throat: it should be the inner bark, and it should be sweetened with honey.

ENDIVE.

Chicorium Endiva. Endive is well known by gardeners and salad eaters.

Medicinal Virtues.—It is a fine cooling and cleansing plant. The decoction of the leaves, or the juice, abate inflammation of the liver, and the heat of the stomach; and it operates powerfully by urine. The seeds have the same property, or are rather more powerful, and are available for faintings and passions of the heart. Outwardly applied, they temper the sharp humours of fretting ulcers, hot tumours, swellings, and remove inflammations of the eyes, and dimness of sight. They allay gouty pains. A syrup made of it is a fine cooling medicine for fevers. Used constantly for some time it cures scurvy, and jaundice.

ERYNGO, OR SEA-HOLLY.

Description.—*Eryngion Campestre.*—A wild plant, growing by the sea-side, and in gardens, for its medicinal uses. It is prickly, like a thistle, and the plant is whitish. The stalk is firm, woody, round, striated and thick, branched and spread irregularly about. The leaves are small, of a pale, bluish green; broad, oblong, jagged and prickly. The flowers grow in little heads at the tops of the stalks, with a circle of small leaves under them. They are of a pale greenish white. The root is long and slender, sometimes from five feet long; its taste is pleasant.

Medicinal Virtues. The plant is venereal, and breeds seed exceedingly, and strengthens the spirit procreative. The decoction of the root in wine, opens obstructions of the spleen and liver, and is good for yellow jaudice, dropsy, pains of the loins, and for colic. The candied roots are most excellent for coughs, and general debility. They possess rare virtues as a diuretic, and are a good remedy for jaundice. They are balsamic as well as diuretic. The roots bruised and applied outwardly, are good for King's evil. The roots bruised and boiled in hog's lard, and applied to broken bones, thorns, &c. remaining in the flesh, they do not only draw them forth, but heal up the place again, gathering new flesh where it was consumed.

EYE-BRIGHT.

DESCRIPTION.—*Euprhasia Officinalis.*—So called from the very bright eye of its flower, and from its efficacy in clearing the eye-sight.

Common Eye-bright is a small low herb, rising up usually with one blackish green stalk, six or eight inches high, spread from the bottom into several branches, whereon are small, almost round, pointed, dark green leaves, finely snipped about the edges, two always set together, and very thick. At the joints with the leaves, are small white flowers streaked with purple and yellow spots or stripes. The root is long, small, and thready at the end. It grows in meadows, and grassy places.

MEDICINAL VIRTUES. If the herb was but as much used as it is neglected, it would half spoil the spectacle-maker's trade. The juice of Eyebright dropped into the eyes, for several days together, relieves infirmities of the eyes that cause dimness of sight. Some make conserve of the flowers to the same effect. Being used any of the ways, it strengthens a weak brain or memory. Tunned with strong beer, and fermented together; or the powder of the dried herb mixed with sugar, a little Mace, and Fennel-seed; or the powder made into an electuary with sugar, has the same powerful effect to restore sight decayed through age; and Arnoldus de Villa Nova says, it has restored sight to them who have been blind a long time.

FENNEL.

Fœniculum.—It is grown nearly in every garden and therefore requires no description.

Medicinal Virtues.—One good old custom is not yet left off, viz. to boil Fennel with fish, for it consumes that phlegmatic humour, which fish copiously produces, though few know why they use it. Fennel is an expellant of wind. It is a good diuretic, and remedy for gravel and urinary diseases. The leaves or seeds boiled in barley water and drunk, are good for nurses, to increase their milk, and make it more wholesome for the child. The leaves or seeds boiled in water, stay hiccough, and remove nausea and heat of the stomach. The seed boiled in wine is good for those who have eaten poisonous herbs, or mushrooms. The seeds and the roots open obstructions of the liver, spleen and gall, and are good in the yellow jaundice. The seed is good in medicines for shortness of breath, and wheezing. It promotes the flow of the menses. The whole plant is a remedy for obesity, or over-fatness. The juice dropped into the eyes, cleanses them from mists and films that hinder the sight. The *Sweet Fennel* is much weaker in physical uses than the Common Fennel. The Wild Fennel is stronger and hotter than the Tame, and therefore most powerful against the stone, but not so effectual to increase milk, because of its dryness.

FENNEL,—HOG'S FENNEL.

Description.—*Hippomarathrum.*—The common Sow-Fennel has several branched stalks of thick and long leaves, about three joined at a place, among which arises a crested straight stalk, less than Fennel, with some joints and leaves thereon, and towards the tops some branches. On the tops of the stalks and branches, are large clusters of yellow flowers; the seed is oblong and flat. At the top of the root is a tuft of hairy matter, made up of the fibres of decayed leaves, which has a singular appearance.

Medicinal Virtues.—The juice of Sow-Fennel (say Dioscorides and Galen) used with vinegar and rose-water, and put to the nose, benefits persons troubled with lethargy, giddiness of the head, the falling sickness, inveterate head-ache, sciatica, and cramp, and all diseases of the sinews, used with oil and vinegar. The juice mixed with wine, or egg, is good for a cough, shortness of breath, and flatulency. It purges gently. A little of the juice dissolved in wine, and dropped into the ears, or put into a hollow tooth, removes the pain. It removes the hardness of the spleen. The powdered root mixed with lard is a good salve for green wounds.

FERN,—MALE.

DESCRIPTION.—*Aspidium Filix Mas.*—Most British Ferns are much alike, and therefore they require some discrimination. It grows at the roots of trees, in dry ditches, on heaths, borders of woods, and in rocky places, and sometimes contiguous to old walls. It has no flower-stalk; but several leaves rise from the root, each a distinct plant. It is two feet high, (the female Fern is much higher,) and nearly a foot broad. The stalk is naked for 6 or 8 inches, above which it has a row of ribs or smaller stalks, each carrying a double row of smaller leaves, with an odd one at the end, the whole forming one great leaf. Round clusters of seeds grow on the back of the smaller leaves.

MEDICINAL VIRTUES.—The root, which is chiefly used, should be collected from July to September, washed and cleared of all decayed parts; dry well quickly and in the open air; powder those parts which are greenish internally, and keep in well-stopped bottles, in a dry place. It is a powerful remedy for worms, and its powder has been sold under a fictitious name as an infallible specific for worms, especially tape-worms. It is an ancient remedy, recommended by Dioscorides, Fragus, and Spigelius. The use of it has been very wisely revived, for it is the best anthelmintic, perhaps superior to the celebrated *Kousso.*

For Tape-worm, of powder, from 1 to 3 drachms, taken on an empty stomach, and followed in 3 or 4 hours, by an aperient, as Castor Oil. A decoction of the fresh root or buds is effectual; dose about 3 ounces. The roots bruised, and boiled in oil, or lard, form a good ointment for healing wounds. The powdered root is also said to cure rickets in children.

FERN,—FEMALE FERN.

DESCRIPTION.—*Felix Fœmina.* It grows on heaths, &c. It grows four feet high, and is called by country people, brakes. The stalks are round, green, and smooth. It is more branching than the Male Fern. The whole plant is often two or three feet broad. On the edges of the little leaves stand the seeds in small clusters, though not so numerous as in the male.

MEDICINAL VIRTUES.—The roots have similar virtues to the male. Fresh gathered, and decocted, they expel long and flat worms from the bowels. No medicine destroys them so effectually. The male Fern is the more powerful.

FERN,—WATER.

DESCRIPTION.—*Osmunda regalis.*—In winter the leaves perish, and in spring it sends forth several rough hard stalks, half round and yellowish, or flat on the other side, two feet high, having several branches of winged yellowish green leaves on all sides, set one against another, longer, narrower, and not nicked on the edges as the former. From the top of some of these stalks grow a long bush of small and more yellow, green, scaly aglets, set in the same manner on the stalks as the leaves are, which are accounted the flower and seeds. The root is rough, thick, and scabby, with a white pith in the middle, called the heart. It grows on moors, bogs, and watery places.

MEDICINAL VIRTUES. It has all the virtues of the former Ferns, is more effectual than they, both for inward and outward ailments, and is good in wounds and bruises. The decoction to be drank; or the root may be made into an ointment for bruises and bones broken, or out of joint, and for ruptures. The decoction of the root in white wine, provokes urine exceedingly, and cleanses the bladder and urinary passages.

FEVERFEW, OR FEATHERFEW.

Description.—*Pyrethrum Parthenium.*—It grows wild about farmers' yards, and is cultivated in gardens, and *ought to be more so*, on account of its medicinal uses. It has divided leaves, and many flowers like daisies. The stalk is round, hollow, upright, branched, two feet high. The flowers stand about the tops of the stalks, white round the edges and yellow in the middle. The root is small, but has strong fibres.

Medicinal Virtues.—The whole plant is to be used. It is to be given in decoction, or infusion. It is very appropriate to female complaints. The infusion is excellent for profuse menstruation. Combined with wormwood and cammomile flowers, it greatly assists in child-birth. Add also St. John's Wort, and you have a capital fomentatiou for severe after-pains, flatulency, and colic. It is beneficial in inflammation and hardness of the womb. With hot water it makes a very good sitz-bath in cases of difficult travail. A decoction with sugar or honey, is good for coughs, wheezing, and difficult breathing. The powder in wine with oxymel of squills, removes phlegm, and oppression of the chest. The herb bruised and applied to the crown of the head, relieves headaches, and swimming in the head.

The decoction drank warm, and the herb bruised with a little bay-salt, and applied to the wrist, previous to the Ague-fits coming on, wards them off. The herb bruised and heated, or fried with a little wine and oil, is a warm external application for wind and colic. It is a good remedy for over-doses of Mercury.

FIG TREE.

Description.—*Ficus.*—A shrub grown in some gardens, especially in the south of England.

Medicinal Virtues. The milk that issues from the leaves or branches when they are broken off, being dropped upon warts, takes them away. The decoction of the leaves is good to wash sore heads with; and there is scarcely a better remedy for the leprosy. It clears the face from scurvy, and the body from scurf, scabs, and running sores. A decoction of the leaves, or a syrup made of them, dissolves congealed blood, caused by bruises or falls, and it allays bloody flux. A syrup made of the leaves, or green fruit, is good for coughs, hoarseness, shortness of breath, and all diseases of the lungs; also dropsy, and falling sickness.

The DRIED FIGS of the grocers are the fruit of the same tree in Spain and Portugal, but they grow larger there, and ripen better. The pulp is wholesome, and rather aperient; but the tough skin should not be eaten by the dyspeptic. Green figs grown in this country are more laxative than the preserved ones from abroad, but they have an unpleasant flavour. The finest come from Turkey. Figs are sometimes used externally, boiled in milk, or roasted. They are applied to boils, or small abscesses, to promote suppuration;—they are very appropriate to gum-boils. They make a *good demulcent gargle* for *sore throats*, thus;—Mallow Roots, 1 ounce; or if they cannot be obtained, Linseed, 1 ounce, 3 figs, split open; water 2 pints; boil to a pint, and strain.

FIG WORT.

DESCRIPTION.—*Scrophularia.*—It is sometimes called *Throat-Wort.*—Fig-wort has several strong, hard, square brown stalks, three or four feet high, on which grow dark green leaves, two at a joint, harder and larger than nettle leaves, but not stinging; at the tops of the stalks stand many purple flowers set in husks, which are sometimes gaping and open, somewhat like those of Water Betony; after which come round heads, a small point in the middle, containing small brownish seed. It is distinguished from Water Betony by not having the round indentings of the leaves, and it does not grow in water. The root is long, white, and thick, with many branches. It grows in moist and shadowy woods, and in the lower parts of fields and meadows.

MEDICINAL VIRTUES.—There cannot be a better remedy for King's evil or Scrofula. The juice of the root is an excellent sweetener of the blood taken in small doses, for a long time together. The fresh roots bruised and applied as a poultice, give ease in the piles. A decoction of the leaves taken inwardly, and the herb bruised applied outwardly, removes congealed blood, within the body, arising from wounds, bruises, or falls. An ointment made of the green leaves is used for the same purposes, and drys up the virulent moisture of hollow and corroding ulcers; it takes away all redness, spots, and freckles in the face, and the scurf.

FLAG,—YELLOW WATER.

DESCRIPTION.—*Iris Luteus Aquaticus, or Flower-de-Luce.* This plant should not be allowed to grow where cattle feed. It grows like the blue Flower-de-luce, but has longer and narrower green leaves, jointed together. The stalk often grows as high, bearing small yellow flowers, shaped like the Flower-de-luce, with three falling leaves, and other three arched, which cover their bottoms; but instead of the three upright leaves, as the Flower-de-luce has, this has only three short pieces standing in their places, after which succeed three-square heads, containing large flat seed. The root is long and slender, of a pale brownish colour, very harsh in taste. It usually grows in watery ditches, ponds, lakes, &c.

MEDICINAL VIRTUES. The root of the Water Flag is very astringent, cooling, and drying, and is good for fluxes, as bleeding at the mouth, nose, or other parts, bloody flux, and the immoderate flux of women's courses. The distilled water of the whole herb, flowers and roots, is a sovereign remedy for watery eyes, to be dropped into them, or to have cloths or sponges wetted therein, and applied to the forehead. The said water fomented on swellings, and inflammations of female breasts, upon cankers also, and spreading ulcers. It cures foul ulcers in the privities; but an ointment made of the flowers is better for those external applications.

FLAX,—COMMON.

DESCRIPTION.—*Linum Usitatissimum.*—This valuable annual plant originally came from those parts of Egypt overflowed by the Nile. It is now extensively cultivated in this country. The seed is what is called Linseed. Linseed contains about one-fifth of mucilage, and one-sixth of fixed oil. The cake which remains after the expression of the oil, contains the farinaceous and mucilaginous part of the seed, and is used in fattening cattle.

MEDICINAL VIRTUES.—Linseed is emollient and demulcent. The entire seeds, or the seeds ground into meal, called Linseed Meal, make very useful cataplasms, or poultices. In ulcerated and inflamed parts, it allays irritation and pain, and promotes suppuration. It is commonly used for abscesses, and other local affections, which require to be brought to a crisis as soon as possible. The infusion of the seed is much employed as a pectoral drink, in scalding urine, nephritic pains, &c.

Linseed Oil mixed with an equal quantity of lime-water is an excellent application for burns.

As a domestic remedy for colds, coughs, and irritation of the urinary organs, *Linseed Tea* is most valuable. Take of Linseed 6 drachms, Liquorice root, 2 drachms; bruise or slice the latter, and pour on both a pint of boiling water; in a covered vessel, let it stand four hours near a fire; strain; when cold it is fit for use. A little honey, and a table-spoonful of lemon juice, make it very agreeable, and more efficacious.—Linseed Oil is sometimes given internally as a laxative, (in milk) from 4 drachms to 1 ounce. It is given in pleurisy and peripneumony with great success; and it is excellent in the gravel and stone.

FLAX,—MOUNTAIN OR PURGING.

DESCRIPTION.—*Linum Catharticum;* or Purging Flax.—A pretty little herb which grows profusely in hilly pastures, in parks, and warrens, about eight inches high. The stalk is round, firm, and at the top divided into small branches. The leaves are little, oblong, and obtuse, two at each joint. The flowers are small and white, and the plant much resembles chickweed; but the seed vessel, on examination, indicates it to be of the flax kind. The root is small and thready.

MEDICINAL VIRTUES.—It makes a strong but safe purge; owing its activity to a peculiar drastic principle, called *Linin*, and which is afforded by the plant after the flower has fallen. The country people boil it in beer, and take it as a remedy for rheumatic pains, for catarrhal affections, as coughs, &c. and dropsy. It has also yielded great relief in biliary disorders. It is useful in all cases where a brisk purgative is required.—Extract, from 4 to 8 grains two or three times a day;—the dried herb, 2 drachms or more, has been found very useful in obstinate rheumatism.

FLAX-WEED, or TOAD-FLAX.

DESCRIPTION.—*Antirrhinon Linarium.*—This weed is reckoned by some to be poisonous; yet it is very useful. Common Flax-weed has various stalks, abounding with long and narrow ash-coloured leaves, and from the middle of them almost upward, stored with a number of pale yellow flowers, of a strong unpleasant scent, with deeper yellow mouths, and blackish flat seed in round heads. The root is a little woody, and white, especially the main down right one, with many fibres, abiding many years, shooting forth roots every way round about, and new branches every year. It grows on dry banks, by the way-sides, in meadows, by hedge-sides, and upon borders of fields. It flowers in Summer.

MEDICINAL VIRTUES.—The tops are used fresh gathered, or the whole herb dried. An infusion is very good against jaundice, and to remove by urine, those watery humours which cause dropsy. A decoction of both leaves and flowers, is rather purgative, and tends to the removal of obstructions of the liver. The herb distilled answers the same purpose. It is very effectual if a little Peruvian Bark, or Solution of Quinine, and a little Cinnamon, be combined with it. The juice of the herb, or the distilled water, is a good remedy for inflammation of the eyes. A fine cooling ointment is made by boiling the fresh plant chopped in lard, till it be crisp—strain, and you will have a fine green ointment good for sores, ulcers, cancers, &c.

FLEABANE.

Description.—*Conyza*, or *Erigeron Canadensis*, belonging to the natural order of *Compositæ*.—It is a pretty wild plant, with whitish leaves, bearing large yellow flowers in Autumn. The stalk is round, erect, strong, and of a reddish colour. It has many leaves which stand irregularly, about an inch long, moderately broad, and of a rough surface. The flowers stand at the top of the branches; they are broader than a shilling, yellow, having many yellow petals. The whole plant has an unpleasant smell. It is found plentifully in the southern counties of England.

Medicinal Virtues.—It possesses diuretic, tonic, and astringent properties, which render it very useful in dropsical complaints, and in diarrhœa. The juice of the plant cures the itch, and the very smell of the herb is said to destroy fleas. For dropsy, or diarrhœa, the dose is, of the flowers in powder, from 30 to 40 grains; of the infusion, from 2 to 4 ounces; of the extract from 5 to 10 grains. For dysentery or bloody flux, infuse the herb in hot water, and give a cupful every hour or two, until a cure is effected. In colic, it affords immediate relief; administering a cupful of the infusion or decoction every half hour. When the case is obstinate, give also an injection of strong infusion. The dose of the powder is from 15 grains to a drachm. The oil is a sure remedy in hemorrhage—five to ten drops.

FLEA-WORT.

Description.—*Psyllium*.—There are two kinds of Flea-wort, differing very little, only the leaves of one kind abide the winter, but the others do not. Ordinary Flea-wort rises up with a stalk two feet high, full of joints and branches on every side to the top, and at every joint two small, long, and narrow whitish green leaves, somewhat hairy. At the top of every branch stand several small, short, scaly, or chaffy heads, from which come forth small whitish yellow threads, like those of the plaintain, which are the bloomings of flowers. The seed enclosed in these heads is small and shining, like fleas, both for colour and size, whence its name. The root is not long, but white, hard, and woody, perishing every year. The whole plant is whitish and hairy, smelling like resin. It is a native of France; and is cultivated in gardens in England. It flowers in July.

Medicinal Virtues.—The seeds fried and eaten, are good in fluxes, and in over-purging caused by mercurial doses. The mucilage of the seed made with rose-water, and a little sugar-candy, is very good in agues and burning fevers, and other inflammations, to cool the thirst, and to remove dryness and roughness of the tongue and throat, hoarseness of the voice, and diseases of the breast and lungs, and the pleurisy. The mucilage of the seed made with plaintain water and the yolk of an egg, is a sure remedy for piles. It relieves inflammations in any part of the body, the headache, and all hot imposthumes, swellings, or eruptions of the skin. It relieves the gout, and sciatica, and the swelling of the navel, applied with oil of roses and vinegar. It is good to heal the nipples and sore breasts of women. The juice of the herb with a little honey put into the ears, cures the running of them, and the worms breeding in them. The juice mixed with lard, is excellent for sores.

FLOWER DE LUCE.

Description.—*Iris.*—A common flower growing in our gardens. The plant grows three feet high. The leaves are a foot and a half long, narrow, flat, and in all respects like the leaves of flags, and of a bluish green. The stalks are round, or a little flatted; thick, firm, upright, and of a greener colour. The flowers are larger, and of a deep blue. The roots spread about the surface, and is thick and of a brownish colour, and marked with rings.

Medicinal Virtues.—The juice of the fresh roots of this plant bruised with white wine is a strong purge; it will sometimes also vomit; but that is not hurtful; it is a cure for dropsies. Gordon, an old physic writer, says if a dropsy can be cured by the hand of man, this root will effect it. I have found it true in practice.

FLUX-WEED.

DESCRIPTION.—*Sisymbrium Sophia.*—There are two kinds; one has broader leaves than the other; the smell is disagreeable. It rises up with a round, hard, erect stalk, four or five feet high, spread into many branches, whereon grow many greyish green leaves, finely cut and severed into a number of short and almost round parts. The flowers are very small and yellow, growing spike fashion, after which come long pods, with small yellowish seed in them. They grow wild in fields, by hedge-sides and highways, among rubbish and in other places. They flower and seed quickly in June and July.

MEDICINAL VIRTUES. The herb and seed of Flux-weed are excellent to stay the flux and diarrhœa. Put the seed and plant into water in which heated steel or iron has been repeatedly quenched. It is effectual to restrain any other flux of blood in man or woman. The juice drank in wine, or a decoction of the herb, kills worms, made into a salve, it quickly heals all old sores, however foul and malignant they may be. The distilled water has the same effects, yet rather weaker. It is called Flux-weed because it cures the flux, and because it unites broken bones, &c. Paracelsus highly extols it.

FOX GLOVE.

DESCRIPTION.—*Digitalis Purpurea*, of the natural order of *Scrophulariaceæ.* Its stalk is erect, tapering, rising four or five feet. The leaves are large, oval, wrinkled, veined, on short wing footstalks, and are downy underneath. The flowers hang down; they are a reddish purple, bell-shaped, marked internally with little dark-coloured spots placed in whitish rings, and long hairs defend the entrance of the tube; so that no insects can enter. The flower-stalks vary in length; at first they depend like the flowers, afterwards they become erect, when they elevate a two-celled capsule containing blackish seeds. This most elegant, but very poisonous plant, unless skilfully and carefully administered, is very common in Britain, in dry sandy soils, by hedge-sides. It flowers in July, and seeds in August.

FOX GLOVE.

Medicinal Virtues.—Its properties are narcoctic, diuretic, and sedative. Useful in inflammatory diseases. The pulse is sometimes remarkably diminished by its use, and sometimes as remarkably resists the powers of this remedy. Dr. Thornton says, "We have seen the pulse sink down, in a patient at Guy's Hospital, to 13 beats a minute, and in other instances, as much as 3 ounces of the tincture have been taken without any alteration in the pulse.

In severe colds, and inflammations of the lungs, the digitalis has been administered instead of bleeding; and also in measles. "Considering that scarlet fever is a mixture of high inflammation and putrid diathesis, confluent, or the one running into the other, this remedy was tried by us in large doses, as 20 drops of the Tincture of Digitalis with ten drops of antimonial wine, in children of twelve years of age and under; and in a large experience in the St. James's Charity School, and in private practice, we have had abundant reason to approve of this discovery, whereby even in the most desperate cases none have died."

In active hæmorrhages, and in phthis, the foxglove has a beneficial effect; it lowers the pulse without at the same time diminishing the strength, and it should be in tincture, beginning with two or three drops at first twice or thrice a day, gradually increasing to twenty or thirty drops. It is also used with great advantage in all kinds of dropsical swellings. Dr. Withering says, "If dropsy can be cured at all, it can be cured by foxglove: for if this fails, there is little chance of any other succeeding." "In dropsy of the chest," says Dr. Graham, "It is considered by some able physicians to be superior to every other remedy. It is of great service in other kinds of dropsy, especially in the dropsy supervening scarlet fever; and its beneficial effects are more certainly obtained in those constitutions, in which there is laxity of fibre, pale complexion, feeble intermitting pulse, cold skin, and where the swelling easily pits. It has been found of great value, when conjoined with nitric acid, in the dropsy which occurs in broken-down constitutions that have been long harassed by mercury."

It has also been used successfully in mania, arising from an effusion of water on the brain. "In paroxysms of insanity," says Dr. Graham," it will act as a valuable narcoctic and sedative, provided the inflammatory symptoms be first controlled by the usual means, and hence also it appears fitted rather for the advanced than the early stages of consumption."

It was in *scrofulous tumours* that foxglove first acquired its reputation. Haller reports that a scorbutic leprosy was cured by a long use of this plant; and that Zeyter, by bruising its flowers, along with lard, cured glandular tumours, and that a deplorable case of *Evil* yielded to this remedy. The expressed juice mixed with linseed meal has been found a successful topical application in several cases when the medicine was also used internally.

In *spasmodic asthma*, the greatest advantage has been realized, probably by producing absorption, and strengthening the habit, for foxglove acts as a tonic. The ancient opinion of *epilepsy* often yielding to the use of foxglove is confirmed by modern experience. Where this disorder has been induced by a determination of blood to the head, modern practitioners have succeeded in removing this afflictive disorder.

The herb is much used by the Italians to heal any fresh and green wound; they bruise the leaves, and bind them on the wound. In the form of ointment (made of the juice and lard) foxglove is applied to scrofulous sores with good effect; and this ointment is one of the best remedies for scabbed head.

For *Pills*, each should contain a grain of powdered leaves—one to be taken twice a day, and gradually increased till its effects are apparent either on the kidneys, the stomach, the pulse, or the bowels; then discontinue.——In dropsy it may be repeated after an interval, if all the water has not left.——*Infusion;*—macerate in a pint of boiling water 2 drachms of the dried leaves, adding 1 ounce of spirit of Cinnamon;—dose from two to six drachms twice or thrice a day.——*Tincture;*—Dried leaves of foxglove, in coarse powder; proof spirit, one pint, digest for 7 to 20 days, and filter; dose, from 6 to 15 drops a day. During the administration, drink freely of diluting drinks. A little sweet nitre with the infusion or decoction counteracts nausea and flatulence.

The Tincture, with Soap Liniment, may be rubbed into the

chest, or other parts to relieve pain; and a strong infusion of the leaves may be applied warm to the abdomen to produce diuresis in dropsy.

To counteract the deleterious effects of an over dose, use laudanum in brandy and water, or ammonia, small doses of opium, or a strong infusion of green tea.

FLUELLEN.

DESCRIPTION—*Antirhinon Elatine.* There are two kinds of Fluellen. The first sends forth many long branches, partly lying upon the ground, and partly standing upright with almost red leaves, a little pointed, and sometimes more long and round, without order, hairy, and greenish white at the joints of the stalks, and with the leaves come forth small flowers, one at a place, upon a very short foot stalk, somewhat like snapdragons, or rather like toad-flax, with the upper jaw of a yellow and the lower of a purplish colour with a small heel or spur behind; after which come forth small brown heads, containing small black seed. The root is small and thready, dying every year.

The other sort has longer branches, wholly trailing upon the ground, two or three feet long, and thinner, set with leaves upon small foot-stalks. The leaves are a little larger and rounder, and cornered sometimes on the edges; but the lower part of them being the broadest, has on each side a small point, like ears, sometimes hairy, but not hoary, and a better green colour than the former. The flowers come forth like the former, but the colours therein are more white than yellow, and the purple not so fair.

They grow in corn-fields, and in borders about them, and in other fertile grounds chiefly in the south of England.

MEDICINAL VIRTUES.—The leaves bruised and applied with barley meal to watering eyes hot and inflamed by defluxions from the head, very much relieve them, as also the bloody-flux, women's courses, and bleeding at the nose, mouth, &c. caused by any bruise or hurt, or bursting a vein; it is very effectual both to heal and close green wounds, to cleanse and heal all foul ulcers, sores, cankers, &c. Made into an ointment with hog's lard, and spermaceti, it is a good remedy for sores, cuts, bruises, &c.

FROG-BIT.

Description.—*Hydrocaris Morcus Ranæ.*—A kind of water-lily; not uncommon on waters; its leaves are round; but it is different from the ordinary water-lily. The leaves are of a roundish figure, and of a dusky green colour; better than an inch broad, and they rise many together in tufts from the same stalk. This stalk runs along a little distance under the surface of the water, and from it descend the roots, loose like the fibres of duckweed. The flowers stand singly upon slender foot-stalks; they are bluish white, and composed of three leaves a-piece, which give them a singular appearance.

Medicinal Virtues.—The fresh leaves bruised are used in external applications, as they are very cooling. The juice mixed with lard makes an excellent ointment for sores, &c.

FUMITORY.

Description.—*Humaria Officinalis.*—It is a beautiful little weed. It shoots forth from one square, slender weak stalk, and leaning downwards on all sides, many branches two or three feet long, with finely cut and jagged leaves of whitish, or rather bluish sea green colour; at the tops of the branches stand many small flowers, in a long spike one above another, made like little birds of a reddish purple colour, with whitish bellies, after which come small round husks containing small black seeds. The root is yellow, small, and not very long. It overspreads the English corn-fields; and it flowers in May.

Medicinal Virtues.—The ancient physicians regarded it as possessing considerable virtues. The expressed juice is excellent against scurvy. It opens obstructions of all the viscera, and is good against the jaundice, and all diseases proceeding from obtsructions. Dr. Cullen says, "This plant is a tonic. I have found it useful in many cases in which bitters are prescribed; but its remarkable virtues are those of clearing the skin of many disorders. I have seen its good effects in many instances of cutaneous affections of the worst character, which I deemed to be *lepra*. I have commonly given the expressed juice, two ounces twice a day; but the virtues remain in the dried plant; so that they may be extracted by infusion or decoction in water. It is best to combine it with other aperient herbs, for it is not strong enough of itself, and either in syrup, or decoction, it will improve the liver, remove jaundice, and clear the blood, and strengthen all the inward parts. The seed is stronger than the leaves. The juice dropped into the eyes, clears the sight, removes inflammation, and redness, though it is rather painful at the first. The juice of Fumitory and Docks, mixed with vinegar, makes an excellent wash for the cure of scabs, pimples, blotches, &c. on the skin.

FURZE, or WHIN.

Description.—*Ulex Europæus.* It is one of the most common of all plants on heaths, and moors. The flowers are very beautiful. Linnæus almost idolized the flower. Some call it Furze, others Gorse, and Whin. It is well known.

Medicinal Virtues.—The virtues are the same as those of the Broom, but in a less degree. A decoction made with the flowers has been found effectual against the jaundice, and to promote urine, and cleanse the kidneys from gravel or stone.

GALLS.

Description.—*Foreign.*—*Quercus Infectoria*, natural order *Corylaceæ.*

Medicinal Virtues.—Galls possess peculiar astringent qualities on account of the large quantity of *tannin* which they contain. They are chiefly used in gargles, lotions, injections, and ointments. Reduced to fine powder, and made into an ointment, with a little powdered opium, and lard, they are a valuable remedy for the piles. The tincture of Galls in mucilage is sometimes given with good effect in cases of diarrhœa; the dose of this preparation is from 1 to 2 drachms. A drachm of powdered galls, with a scruple of Sulphate of copper, and 1 ounce of lard, makes a good ointment for ringworms. They form a useful injection in whites and gleet, and are of much use as an astringent in prolapsus of the anus and womb. In bleeding from the bladder, Gallic acid is the best remedy—5 grains in solution of Gum Arabic, repeat as required.

GARLIC.

Allium Sativum. It needs no description; it is so well known.

MEDICINAL VIRTUES.—Applied externally it acts as a stimulant, rubefacient, and blister. Internally, it is often useful in diseases of languid circulation, and interrupted secretion. In cold leuco-phlegmatic habits it is a powerful expectorant, diuretic, and if the patient be kept warm, sudorific. It is thought to be an emenagogue. But in cases where irritability prevails, large doses may be injurious. As a condiment, taken in moderation, it promotes digestion; taken in excess, it produces headache, flatulence, thirst, &c. In fevers of the typhoid kind its virtues have had a good effect. It has succeeded in curing obstinate quartanagues. In catarrhal disorders of the breast, spasmodic and pituitous asthma, flatulent colics, hysterical and other diseases, proceeding from laxity of the solids, it has good effects. Sydenham says that he has known the dropsy cured by the use of Garlic alone.

Cotton saturated with the juice, and put into the ear is good for deafness. Renew it several times a day. Applied as a poultice to the pubis, it has promoted the flow of urine. Sydenham regarded Garlic as a powerful means of causing a derivation or revulsion from the head, applied to the soles of the feet. For this he used it in the confluent smallpox, about the seventh or eight day, after the face began to swell. The root cut small, and tied in a linen cloth, was applied to the soles of the feet, and renewed every day till the danger was over.

A dose or two of the juice of Garlic may be taken in the morning for *worms*. An infusion of Garlic, made of half a pound of the bruised roots to a pint of boiling water, two spoonfuls before and after every meal, for *epilepsy*. Of the syrup of Garlic, made of one ounce of the expressed juice, to 1½ ounce of lump sugar, a tea-spoonful taken occasionly by children, for *coughs*, without inflammation. Of the milk of Garlic, 2 drachms, of the bruised bulbs boiled in 6 or 8 ounces of milk, useful as a clyster for *thread-worms* in children. Wine of Garlic, three or four bulbs bruised and macerated in a quart of proof spirits, is a good stimulant lotion for *baldness of the head*.

If you are troubled with *asthma*, take a number of bulbs, and boil till they are soft; then dry them well. Put an equal quantity of good vinegar to the water in which the bulbs of Garlic have been boiled, add sugar, and boil into a syrup. Pour the syrup over the dried bulbs, and secure in a jar for use. Take a bulb or two in a morning fasting, with a little of the syrup, and you will find relief. We are informed that Dr. Bowles secured a large fortune by this remedy.

GENTIAN,—BRITISH.

Description.—*Gentiana.*—Sometimes called Felwort, or Baldmony. Though the foreign Gentian is principally used, yet there are two kinds in this country, which equal that imported. The greater of the two has many small long roots deep in the ground, and abiding all the Winter. The stalks are of a brownish green colour, two feet high if the ground be fruitful, having many long, narrow, dark green leaves, in couples up to the top; the flowers are long and hollow, purple, ending in fine corners. The smaller sort grows with several stalks, not a foot high, parted in several small branches, whereon grow small leaves together, very like those of the lesser centuary, of a whitish green colour; on the tops of these stalks grow blue flowers, standing in long husks, but not so large as the other; the root is very small, and full of threads.

Both grow in several places both of the East and West countries, near Gravesend, in Kent, and in Bedfordshire. They flower in August.

MEDICINAL VIRTUES.—They resist putrefactions, poison, and a surer remedy cannot be found to prevent the epidemic diseases; it strengthens the stomach exceedingly, helps digestion, comforts the heart, and preserves it against faintings. The powder of the dry roots opens obstructions of the liver, and restores the loss of appetite. The herb steeped in wine, and drank, refresh such as be overweary with travel, and lame in their joints. It relieves stitches, and griping pains in the sides; it is an excellent remedy for such as are bruised by falls; it provokes urine and the terms; but should not be given in pregnancy. A decoction of it is very useful in cramps, convulsions; in stone, rupture, and in cold diseases, and to such as are troubled with tough phlegm, scabs, itch, or sores and ulcers. It is an admirable remedy to kill the worms, by taking half a drachm of the powder in a morning in any convenient liquor; taken inwardly it is good for the king's evil. It relieves agues, and the yellow jaundice, as also the bots in cattle: when kine are bitten on the udder by any venemous beast, only stroke the place with the decoction of any of these, and it will instantly heal them.

GENTIAN,—FOREIGN.

It is obtained from the *Gentiana Lutea*, or yellow Gentian. It is a native of the Alps, Pyrenees, &c. The root is used. It is one of the most useful of our bitter vegetable tonics. It is especially useful in states of exhaustion, from chronic disease, and all cases of debility, unconnected with excessive irritability of the stomach. It possesses febrific, anthelmintic, and antiseptic properties, and as a warm stomachic tonic, it is unrivalled. It is an excellent tonic to combine with a purgative, to prevent its debilitating effects.—☞ All purgatives ought so to be compounded. The *extract*, which may be purchased at the shops, is used in from 5 to 10 grains, or more made into pills. The *compound tincture* may be taken in one or two spoonful doses, in water. The *root powdered* may be taken; dose, from 10 to 20 grains—this is sometimes sprinkled on foul sloughing ulcers. The best preparation, however, for general use, is the *concentrated infusion*,—thus prepared:—

To every ounce of sliced Gentian root, add a quarter of an ounce of dried orange peel, and infuse these—not boil, with successive quantities of boiling water poured over them, until their strength is exhausted. Strain the liquor from the root, and concentrate by boiling in a well-tinned or porcelain-lined saucepan, until the quantity is so far reduced, that there is left half a pint of the concentrated infusion for every ounce of Gentian used. Then to each half pint, half an ounce of alcohol is to be added. The effect of the alcohol is to coagulate it from a quantity of jelly-looking substance, which must be separated by straining. This infusion will keep a long time—the dose being one tea-spoonful in an ounce of water. This is one of the best strengtheners of the human system.

GERMANDER.

DESCRIPTION.—*Teucrion, vel, Chamædrys.*—This celebrated plant is cultivated chiefly for medical purposes. It has several stalks with small round leaves dented at the edges. The flowers stand at the tops, of a deep purple colour. It is cultivated in gardens. It flowers in June and July.

MEDICINAL VIRTUES.—It strengthens the brain and apprehension exceedingly when weak, and relieves them when drooping. Taken with honey (says Dioscorides) it is a remedy for coughs, hardness of the spleen, and difficulty of urine, and gives relief to dropsy, especially at the beginning of the disease, a decoction being made of the green herb. Used with honey it cleanses old ulcers; and made into an oil, and the eyes anointed therewith, it removes dimness and moisture. It is likewise good for pains in the sides and for cramps. The decoction taken for four days together, cures both tertian and quartan agues. It is also good against all diseases of the brain, as continual headache, falling-sickness, melancholy, drowsiness, lowness of spirits, convulsions, and palsies. A drachm of the seed taken in powder, is good against the yellow jaundice as it promotes urine. The juice of the leaves dropped into the ears, kills worms in them. The tops when in flower, steeped twenty-four hours in white wine, destroy worms.

GERMANDER,—WATER.

DESCRIPTION.—*Teucrium Scordium.*—It is an insignificant looking plant, growing wild, and cultivated in gardens for its medicinal uses. The stalks are square, hairy, of a dirty green, and very weak. The leaves are short, broad, indented at the edges, woolly and soft. The flowers are small and red, standing in little parcels on the upper joints of the stalks. The smell of the plant is unpleasant.

MEDICINAL VIRTUES.—Used as a decoction, it is sudorific. It is good against fevers. The Tincture, in small doses, is a good remedy for exhilarating and rousing torpid faculties.

GINGER.—FOREIGN.

Amomum Zingiber. It is a perennial plant, indigenous in the East and West Indies, having stimulent, carminative, and tonic properties, which render it extremely valuable. It is very useful in cold flatulent colics, and in laxity and debility of the intestines, not heating so much as the peppers, and its effects are more durable. Persons subject to indigestion, flatulency, and gout, have been known to receive great benefit from the use of Ginger tea. Many gouty patients have for years been in the habit of taking a tea-spoonful of powdered Ginger, mixed in any liquid, an hour before dinner, with considerable advantage. When employed with food, it is called a condiment, and by stimulating the stomach and bowels, it may be considered as one of the most useful. Combined with purgatives, it corrects their griping tendency, and it acts externally, like mustard, as a rubefacient, even raising a blister.

As Ginger promotes the circulation through the extreme vessels, it is to be advised in torpid and plegmatic habits where the stomach is subject to be loaded with slime, and the bowels distended with flatulency.

GILLIFLOWERS,—CLOVE.

It is in vain to describe a plant so well known. It is sometimes called *Gilliver.*

MEDICINAL VIRTUES. They are gallant, fine, temperate flowers, yea, so temperate, that no excess, neither in heat, cold, dryness, nor moisture, can be perceived in them; they are great strengtheners both of the brain and heart, and will therefore serve either for cordials or cephalics, as your occasion will serve. There is both a syrup and a conserve made of them. To take now and then a little of either, strengthens nature much in such as are in consumptions. They are good in hot pestilential fevers, and expel poison. One ounce of the flowers, in one pint of boiling water constitutes the infusion. For the Syrup, flowers, 1 ounce, boiling water, 4 ounces, refined sugar, half a pound. Let the flowers infuse half-a-day; then very gently boil down to one-fourth the quantity. The vinegar of cloves is a cephalic, the smell removing headache, sickness, &c. It is an excellent deodoriser for sick rooms. It is made by merely steeping one ounce of petals in a pint of best vinegar for 14 days.

GLADWIN,—STINKING.

DESCRIPTION.—*Iris Fœtidissima.*—It is a wild plant of the Iris kind. Its leaves are very like a Flower-de-luce but sharp-edged on both sides, and thicker in the middle, of a deeper green colour, sharper pointed, and have a strong ill scent, if bruised. In the middle rises up a strong stalk, a yard high, bearing three or four flowers at the top, like the flower-de-luce, with three upright petals, of a dead purplish ash colour, with some veins discoloured in them; the other three do not fall down, nor are the three other small ones so arched, nor cover the lower leaves like the flower-de-luce, but stand loose from them. The root is like that of the flower-de-luce, but reddish on the outside, and whitish within, very hot in the taste, of a bad scent.

It grows in high lands, in moist places, woods, and shadowy places, and by the sea-side, and is cultivated in gardens. It flowers in July, and the seed is ripe in August.

MEDICINAL VIRTUES. It is used by country people to purge corrupt phlegm and choler, by drinking the decoction of the roots; or by infusing the sliced roots in ale; and some use the leaves.

The juice snuffed up the nose, causes sneezing, and draws from the head much corruption; the powder has the same effect. The powder drank in wine, relieves cramps and convulsions, the gout and sciatica, and griping pains. It is given with much profit in fluxes which it stops, having first cleansed and purged them by its astringent qualities. Half a drachm of the seed beaten to powder, and taken in wine, promotes a flow of urine. Taken with vinegar, it removes the hardness of the spleen. The root is effectual in all wounds especially of the head; and to draw forth splinters, thorns, or broken bones, or any thing sticking in the flesh, without causing pains, being used with a little verdigrease and honey, and the great Centaury root. Boiled in vinegar, and laid upon any tumour or swelling, it removes them. It is a fine remedy for the king's evil. The juice of the leaves or roots heals the itch, and all running sores, blemishes, or scars in the skin.

GOLDEN ROD.

Description.—*Solida Virga-Aurea.*—By some it is called Woundwort. It has small round stalks, two feet high, having many narrow and long dark green leaves, undented about the edges, and without stalks or white spots therein, yet they are sometimes divided at the tops into many small branches, with small yellow flowers on every one of them, which are all turned one way. The seeds are downy. The root consists of many small fibres. It grows in the open places of woods and copses, on heaths, and it is cultivated in gardens.

Medicinal Virtues.—Arnoldus de Villa Nova commends it much against stone, and to provoke urine in abundance, by which gravel and stone may be voided. The decoction of the herb, green or dry, or the distilled water, is very effectual for inward bruises; outwardly applied, it arrests bleeding in any part of the body, and of wounds; also the fluxes of humours, the bloody flux, and women's courses; and is no less prevalent in ruptures or burstings, drank inwardly and outwardly applied. It is a sovereign wound herb, inferior to none for inward and outward hurts; green wounds, old sores and ulcers, are quickly cured with it. It makes an excellent lotion for sores or ulcers in the mouth, throat, or privy parts in man or woman. The decoction tends to fasten loose teeth.

GOLD OF PLEASURE.

Description.—*Camelina Sativa.* It is a pretty plant growing in some parts of England, and easily known by its numerous seed vessels. It grows two feet high; the stalk is round, thick, erect, having many erect branches at the top. The leaves are long, not very broad, of a pale green, few and irregular, indented, and encircle the stalk at the base. The flowers are small and white. The seed vessels, short and roundish, and they appear in great quantities, resembling a spike to the very top of the branches.

Medicinal Virtues.—The fresh tops of the plant should be used before the flowers are gone. The flowers make an excellent poultice for inflamed parts. An infusion of the fresh tops sweetened with honey, is excellent for sore throats, and ulceration of the mouth. From the seed a great quantity of oil may be expressed; and probably the plant would pay for cultivation, on account of its great yield of oil. The oil is pleasant, well-tasted; and it makes an excellent rubefacient.

GOOSEBERRY-BUSH.

Description.—*Ribes Gros-sularia.*—It is well known.

Medicinal Virtues.—The fruit is most wholesome. The berries are aperient, and the seeds add to this property, by their mechanical action upon the bowels. The green berries being scalded, or baked, are good to stir up a fainting or decayed appetite, especially in persons afflicted by choleric humours. The decoction of the leaves cool hot swellings and inflammations, and St. Anthony's fire. The ripe gooseberries are an excellent remedy to allay the violent heat of the stomach and liver. The young tender leaves expel the gravel both from the kidneys and bladder.

GOUTWORT.

Description.—*Podograria.*—It is also called Gout-weed, Herb-gerrard, Ash-weed, and Ground-ash. It is a low herb, seldom rising half a yard high, having many leaves standing on brownish green stalks by three, snipped about, and of a strong and unpleasant savour; the umbels of the flowers are white, and the seed blackish, the root runneth in the ground, taking a great deal of room. It grows by hedge and wall-sides, and in the border and corners of fields, and in gardens also.

Medicinal Virtues.—Goutwort has not its name for nothing for it heals the gout and sciatica; as also joint-aches, and other pains. The root and leaves boiled together, and applied to the hip, and occasionally renewed, has a wonderful effect. The plant makes an excellent fomentation for pained and inflamed parts.

GRAINS OF PARADISE.

The seeds of the *Amomum Granum* Paradisæ, belonging to a genus of plants, all of which bear aromatic seeds. These grains are stimulant, aromatic, and tonic, and have been given in large doses with good effect in agues, and paralysis. They are also used to give strength to beer, wine, &c. In moderation, they certainly improve those beverages, and act as a tonic. In veterinary practice, they are very serviceable in the diseases of animals, as a permanent stimulant.

GROMWELL.

Description.—*Lithospermon Officinale.*—Of this plant there are several kinds:—

The *greater Gromwel* grows up with slender and hard hairy stalks, trailing and taking root in the ground, and is parted into many other small branches, with hairy dark green leaves thereon. At the joints with the leaves come forth very small blue flowers, and after them hard stony roundish seed. The root is long and woody, and perennial.

The *smaller wild Gromwel* has several upright hard branched stalks, two or three feet high, full of joints, at every one of which grow small, long, hard, and rough leaves like the former, but less; with small white flowers, and after them greyish round seed like the former, the root is not large, but has many fibres.

The *garden Gromwel* hath various upright, slender, woody hairy stalks, blown and cressed, very little branched, with leaves like the former, and white flowers; after which in rough brown husks, is contained a white hard round seed, shining like pearl, larger than both the former; the root is like the first.

The great and the small Gromwell grow wild in barren or untilled places, and by the way-sides. The last is cultivated in gardens.

Medicinal Virtues.—The seed powdered and taken in barley water, is excellent to dissolve the stone, and to remove gravel from the kidneys. It must therefore be very diuretic, powerfully promoting urine. The herb itself (when the seed is not to be had) either boiled, or the juice thereof drank, is effectual, but not so powerful as the seed.

GROUND PINE.

Description.—*Ajuga Chamæpitys.*—A small wild mossy plant, of a resinous smell. It grows four inches high. The stalks are hairy, the leaves close set; the young shoots obscure the stalk, in the form of a thick round tuft. The leaves are short, narrow, and divided into three parts at the end, rough and hairy. The flowers are small and yellow, standing at the joints.

Medicinal Virtues.—The whole plant is to be powdered for infusion. It is a powerful diuretic, promoting urine, and removing obstructions of the liver and spleen; therefore valuable in jaundice, rheumatism, and most of the chronic diseases. Take, for a dose, a small teaspoonful of the powder. A decoction of this plant, Dandelion, and Agrimony, is a great remedy for liver complaints, and obstructions.

GROUNDSEL.

Description.—*Senecio Vulgaris.*—This plant is well known; and it grows everywhere.

Medicinal Virtues.—Groundsel is now chiefly used as food for birds. It was formerly much used for poultices; and it was reckoned as good for sickness of the stomach. A weak infusion of the plant is now sometimes given as a purgative, and a strong infusion as an emetic, as it causes no irritation and pain. As a weak decoction it is safe and friendly to the body of man. It is a great cooler. It relieves pain at the stomach arising from choler or bile. The juice taken in weak wine has the same effect.

GROUND-IVY.

Glechoma Hederacea.—It is also called Cat's-foot, Alehoof, Gill-go-by-ground, and Gill-creep-by ground, Turnhoof, Hay-maids, and Jack-by-the-Hedge.

Description.—It creeps upon the ground, sends forth the roots at the corners of tender jointed stalks, and has two round leaves at every joint, crumpled, and dented about the edges. The stalks are hollow and square, a foot or more in length. It has hollow long flowers of a blueish purple colour, with small white spots upon the lips which hang down. The root is small and fibrous. It is found under hedges, and on the sides of ditches, in shady lanes, and waste grounds. The plant has a peculiar smell; it flowers early, and it should be gathered when in flower.

Medicinal Virtues.—It is known to be gently stimulant, and tonic, aperient, diuretic, and corrobarant, with a particular action on the lungs and kidneys, and it has long been a popular remedy for coughs, pulmonary complaints, and urinary affections. A conserve of it may be made in spring, and it may be made into tea. The expressed juice snuffed up the nose is curative of headache, when all other medicines have failed. It may also be taken with great benefit, conjoined with Elecampane leaves, Liquorice root, equal quantities, infused in boiling water. It is a very good remedy for inward wounds, for colic, griping pains, and the yellow jaundice, by removing obstructions of the gall and liver; it removes melancholy by opening the spleen. A decoction of it in wine is good for sciatica, or hip-gout, and for gout in the hands, feet, and other joints. If some honey, and a little burnt alum be added to the decoction, it is useful as a gargle for a sore mouth or throat. The juice boiled with honey and a little verdigrease, cleanses fistulas, and ulcers. The juice of Celandine, of Field Daisies, and of Ground Ivy clarified with a little sugar dissolved therein, and dropped into the eyes, is a sovereign remedy for inflammation, watery humours; and dropped into the ear, it is good for deafness.

In short, this is a valuable herb, and ought to be gathered in the season by every family for use. Such a step would never be regretted.

GUIACUM.

Foreign; Guiacum Officinalis.—Lignum Vitæ is a West Indian tree. The wood and gum are both used for the cure of chronic cutaneous and syphilitic diseases, for gout and rheumatism. From the rasped wood is prepared a decoction, to be taken from 2 to 4 ounces at a time. It is also one of the ingredients of the Compound decoction of Sarsaparilla, and other diet drinks for purifying the blood. Guiacum is often *extremely useful* in rheumatism.

Dr. Graham thus describes a compound by which Lord Amherst was cured of rheumatism. Guiacum, 1 drachm; powdered rhubarb, 2 drachms; cream of tartar, 1 ounce; flowers of sulphur, 2 ounces; one nutmeg finely powdered, made into an electuary with 1 pound of honey. Two large spoonfuls to be taken night and morning. The best form of administration is the Tincture, which may be given in one or two teaspoonful doses at bed-time. Milk is the best vehicle for its administration. The tincture is excellent for painful menstruation.

HART'S TONGUE.

DESCRIPTION.—*Scolopendrium Vulgaris.*—It is always green, though it has fresh leaves in Spring. It has several leaves arising from the root, which fold themselves in their first springing and spreading : when full grown they are about a foot long, smooth and green above, but hard, with little sap, and streaked on the back, thwart on the sides of the middle rib with small and rather long brownish marks ; the bottoms of the leaves are a little bowed on each side of the middle rib, rather narrow and small at the end. The root has many black threads interlaced together. It is green all the Winter ; but new leaves spring every year.

MEDICINAL VIRTUES.—It is an excellent purifier and strengthener of the liver, and it ought to be more extensively known.

HAWK-WEED.

DESCRIPTION.—Of this plant there are several kinds, as MOUSE-EAR HAWK-WEED, *Hieracium Dubium;* and LUNG-WORT HAWK-WEED, *Hieracium Pulmonarium,* but their virtues are the same. It has many large leaves lying upon the ground, much rent and torn on the sides into gashes like Dandelion, but with greater parts, more like the smooth Sow Thistle, from among which rises a hollow rough stalk, two or three feet high, branched from the middle upward, whereon are set at every joint longer leaves, little or nothing rent or cut, bearing on their top beautiful pale yellow flowers, consisting of many small, narrow leaves, broad pointed and nicked at the ends, set in a double row or more, the outer-most being larger than the inner, which turn into down, and with the small brownish seed is blown away with the wind. The root is long, and rather large, with many small fibres thereat. The whole plant is full of bitter milk. It grows in many places about the field-sides, and the path-ways in dry grounds. It is now cultivated in gardens.

MEDICINAL VIRTUES.—Hawk-weed is cooling, drying and binding, and therefore good for the heat of the stomach, and gnawings therein; for inflammations, and the hot fits of agues. The juice in wine, promotes digestion, expels wind, and neutralizes acidity in the stomach. A scruple of the dried root given in wine and vinegar, is good for the dropsy. The decoction taken with honey, and with hyssop, promotes expectoration and allays cough. The decoction with a little wild succoury, made with wine, relieves colic, and hardness of the spleen: it procures rest and sleep, purges the stomach, increases and purifies the blood. It is also good for bleeding piles, and the leaves boiled in milk may be applied outwardly. In many parts of Europe it is a constant medicine in diseases of the lungs, asthma, and incipient consumption. The juice mixed with milk is good for inflamed eyes. The green leaves bruised and mixed with salt make a good ointment for burns, erysipelas, and inflamed parts.

HAZEL-NUT.

Corylus Avellana.—Hazle Nuts are so well known that they need no description.

Medicinal Virtues.—The parted kernels made into an electuary, or the milk drawn from them, with honey water, relieves an old cough. The dried husks and red skin of the kernels to the weight of two drachms, taken in red wine, restrain profuse menstruation. Nuts do not cause shortness of breath. For how can that which strengthens the lungs cause shortness of breath? If any thing of the Hazel-nut be stopping, it is the husks and shells, and nobody is so mad as to eat them, unless medicinally; and the red skin which covers the kernel, you may easily pull off.

HEART'S EASE.

Description.—*Viola Tricolor.*—It is also called Pansy. Some of them grow wild in fields, and they are extensively cultivated in gardens.

Medicinal Virtues.—It is anti-venereal, made into a decoction. The spirit of it is good for convulsions in children, for falling-sickness, and for inflammation of the lungs and breast, pleurisy, scabs, itch, &c.

HEDGE HYSSOP.

DESCRIPTION,—*Gratiola Officinalis*,—There are several kinds of this plant; the first is Italian, and cultivated in gardens. Two or three sorts grow wild. The first is a smooth, low plant, not a foot high, very bitter in taste, with many square stalks, diversly branched from the bottom to the top, with several joints, and two small leaves at each joint, broader at the bottom than they are at the end, and full of veins. The flowers stand at the joints, of a fair purple colour, with white spots, like those of dead nettles. The seed is small and yellow, and the roots spread much under ground.

The second seldom grows half a foot high, sending up many small branches, whereon grow many small leaves, set one against the other, somewhat broad, but very short. The flowers are like the flowers of the other in fashion, but of a pale reddish colour. The seeds are small and yellowish. They grow in wet low grounds, and by the water sides. They flower in June and July.

MEDICINAL VIRTUES.—They are violent purgatives especially of choler and phlegm. They assist in the cure of dropsy, gout, and sciatica, outwardly used in ointments; they kill worms, and are good to cleanse old ulcers. The best mode to use them is:—put 2 drachms of the fresh leaves, into 6 ounces of boiling water, and let it stand 12 hours, and then add 6 blanched almonds, and 1 ounce of syrup of violets. A tablespoonful to be taken every hour, until it vomits or purges.

HELLEBORE,—BLACK.

DESCRIPTION.—*Heleborus Niger*.—It is also called Setterwort, Setter grass, Bear's-foot Christmas-herb, and Christmas-Rose.

It has fair green leaves rising from the root, each of them

standing about a handbreadth high from the earth; each leaf is divided into eight or nine parts, dented from the middle of the leaf to the point on both sides, abiding green all the winter; about Christmas, if the weather be temperate, the flowers appear upon footstalks, consisting of five large, round, white leaves a-piece, sometimes purple at the edges, with many pale yellow threads in the middle; the seeds are divided into several cells, like those of Columbines, but are larger, they are black, long, and round. The root consists of numberless blackish strings, all united into one head. They are found in some woods.

Medicinal Virtues.—It is an irritant poison, although sometimes given medicinally. In large doses both black and white Hellebore are drastic purgatives; in smaller doses, they are diuretic and emmenagogue. They are principally used as purgatives in case of mania, melancholy, coma, dropsy, worms, and emmenagogue. It ought not to be given except under skilful direction. The *Helleborus Foetidus*, Stinking Hellebore is given to expel worms; the dose of the Powdered Leaves being for a child 4 to 20 grains, or a fluid ounce of the decoction. The *Helleborus Viridens*, Green Hellebore, has been employed in America as a remedy for typhus fever, and for some convulsive diseases of children. But its administration requires both skill and great care.

HEMLOCK.

Description.—*Conium Maculatum.*—The common great spotted Hemlock has a green stalk, four or five feet high, or more, sometimes full of red spots, and at the joints very large winged leaves which are divided into many other winged leaves, one set against the other, dented at the edges, of a sad green colour, branched towards the top, where it is full of umbels or white flowers which produce whitish flat seed; the root is long, white, crooked, and hollow within. It has a very disagreeable smell. It grows throughout the land, by walls and hedge sides, in waste grounds and untilled places.

Medicinal Virtues.—Hemlock is very cold, and very dangerous, especially to be taken inwardly. It may safely be applied to inflammations, tumours and swellings in any part of the body, (save the private parts) as also to St. Anthony's fire, ulcers that arise from hot humours, by cooling and repelling the heat; the leaves bruised and laid to the brow or forehead are good for eyes red and swollen; and to take away films, specks, &c. in the eye; this is a tried medicine.

The ancients regarded it as a good discutient and anodyne external application, and used it both for fomentations and poultices. The dried leaves mixed with a carrot, or other poultice, and applied twice a day, correct the fœtor of a cancerous discharge in a very short time, and alter the discharge into a salutary pus. The decoction is good for swelled testicle. This is also a valuable remedy for ulcers, and glandular tumours. It allays pain and irritation in palsy and rheumatism. The powdered leaves and the extract are the forms in which it is given. The dose of the powder is three grains twice or thrice a day. It has been regarded as valuable in scrofula, in the latter stage of hooping cough, and in pulmonary consumption. The extract of Hemlock and Henbane in mucilage, subdues cough and pulmonary irritation, or they may be made into pills. Dose of extract, 2 to 3 grains once a day; (increase if necessary,) of the Compound Pill from 3 to 5 grains. For poisoning by Hemlock, the antidote is vinegar, taking previously as an emetic 20 grains of Sulphate of Zinc.

HEMP.

Cannabis Sativa.—It is too well known to require description.

MEDICINAL VIRTUES.—It has narcotic properties. The Hindoos prepare from it an intoxicating liquor called Banga, and so do the Turks, Arabians, and others. These properties are not quite so strong in the European Hemp. The seed boiled in milk, relieves a hot dry cough; strain and drink. The Dutch make an emulsion of the seed, and give it with good success in jaundice, for it opens obstructions of the gall and bile. The emulsion or decoction of the seed restrains fluxes, eases the colic, and removes humours in the bowels, and arrests bleeding at the mouth, nose, and other places. It is good to kill worms, and the juice dropped into the ears, kills the worms and other insects which may have entered. The decoction of the root eases gouty pains, the hard humours of knots in the joints, the pains and shrinking of the sinews, and the pains of the hips. The fresh juice mixed with a little oil and butter is good for burns.

HENBANE.

DESCRIPTION.—*Hyoscyamus.*—Henbane has very large, thick, soft, woolly leaves, lying on the gound, indented or torn on the edges, of a dark, ill greyish green colour, among which rise up several thick and short stalks, two or three feet high, spread into several small branches, with smaller leaves on them, and many hollow flowers, scarcely appearing above the husk, and torn on one side, ending in five round points of a dead yellowish colour, paler towards the edges, with purplish veins; and a dark yellowish purple in the bottom of the flower, with a small point of the same colour in the middle, each of them standing in a hard close husk, which after the flowers are past, grows very like the husk of Asarabacca, and somewhat sharp at the top points, having much small seed, like Poppy seed, of a greyish colour. The root is great, white and thick, so like a Parsnip root (but not so white) that it has deceived others. It commonly grows by the way-sides, under hedges and walls, and on ditch banks.

MEDICINAL VIRTUES,—It is a strong narcotic poison; the leaves and seeds being chiefly used in medicine. It is found to allay pain, and subdue nervous excitement without confining the bowels, and acting otherwise prejudicial, as opium often does. In irritable affections of the lungs, bowels, and other organs, its sedative properties make it very valuable. Like Hemlock, it favours the natural action of the bowels. It is useful in red gravel and stone, as it allays irritation and pain. It is a valuable addition to purgatives which are apt to gripe. It may be given in the form of extract or tincture. *Extract*, from 4 to 20 grains made into pills, twice or thrice in 24 hours. Tincture from half a drachm to 1 or 2 drachms. The dose of the *powdered leaves* is from half a drachm to 2 drachms—of the *fresh juice* from half a drachm to 1 drachm.

In his *Elements of Materia Medica*, Dr. Thompson says, "In my own practice, I have seen more good derived (in *mania*) from 8 or 10 grains, combined with 10 grains of camphor, and given at bed-time, than from the repetition of smaller doses." It forms a valuable ingredient in *Cough Pills*. The seeds sometimes relieve toothache:—Heat a small piece of metal nearly red-hot; and place the seed upon it; inhale the vapour, but not too much. The remedy for an overdose, is vinegar, as prescribed under *Hemlock*.

HOLLYHOCK.

Altheæ Rosea. It is well known as a beautiful garden plant.

Medicinal Virtues.—The root is white, long, and thick, and of a slimy nature. This is the part to be used. A decoction of it operates by urine; it is excellent for gravel. It has nearly the same virtues as the Mallow, and Marshmallow. The flowers are rather astringent.

HOLLY.

Description.—*Ilex Aquifolium.* Belonging to the natural order *Aquifoliaceæ* the only British member of the genus *Ilex*. It is well known. It is sometimes called Holm, or Hulm, or Hulver Bush. Holly is probably a corruption of *Holy*.

Medicinal Virtues.—The leaves are bitter, mucous and astringent, having an austere taste. The berries expel wind, and therefore good for the colic, They are very purgative, 10 or 12 being generally sufficient to act on the bowels. Used when ripe, they are efficacious in cleansing from morbid matter. They also act as an emetic and diuretic. The expressed juice is said to be beneficial in jaundice. A decoction of the bark and leaves makes an excellent fomentation for broken bones, &c. The berries dried, and powdered, are astringent and stay fluxes. The leaves were formerly used as a diaphoretic, and an infusion of them was given in catarrh, gout, pleurisy, and small-pox. In France, a few years ago, some physicians pronounced it to be a very superior febrifuge, being equal, if not superior to Peruvian bark, their virtues being dependant on a better principle called *Tlicin*. Pliny *absurdly* says the branches of the tree defend houses from lightning, and persons from witchcraft! From the inner bark *bird-lime* is prepared; it is steeped in cold water for a few hours, and then beaten in a mortar, washed in cold water, left to settle a day or two, the scum taken off, and the bird-lime is ready for use.

HONEYSUCKLE.

Periclymenos.—It is so well known as to forbid description. It is known also by the names of Woodbine, Meadow Trefoil.

MEDICINAL VIRTUES.—A decoction of the leaves removes obstructions of the liver and spleen; and is a good gargle for sore throats. It promotes urine. The seed and flowers boiled in water, made into a poultice, with a little oil, and applied, cures hard swellings and imposthumes. The juice dropped into the eyes, is a familiar medicine, to take away specks, &c.

HONEWORT.

DESCRIPTION.—*Sison Segetum.*—A common plant in corn-fields and dry places. It has pretty leaves, and little umbels of white flowers. From the root arise six or more leaves, which are beautifully spread on the ground. The stalks do not appear till the end of summer, and by that time the leaves decay, so that they are not known to belong to it. These leaves are eight inches long, and nearly two inches broad. Each is composed of a double row of smaller leaves, on a common rib with an odd leaf at the end; they are nicely indented, and of a fresh green colour. The stalk is two feet high, upright, round, hollow, not very firm, and branched at the top.

MEDICINAL VIRTUES.—Its name is derived from its virtues. In some parts painful swellings are called hones, and the herb from its efficacy in curing them, has received the name of *hone-herb*, or *honewort*. The leaves are to be used, fresh gathered, and reduced in a mortar to a kind of paste. Applied to red and painful swellings, it is effectual in dispersing them. Some say it is good for scrofula.

HOP.

Humulus Lupulus.—This plant is well known, and requires no description. It is cultivated, and also grows wild.

MEDICINAL VIRTUES.—Hops are used to impart a bitter flavour to ale and beer. The bitter principle is tonic, the aromatic warm and stimulating; they are also astringent and slightly anodyne. A pillow stuffed with hops has been found to promote sleep, and a fomentation to allay the pain and irritation of angry tumours. A teaspoonful of the Tincture of Hops will often induce sleep when opium has failed, and without the injurious effects of the drug. Herophilus Lobbuis says that by a decoction of Hops he has softened the hardest urinary calculi; and Darelius says that half a pint, or more, of the decoction, taken in the morning, expels worms. Dr. Thornton says, the Hop merits regard in consumption, disorders arising from weakness of the primæ viæ, gout, and especially calculous complaints. They are good to remove obstructions of the liver and spleen, and to cleanse the blood. In cleansing the blood they help to cure scabs, itch, ring-worms, and spreading sores. A bread poultice well saturated with strong Hop decoction, is a powerful remedy for bad ulcers. Half a drachm of the seed in powder taken in drink, destroys worms. A syrup made of the juice and sugar, cures the yellow jaundice, and tempers the heat of the liver and stomach. Hops heated in a flannel bag, are a common remedy for toothache, and neuralgic pains. The Tincture is made by macerating for eight or nine days six or seven ounces of Hops in two pints of proof spirit. Begin with half a drachm.

HOREHOUND.

Marrubium Vulgare.—There are two kinds of Horehound, white and black; the latter is also called Hen-bit; but the white is the one here recommended.

Common Horehound has square hairy stalks, half a yard or two feet high, set at the joints with two round crumpled rough leaves, of a sullen hoary green colour, of a moderate scent, but a very bitter taste. The flowers are small, white and gaping, set in a rough, hard prickly husk round the joints, with the leaves in the middle of the stalk upwards, after which follow small round black seed. The plant is well known.

Medicinal Virtues.—A decoction of the dried herb, with the seed, or the juice of the green herb taken with honey, is a remedy for difficult breathing, cough, and consumption, through thin distillations of rheum upon the lungs. It promotes expectoration of tough phlegm, taken with the roots of Iris or Orris. As a decoction, it is useful in female weakness, removing obstructions, &c. The dose is an ounce or two of the expressed juice, or the infusion of half a handful of the fresh leaves in a sufficient quantity of boiling water. Sweetened with sugar or honey, and a little ginger, it becomes more efficacious. The best part of the plant for medicinal use is the tops of the young shoots. It is an excellent drink in winter for hoarseness, coughs, &c. A handful of the leaves of White Horehound, one of Black and one of Betony in 5 or 6 pints of boiling water is a serviceable drink for gouty and rheumatic subjects. *Syrup of Horehound* is made by boiling a pound of Lump Sugar with the same quantity of a strong decoction of the leaves, until it assumes the proper consistency. *Candied Horehound* is made by evaporating the Syrup until it becomes thick enough, on cooling, to eat as a lozenge. Galen says, it opens obstructions of the liver and spleen. The powder, or the decoction, destroys worms. The green leaves bruised, and boiled in lard, and made into an ointment, is good for wounds. There is a syrup made of Horehound to be had at the apothecaries, very good for old coughs.

HORSE RADDISH.

Cochlearia Armoracea.—It is well known. It belongs to the Scurvy-grass tribe of plants.

Medicinal Virtues.—It is a powerful stimulant, whether taken inwardly, or applied outwardly. A poultice of the scraped root serves instead of a Mustard plaister. Its therapeutic effects are, diuretic, emetic, sudorific, and stimulant. It is chiefly administered in paralytic affections, and chronic rheumatism, and in scurvy. As it operates powerfully by urine it is good for the jaundice and dropsy. The decoction is a great purifier of the blood. It destroys worms in children &c. The root bruised and applied to any part affected with sciatica, joint-ache, &c. or to hard liver and spleen, gives great relief.

Dr. Cullen says, "I have found that one drachm of the root fresh scraped down was sufficient for four ounces of water, to be infused two hours in a close vessel, and made into syrup with double its weight in sugar. A teaspoonful or two, occasionally repeated, and swallowed leisurely, is very effectual in hoarseness. As a condiment, it stimulates the stomach, and promotes digestion. I have known a strong decoction of this root drunk as an emetic, which has relieved pituitous asthma more than by any other means. It should be much used in diet by persons of phlegmatic habits, especially if afflicted with dropsy.

HORSETAIL.

Description.—*Hippurus.*—There are many kinds of this plant. As it rises up, it has heads like those of asparagus, which grow to be hard, rough, hollow stalks jointed at various places up to the top, a foot high, as if the lower parts were put into the upper, where grow on each side a bush of small long rush-like hard leaves, each part resembling a horse-tail, from whence it is so called. At the tops of the stalks come forth small catkins, like those of trees. The root creepeth. It grows in wet grounds. They spring up in April, and produce catkins in July.

Medicinal Virtues.—Horsetail, the smooth rather than the rough, and the leaved rather than the bare, is most medicinal. The juice or decoction is very powerful to staunch bleeding either inward or outward, or the juice or distilled water applied outwardly. It is astringent, and restrains bloody flux, and bloody urine; and it heals inward and outward ulcers, excoriation of the entrails, bladder, &c. and soon closes and heals green wounds. The decoction in wine is diuretic and relieves the stone and stranguary. A small quantity of the distilled water drunk two or three times a day, eases and strengthens the intestines. A drachm of the dried leaves powdered taken three or four times a day, is very effectual in spitting of blood.

HOUND'S TONGUE.

Description.—*Cynoglossus Vulgaris.*—The great Hound's tongue, or Dog's Tongue, has a disagreeable scent, resembling that of mice.

The great ordinary Hound's Tongue has many long, and narrow, soft, hairy, darkish green leaves lying on the ground, resembling Bugloss leaves, from which rises a rough hairy stalk, two feet high, with smaller leaves thereon, and branched at the tops into several parts, with a small leaf at the foot of every branch, somewhat long, with many flowers set along the same; they are small, and of a deep purple. It has sometimes a white flower. The seeds are rough, flat, with a small point in the middle, easily cleaving to any garment. The root is black, thick, and long, hard to break, and full of clammy juice. It grows in moist places, in waste grounds, and untilled places, by highway-sides, lanes, and hedge-sides. It flowers about May or June.

Medicinal Virtues.—The root is principally used, and is very effectual in pills, as well as the decoction, to stay all sharp and thin humours from the head into the eyes or nose, or upon the stomach or lungs, and for coughs, and shortness of breath. The leaves boiled in wine are good for purgings, retchings, and violent pains in the stomach and intestines. The decoction relieves the piles, and stops their bleeding. The leaves bruised, or the juice boiled in lard, and applied, stops falling away of the hair. The root baked under the embers, wrapped in a wet double cloth, and applied to the fundament, effectually relieves piles. An ointment made of the leaves with honey and turpentine, makes an excellent ointment for dressing old ulcers, sores, &c. Let the decoction be drank freely at the same time. I cured the biting of a mad dog with this only medicine.

HOUSELEEK, OR SENGREEN.

Sedum, vel Sempervivum Lectorum.—No description is needed. It grows on the tops of walls and houses.

Medicinal Virtues.—It contains malic acid, in combination with lime, and is cooling, astringent, and diuretic. Its thick succulent leaves are sometimes applied to burns with success, stings of insects, ulcers, and inflammatory swellings, and to corns and bunions with good effect. A posset made with the juice of Houseleek is good in hot agues, for it cools the blood and spirits, and quenches thirst; it is good to stay hot and salt rheums in the eyes, the juice being dropped into them. It is good in Erysipelas, called St. Anthony's fire, and eases the pain of the gout. The juice takes away warts and corns, the skin and leaves being laid on them afterwards; applied to the temples and forehead, it eases the headache, and heat of the brain in frenzies, or through want of sleep.

HYACINTH,—WILD.

Hyacinthus.—The common Wood Hyacinth is a native of Persia, and of many parts of Europe. In the spring it is very common in our woods, hedges, &c. It is familiarly called, Blue-bells, and the Harebell:—

> "In the lone copse, or shadowy dell,
> Wild cluster'd knots of harebells blow."

Medicinal Virtues.—It abounds with a slimy juice. But it is to be carefully dried. The decoction of the roots is diuretic, promoting the flow of urine. The powder is balsamic, and rather styptic. A more powerful remedy for the whites can scarcely be found. It ought to be better known.

HYSSOP.

Hyssopus Officinalis.—A very pretty garden plant requiring no description.

Medicinal Virtues.—It should be gathered when just

beginning to flower, dried, and placed in bags. An infusion of Hyssop sweetened with honey is good for hoarseness, and obstructions in the breast. Made into a Syrup with honey, it has the same effect. Some persons add a little Oil of Almonds. It makes a wholesome tea combined with Balm as the principal, and a very small quantity of Mint. Hyssop is a vermifuge expelling worms from children. A handful of dried Hyssop in a linen cloth immersed in boiling water, is the best application to a black or blood-shot eye. Boiled with Rue and honey, it relieves cough, wheezing, shortness of breath. With bruised figs it is an easy purgative. It improves the natural colour, spoiled by the yellow jaundice; and taken with figs and nitre, relieves dropsy and spleen. Boiled with wine it is good to wash inflammations. It takes away black and blue spots caused by strokes, bruises or falls, applied with warm water. It is excellent for the quinsy, to wash and gargle the throat, being boiled with figs. The hot vapours of the decoction forced by a funnel in at the ears, ease inflammations and singing noises. It assists to expectorate tough phlegm, and is effectual in all diseases of the chests or lungs. The green herb bruised, and a little sugar, quickly heals cuts or green wounds.

ICELAND MOSS.

Cretaria, or Lichen Islandica.—It belongs to the class of *Lichens.* It is a parasite, growing upon the trunks and branches of trees. It is found abundantly in Iceland, and also in Northern Europe, and amid the higher mountains of North Britain. It is generally sold by Druggists in a dried state. The taste is bitter and unpleasant. The Icelanders use it as an article of food, and denominate it "the gift of a bountiful providence, affording them bread out of the very stones." Its preparation is by repeated steepings in cold water, drying, and powdering, after which it is made into cakes, or boiled in milk. Washing, of course, deteriorates its tonic properties, though it may retain a part, and all its demulcent and nutritive properties.

Its medicinal virtues in consumption have been highly commended, perhaps too much so; yet it is unquestionably of much service in *catarrhal* consumption, which has its seat in the windpipe and its terminations. It allays the tickling cough, relieves the oppressed breathing, arrests the hectic fever, strengthens the digestive organs, it has a soothing influence on the bronchi, and helps to sustain the system by the nutrition which it contains. It may be administered by decoction, by 1 or 2 ounces in a quart of water till it becomes a jelly, adding sugar, and straining. A wineglassful may be taken twice or thrice a day either alone or mixed with milk. *Olasson* asserts that a soup made with the meal or powder is twice as nutritious as that prepared with flour.

IPECACUANHA.

Cephaelis Ipecacuanha.—It is a Brazilian plant of the order *Chinchonaceæ.* The root is used, of which there are three kinds, the brown, the grey, and the white. The brown is the best. As an *emetic* Ipecacuanha is the most certain, safest, and the best that we have. It is also a valuable expectorant and diaphoretic remedy, and greatly aids the action of aperients. It has a specific action on the Bronchial mucous membrane, so as to excite its secretion when too dry; it relieves the system, and causes perspiration. As an emetic it does not nauseate, and reduce the system so much as Tartar Emetic, nor is its action so irritating as Sulphate of Zinc. An emetic given at the commencement of fevers will arrest their course; and if it fail, it is sure to give to the disease a milder form; say from 10 to 20 grains of Ipecacuanha powder. Dr. Graham says, "In doses of two or three grains, repeated every 3 or 4 hours, till it operates by vomiting, sweating, or purging, it is found of great utility in dysentery and chronic looseness: indeed its effects in these severe complaints are often invaluable, and it is perhaps the most beneficial aperient in dysentery; for when we can bring it to act in this way, it produces a steady determination of the peristaltic motion of the bowels downwards, at the same time that it strengthens their internal surface, and relaxes the skin."

Where it is necessary to excite nausea and vomiting in children and delicate persons, Ipecacuanha is the best; its expectorant property renders it very useful in catarrhal affections, when it is frequently combined with squills. In hooping cough and in asthma, it relieves spasmodic restriction, and to clear the chest of phlegm by vomiting. In spitting of blood it is invaluable, arresting its progress, and preventing its return. In dyspepsia, or indigestion, bilious, and liver complaints, it has great efficacy.—*Dose;* of powder, as an *expectorant*, from 1 to 2 grains; as a *diaphoretic*, from 2 to 4 grains; as an *emetic*, from 10 to 20 grains, according to the age and strength of the patient. The vomiting is promoted and facilitated by drinking copiously of warm watery fluids. The Ipecacuanha Lozenges are useful in cough, and may be taken also to the extent of an emetic, even one or two sometimes being sufficient for that purpose.

The compound powder, or the celebrated *Dover's Sudorific Powder.* Ipecacuanha, in powder, and purified opium, of each one part; sulphate of potass, eight parts, triturate them together into a fine powder. This powder is one of the most certain sudorifics, recommended by Dr. Dover as an effectual remedy in rheumatism; it is useful also in dropsy, and several other diseases, where it is difficult, by other means, to produce a copious sweat. The dose is from 2 to 5 grains repeated as the patient's stomach and strength can bear it. Avoid much drinking immediately after it, to avoid vomiting before the other effects are produced.—"It is a valuable anodyne, sudorific, and alterative, of great service in acute and chronic rheumatism, and in other complaints; it relieves pain, procures sleep, and relaxes the skin."—It is the best to buy the root, which is soon powdered. The *wine* may be made by steeping well half an ounce of the root, bruised in half a pint of sherry for two or three weeks, and then filtering. *Dose; expectorant,* 10 to 20 drops; as an *emetic*, 2 to 4 drachms; for a child from 10 drops.

IVY.

Hedera Helic.—Ivy is known by all.

MEDICINAL VIRTUES. A drachm of the flowers decocted in wine, restrains dysentery, or bloody flux. The yellow berries are good against the jaundice; and for those who spit blood, and the white berries being taken inwardly, or applied outwardly, destroy worms. Taken in wine, they help to break the stone, provoke urine, and women's courses. The fresh leaves of Ivy boiled in vinegar, and applied warm to the sides of those who are troubled with the spleen, ache, or stitch in the sides, give much ease. The same applied with Rose-water, and oil of Roses, to the temples and forehead, eases the head-ache. The leaves boiled in weak wine form an excellent wash for ulcers, sores, burns, scalds, &c. The juice of the berries or leaves snuffed up into the nose, purges the head and brain of rheum, which causes defluxions into the eyes and nose; the same dropped into the ears, cures sores therein. The fresh leaves applied to corns and bunions effectually cure them. Intoxication by wine, the effects are removed by a handful of leaves bruised, and gently boiled in wine, and the liquor drank.

JALAP.

Convolvulus Jalapa.—It is a plant of Mexico and Vera Cruz. The root is used. Half a drachm of Jalap proves an effectual, and in general, a safe purgative, operating mildly. But in hypochondriacal disorders, and in hot bilious temperaments, it gripes violently, if the jalap be good, and rarely takes due effect as a purge. The best form for its administration is the compound powder, composed of jalap in powder, 3 ounces, cream of tartar, 6 ounces, and ginger, 2 drachms, well rubbed up together;—dose, half a drachm to a drachm.

Jalap accelerates the action of rhubarb, and in this form it expels worms. Some, for that purpose, add a little calomel; but powdered Wormwood would be better. In rheumatism jalap is an excellent purge. When triturated with sugar, in small doses, it is a safe purge for children; they will receive it in this way, the jalap having but little taste.

JUNIPER BUSH.

Juniperis Communis.—It is needless to give a description of a bush so commonly known.

It grows plentifully in several woods in Kent; Warney Common, near Brentford, in Essex; upon Finchley Common, Newfound wells, near Dulwich, upon a common between Mitcham and Croydon; and other places. The berries, however, are chiefly brought from Holland.

The berries continue green two Summers and one Winter before they are ripe, at which time they are of a purplish black colour, and therefore you will always find upon the bush green berries.

Medicinal Virtues.—The berries have a strong aromatic odour peculiar to themselves, and a flavour much like that of turpentine. They are aromatic, stimulating, diuretic, and diaphoretic, and are chiefly employed as a combination with other remedies, and to increase the discharge of urine in dropsy. The oil of juniper is an effective expellant of wind, and it quickly relieves colic. It is a good stomachic. An infusion of the berries will have a similar effect; say a pint of boiling water poured on 2 or 3 ounces of the berries, taking a cupful every three hours. From 6 to 12 berries eaten will have a similar effect. They are very good for a cough, shortness of breath, and pains in the belly. They are good in all kinds of agues, are good for gout, sciatica, and they give strength to the limbs. The ashes of the wood make an excellent dentrifice for scurvy in the gums. They are useful in dysentery, stone, and diseases of the kidneys.

The essential oil of Juniper is a prime ingredient in Geneva or Hollands Gin, and upon which its flavour and diuretic properties depend. English Gin, however, has more of turpentine than of this oil in it.——The dose of the oil is from 3 to 6 drops.

KIDNEYWORT.

Description.—*Cotyledon Umbilicus.*—It is also called Navel Wort, Wall Pennyroyal, and Wall Pennywort. It has many thick, flat, and round leaves growing from the root, each having a long footstalk, fastened underneath, about the middle of it, and a little unevenly weaved sometimes about the edges, of a pale green colour, and rather yellow on the upper side like a saucer; from which arise one or more smooth, hollow stalks, half a foot high, with two or three small leaves thereon, rather long, and divided at the edges; the tops are divided into long branches, bearing a number of flowers, round a long spike one above another, which are hollow like a little bell, of a whitish green colour, after which come small heads, containing small brownish seed. The root is round and smooth, greyish without, and white within. It grows upon stone or mud walls, upon rocks, and in stony places upon the ground, at the bottom of old trees, and on those that are decayed. It flowers in May.

Medicinal Virtues.—The juice and the extract are reputed for the cure of Epilepsy. The juice allays inflammations and heat of the liver, stomach, and strengthens the bowels. The juice of the herb outwardly applied restrains St. Anthony's fire, or erysipelas. It heals pimples, sores, &c; and taken inwardly it relieves inflamed kidneys, and is good in all gravelly complaints. Made into an ointment, it is good for the piles, for gouty pains, sciatica, and swelled testicles; the ointment, or the juice alone is good for scrofula sores, chilblains. It stops the bleeding of green wounds.

KINO.

This is an extract obtained from several trees of the genus *Pterocarpus*. It has been regarded as the most powerful of all the vegetable astringents, containing 70 per cent of tannic acid. Hence it has been found eminently useful in diarrhœa, dysentery, gonorrhoea, leucorrhœa, internal bleedings, and discharges generally. Externally, it is a good application to foul ulcers. It makes an excellent gargle for sore throats, and diseased uvula. It is useful as a styptic. The dose of the powder is from 12 grains to 1 drachm; of the tincture from one to two drachms. The compound powder contains one grain of opium to 20 grains of Kino;—take from 10 to 20 grains.—

KNAPWEED.

DESCRIPTION.—*Centaurea Jacea.*—It has many long and rather broad dark green leaves, dented about the edges, sometimes a little torn on both sides, and rather hairy; amongst which arises a long round stalk, four or five feet high, divided into many branches, at the tops stand great scaly green heads, enclosing a number of dark purplish red thrums or threads; which after they are withered, come black seeds wrapped in down, resembling thistle-seed, but smaller. The root is white, hard, and woody. The flowers appear in June and July. It is found in fields and meadows, and on the road sides.

MEDICINAL VIRTUES.—It stays dysentery, or bloody flux, bleeding at the nose, and inward bleedings. It is good in catarrhal affections, restraining distillations of thin and sharp humours from the head upon the stomach and lungs. It is strongly recommended for cuts and bruises, and running sores, as it dries them up, and heals them gently. It may be taken in decoction, or be made into an ointment for outward application.

KNOTGRASS.

DESCRIPTION.—*Polygonon.*—A very common wild plant growing in fields, pathways, and hedges. The stalks of Knotgrass are ten inches long, round, jointed, and of a dusky green. The leaves are oval, of a bluish green, not indented. The stalks lie upon the ground, and only one of these grows at each joint. The flowers are small and white, with a slight red tinge.

MEDICINAL VIRTUES.—It is an excellent astringent. The juice is effectual to stay bleeding of the mouth, drunk in steeled or red wine; and bleeding at the nose, to be applied to the forehead or temples, or to be squirted up into the nostrils. It cools the blood, and the stomach. It restrains bloody flux, profuse menstruation, and running of the reins. It is useful in that distressing complaint strangury, provoking urine, and easing pains in the bladder, and it is an expellant of stone, &c. Take a drachm of the herb powdered in wine, twice a day. The decoction destroys worms. A decoction of the roots, stalks, and leaves, is a first-rate astringent, applicable to all bleedings, and especially to the bleeding piles; and the juice made into an ointment, it is a sovereign remedy for inflammations, breakings out, hot swellings and imposthumes, gangrene, canker, and green wounds. The juice is good for sores in the ears.

KOUSSO.

The dried flowers and unripe seeds of the *Brayera Authelmintica*, obtained from Abyssinia. It is a most efficient cure for the tapeworm. Dr. S. Thompson says, "In two cases which had resisted all previous treatment, I found the Kousso perfectly successful." It should be taken in the morning fasting; no *solid* food to be taken for 24 hours before taking it, and a dose of castor oil administered the previous evening. Half an ounce of the powder must be taken, which must be infused in warm water, and taken unstrained; it will be more palatable with honey and lemon juice; and if it does not operate in 10 or 12 hours follow with a dose of castor oil. It is very seldom that a second dose is required; if it is, repeat in a day or two after the first, taking only very simple food.

LADIES' BED STRAW.

Description.—*Galium Verum.*— It is also called Cheese Rennet, because it performs the same office as Rennet; Maid Hair, and Wild Rosemary. *Galium Verum.* It grows in meadows and pastures, and by hedges. It rises up with small, brown, and square upright stalks, two or three feet high; sometimes it branches forth into divers parts, full of joints, with several very small leaves at every one of them. At the tops of the branches grow very thickly many yellow flowers from the several joints, which consist of four leaves each, which smell strong, but not unpleasant. The seed resembles poppy seeds. The root is reddish, having many small fibres. The branches bend to the ground, and take root at the joints, by which it is increased.

There is another kind which bears white flowers; but the branches of this are so weak, that, unless supported by the hedge, &c., it lies on the ground. The leaves are larger than the former, but the flowers are not so numerous.

MEDICINAL VIRTUES.—This herb possesses very great virtues. It is a popular remedy for hysterical complaints and epilepsy, and has been given in inflammations of the brain, as an infusion, made by pouring 1½ pints of boiling water on 2 drachms of the herb, taking a wineglassful several times a day. The decoction is good to dissolve stone, to provoke urine, to stop inward bleeding and bleeding at the nose, and to heal inward wounds. The herb and its flowers made into an ointment, by boiling with sallad oil, and adding a little wax, then straining, is a remedy for burns and scalds, and especially for scrofulous sores. The decoction of the herb and flowers refreshes the feet after long walking. The ointment removes the dry scab and itch.

LADIES-MANTLE.

DESCRIPTION.—*Alchemilla Vulgaris.*—It is a beautiful plant, common in gravelly fields, and by road sides. It has many beautiful broad roundish leaves, divided into eight parts, each prettily indented at the edges. They are of a yellowish green colour, nearly as broad as the palm of the hand. They look plaited at first, and then a little crumpled, a little hairy, as is the stalk also. The stalks are round, eight inches long, or more, not very upright, and of a pale green colour. The flowers stand abundantly at the top, and they are white, proceeding from small yellowish green heads. The root is long, thick, and dark coloured. It flowers in May and June.

MEDICINAL VIRTUES.—Ladies-Mantle is very proper for inflamed wounds, and is very effectual to stay bleeding, vomitings, fluxes of all sorts, bruises, and it relieves ruptures. Some females apply the leaves to enlarged breasts, in order to reduce them, and give them their proper form. As a decoction it is useful in conception, by its retentive influence. It is a most valuable wound herb; highly prized by the Germans, who use it in all inward and outward wounds. They drink the decoction, and wash the wounds with it, and it effectually heals them. The herb and the root powdered, is good for violent purgings.

LADIES' SMOCK.

Description.—*Cardamine Pratensis.* It is also called Cuckoo-flower. It is a beautiful wild plant, frequent in meadows in Spring. The root is composed of many small white threads, from whence spring long stalks of winged leaves consisting of round, tender, dark green leaves, set one against another upon a middle rib, the greatest being at the end, amongst which rise up weak, round, green stalks, streaked, with longer and smaller leaves upon them; on the tops of which stand flowers almost like the Stock Gilliflowers, but rounder, and not so long, of a blushing white colour; the seed is reddish, and of a sharp biting taste, and so also the herb.

Medicinal Virtues.—The plant has the same virtues as Water-Cresses, and is good for the scurvy. It provokes urine and breaks the stone, and warms a cold and weak stomach, restoring lost appetite, and promotes digestion. It is very useful in jaundice, and green sickness.

LAVENDER.

Description.—*Lavendula Vera.*—It is a well-known, small, shrubby, perennial plant, a native of the South of Europe, and cultivated in our gardens for the sake of its perfume.

Medicinal Virtues.—Its flowers contain a volatile oil, obtained by distilling. It is warm, aromatic, and carminitive. It is used as a stimulant in debility, lowness of spirits, and other nervous affections. It invigorates the stomach, and removes obstructions from the liver and spleen. The oil is good for toothache. The distilled water removes hoarseness, loss of voice, faintings, trembling, &c. It removes obstruction of urine, and flatulency. The Oil and also the Compound Tincture may be obtained at the shops; the latter preparation is known by the name of "Lavender Drops," which are very useful in languors and faintings. It is a useful addition to stomachic infusions, as infusion of gentian, cascarilla, &c. The oil of Lavender, with equal quantities of Lard and Butter of Cocoa, makes a good application to stimulate the growth of the hair.

LEADWORT.

DESCRIPTION.—*Plumbago Europœa*—This is a small garden plant, growing two feet high. The stalks are slender, tough, yet weak, not able to support themselves. The leaves are a pale bluish green colour, oblong, but not broad, growing round the base of the stalk. The flowers are red, very small, in thick oblong clusters, standing on the tops of the stalks.

MEDICINAL VIRTUES.—Every part of this plant is acid, particularly the root; which when chewed excites a flow of saliva, and it has been recommended for toothache. Slightly boiled in Olive oil it is a successful application for the itch, old ulcers, and even cancers. It is excellent for headache. It is more acrid and fiery than even Pelitory of Spain. It makes a first rate rubefacient for pained limbs.

LEMON.

Citrus Communis.—It is cultivated chiefly in France, Spain, Italy, Sicily &c. It is common in the green-houses of this country. The acidity in the juice is owing to the presence of Citric Acid, the most agreeable acid for effervescing draughts. Lemon juice is a powerful and pleasant *antiseptic*. Dr. Wright says, its powers are much increased by saturating it with Muriate of Soda. This mixture he recommended as very efficacious in dysentery, remittent fever, bellyache, putrid sore throat, and as being perfectly specific in diabetes.

Citric Acid is often successfully used for allaying vomiting; it is mixed with carbonate of potash, from which it expels the carbonate acid with effervescence. It should be drank *as soon as it is made;* if not it would do harm instead of good. The doses are about a scruple of the carbonate dissolved in eight or ten drachms of water, and an ounce of lemon juice, or an equivalent quantity of Citric Acid. It is one of the greatest sick-room luxuries that we know; it is of great use in allaying febrile heat, and thirst.

The chief medical use of Lemon-juice has hitherto been in scurvy, in which it is a curative medicine, and a *preventive;* and therefore it is most useful in long sea-voyages. The best way to preserve it for keeping, is to add to it about one-tenth of Spirits of Wine, which coagulates the gummy matter, which would be likely to cause fermentation; and it should therefore be seperated from the clear juice by straining. A little of it should be taken every day when at sea, when fresh vegetables cannot be obtained, during the use of salt provisions. Lime-juice is sometimes used as a substitute, but with less effect.

Latterly, Lemon-juice has been employed for the cure of gout and rheumatism with great success. The author has reason, from his own experience, to speak favourably of its remedial power in rheumatic fever. The dose is half an ounce every half hour, or hour on an empty stomach. Besides being anti-scorbutic and antiseptic, it is *tonic* and *diaphoretic.* As a *tonic,* it forms with Orange peel an ingredient in the Compound Infusion of Gentian.

Lemon-juice also counteracts the effects of Opium.

"*Salts of Lemon,*" sold for removing the stains of ink or iron from linen, is wrongly named; for it is a salt of Oxalic Acid, and a rank *poison.*

LENTIL.

Ervum Lens.—Lentils belong to the Pea tribe, and are used as food all over the south of Europe, in the East, and in Egypt. The flour is very wholesome and nutritious, and Dr. Playfair found that it contained more nutritious matter than any other Pea or Bean meal. In addition to their rice the Hindoos take Lentils when engaged in hard labour. The Egyptian Lentil meal known as Revalenta and Ervalenta Arabica is very nutritious, easy of digestion, and possesses aperient properties, and therefore very suitable for the diet of invalids, especially for the dyspeptic.

LETTUCE,—GARDEN.

Lactuca Sativa.—As an article of diet, Lettuce is extensively cultivated in the kitchen garden. The botanical name, *Lactuca*, from *Lac*, milk, is given on account of the milky juice which exudes from the plant when cut, this milky juice turns brown, and dries on exposure to the air, and is then called Lactucarium, or Lettuce-opium. It is narcotic, but less powerfully so than opium, and it does not confine the bowels as that gum is apt to do. It is recommended in phthisis and catarrh. It is given to ease coughs, and to procure sleep; the dose is from 1 to 6 grains.

The juice mixed with oil of roses promotes sleep, and relieves headache. It is gently aperient, and aids digestion. It is also a good application for inflamed parts.

LETTUCE,—WILD.

Lactuca Virum.—It is found in many parts of Britain, in hedges. It resembles the Garden Lettuce in its flowers, though not in the manner of its growth. It rises four or five feet, and has three different kinds of leaves. They are very large, a foot long, and five inches broad, of a pale green colour. Those proceeding from the root are slightly toothed; those from the stem are cut into pinnated lobes; and those attached to the flower-stalks are arrow-shaped, pointed entire, and minute. The flowers are pale yellow.

MEDICINAL VIRTUES.—An extract prepared from the expressed juice of the leaves; gathered when in flower, in small doses is good in dropsy; two grains at first, twice a day, and gradually increased till two scruples, or more, are given daily. In dropsies of long standing, proceeding from visceral obstructions, it has been given to the extent of half an ounce a day. A syrup made from a strong infusion of it, is a good anodyne;

it eases the most violent pain in colics, and other disorders, and gently disposes to sleep. It is said to agree with the stomach, to quench thirst, to be gently aperient, very diuretic, and rather diaphoretic. Plentiful dilution must be allowed during its operation. Dr. Cullen, of Vienna, asserts that out of 24 dropsical patients, all but one were cured by this medicine.

LILY OF THE VALLEY.

DESCRIPTION.—*Lilium Convallium.*—It is also called Male Lily, and Lily Confancy. The root is small, and creeps far in the ground, as grass roots do. The leaves are large, long, and broad, of a dark green colour and full of very thick ribs and veins, from which rises a stalk half a foot high, with many white flowers, like little bells with turned edges, of a strong, though pleasing smell; the berries are red, not much unlike those of Asparagus.

MEDICINAL VIRTUES. A decoction of the flowers is said to be useful in removing obstructions in the urinary canal. Powdered, they are serviceable in headache, earache, and apoplexy. But they must not be used when there is a tendency to inflammation of the brain. Mixed with lard it strengthens the spine. Equal quantities of the leaves, and of the leaves of marjoram, and 12 drops of the essential oil of marjoram, form an excellent cephalic snuff. The distilled water dropped into the eyes, helps inflammations there, as also that infirmity which they call pin and web. The spirit of the flowers distilled in wine, restores lost speech, helps the palsy, and is exceeding good in the apoplexy, it comforts the heart and vital spirits. Gerrard says, that the flowers being close stopped up in a glass, put into an ant-hill, and taken away again a month after, you shall find a liquor in the glass, which being outwardly applied, helps the gout.

LILY,—WATER.

Of these there are two kinds, viz. the White and the Yellow

DESCRIPTION.—*Nymphæa Alba.*—The White Lily has very large and thick dark green leaves lying on the water, sustained by long, and thick foot-stalks, arising from a great, round, and long tuberous black root, spongy or loose, and internally white; from which rise other similar thick green stalks, sustaining one large flower, green on the outside, but as white as snow within, consisting of several rows of long, thick and narrow leaves, encompassing a head with many yellow threads in the middle. The seed vessel is large and roundish, abounding with seeds.

The Yellow kind is little different from the former, save only that it has fewer leaves on the flowers, greater and more shining seed, and a whitish root both within and without. They grow in pools and standing waters, and in slow running rivers, and ditches of water.

MEDICINAL VIRTUES. The fresh root is the part chiefly used, given in a strong decoction. The leaves and flowers are cold and moist, but the roots and seeds are cold and dry. The leaves cool inflammations, and the heat of agues; and so do the flowers, either in syrup or conserve. The seed is effectual to stay fluxes of blood or humours of wounds, and severe purgings. But the roots are more effectual to restrain all fluxes in men and women. Its frequent use extinguishes venerous actions. The root is likewise very good for those whose urine is hot and sharp, to be boiled in wine and water, and the decoction drank. The distilled water of the flowers has the same effect taken inwardly, or applied outwardly; and it is said to take away freckles, spots, sunburn, and morphew from the face, and other parts of the body. The oil made of the flowers, as Oil of Roses is made, is profitably used to cool hot tumours, and to ease painful sores.

LILY,—WHITE.

Lilium Album Hortense.—This is a well known garden flower, needing no description.

MEDICINAL VIRTUES.—This plant is good in pestilential fevers, the roots being bruised and boiled in wine, and the decoction drank; for it expels the venom to the exterior parts of the body. The juice being mixed with barley-meal, baked, and eaten for ordinary bread, is an excellent cure for dropsy. An ointment made of the root and lard is good for scald heads, and for cleansing ulcers. The root roasted, and mixed with a little lard makes a gallant poultice to ripen and break plague-sores. The ointment will cure burnings and scaldings without a scar and trimly deck a blank place with hair.

LIME TREE.

Tilia Europœa. The Linden or Teil tree, common in parks and in some gardens. The trunk is thick, the branches pretty regular, the leaves short, broad, nearly round in figure, pointed, and serrated at the edges. The flowers are yellowish white, of a sweet smell, and delicate.

The flowers are useful in Epilepsy and nervous fevers, made into a decoction or infusion; they are useful in asthma and irritable coughs. The tree, and especially the inner bark abounds with a soft mucilage, which is very useful in burns, scalds, and gouty swellings. The leaves powdered, and half a drachm taken in treacle, or in tea, subdues urinary heat and inflammation.

LIQUORICE.

The root of the *Glycyrrhiza Glabra.*—It grows wild in many countries, and is cultivated in some parts of England, as Pontefract, &c. Its virtues are very great. It is the principal constituent part in Spanish Juice, or Spanish Liquorice. Its demulcent properties render it very useful in coughs and bronchial irritation, and in some stomach complaints, arising from a deficiency of the natural mucus which should defend the stomach against the acrimony of the food, and the fluids secreted in it. It is also used in heartburn, and may be taken in considerable quantities without disordering the stomach, or causing thirst. The Pontefract cakes, lozenges, and Bath-pipe, are very useful in coughs, shortness of breath, and hoarseness. Liquorice also works gently by urine, and is very soothing to ulcerated kidneys or urinary passages. The extract is employed to cover the taste of nauseous drugs, as aloes, &c. The powdered root is much used.

LIVERWORT.

DESCRIPTION.—*Lichen Vulgaris.*—Botanists reckon on upwards of 300 species of Liverwort.

Common Liverwort grows close, and spreads much upon the ground in moist and shady places, with many small green leaves, or rather sticking flat to one another, very unevenly cut in on the edges, and crumpled; from among which arise small slender stalks an inch or two high at most, bearing small star-like flowers at the top; the roots are very fine and small.

MEDICINAL VIRTUES.—It is a singular good herb for all diseases of the liver. It is to be given in strong decoction, and is very effectual in yellow jaundice. Bruised and boiled in small beer, it has the same effect. It is a good remedy for diseased kidneys, the whites, and very appropriate in the first stages of consumption. It is good to stay the spreading of ringworms, and other running sores and scabs, and is an excellent remedy for those whose livers are corrupted by surfeits, which causes their bodies to break out, for it fortifies the liver, and makes it impregnable. It grows on old walls, in wells and other damp places.

LIVERWORT,—ASH COLOURED.

Lichen Caninus.—It spreads on the ground, consisting of a leather-like substance, ash-coloured, and appears as if covered with farina, divided into lobes, woolly underneath, and veined. It is found in dry pastures, woods, and on heaths.

It has been used for the bite of a mad dog, ending in hydrophobia. It was combined with black pepper, one part of the latter to two of the former. By the authority of Sir Hans Sloaane, it was published in the Philosophical Transactions, and afterwards, at the request of Dr. Mead, it was adopted in the London Pharmacopœia.

LOBELIA.

Lobelia Inflata.—It is a native of America; where it is much used as medicine, its use having been derived from the Indians. It is recommended for spasmodic Asthma. In small doses it is a good diaphoretic, and expectorant; in large doses, it is antispasmodic, sedative, and emetic. Sometimes it is of extraordinary efficacy in Asthma, and if other prescriptions have failed, this has been found efficacious. The tincture is the form in which it is used, which is made by digesting for a few hours two ounces of the dried plant in a pint of diluted spirits of wine. A tea-spoonful taken in water, to be repeated three times a day; or the powder from 4 to 10 grains, beginning with the smallest, and gradually increasing, in plenty of warm water.—☞ Always commence with *small* doses.

LOGWOOD.

Hæmatoxylon Campechianum, or Logwood, is used medicinally in the form of decoction, and Extract, for diarrhœa, or looseness, and dyssentery, or bloody flux. It acts as an astringent, without irritating the coats of the stomach. For extreme diarrhœa, Logwood decoction, a few raspberry leaves, and a few drops of Laudanum, will effect a cure.

For the ordinary decoction, Buchan says, "Boil three ounces of the shavings or chips of Logwood, in four pints of water, to one half; two or three ounces of Cinnamon water may be added. In fluxes of the belly, where the stronger astringents are improper, a tea-cupful of this decoction may be taken with great advantage three or four times a day.

LOOSESTRIFE,—PURPLE.

DESCRIPTION.—*Lythrum Salicaria.*—It is also known by the name of Grass-polly. It grows with many woody square stalks full of joints, three feet high, on each stand two long leaves, shorter, narrower, and a greener colour than the former. The stalks branch into long stems of spiked flowers half a foot long, growing in bundles, one above another, out of small husks, like the spiked heads of lavender, each of which flowers have five round pointed leaves of a purple violet colour. The seeds are small and brown. The root creeps like the yellow, but it is larger. It grows by rivers, and ditch-sides, in wet grounds. It flowers in June and July.

MEDICINAL VIRTUES.—For preserving the sight, and for the cure of sore eyes, this herb is fully, if not superior to Eyebright. This I have found by experience. The distilled water is a present remedy for hurts and blows on the eyes, and for blindness, provided the crystalline humour be not injured or destroyed. This was experienced by an intelligent man, who kept it long as a great secret. It clears the eyes of dust, or any thing got into them, and preserves the sight. It is also very available against wounds, made into an ointment. To every ounce of water, add two drachms of May butter without salt, sugar and wax of each as much, boil them gently together; after it is cold, apply it on cloths to the wounds. It cleanses and heals ulcers and sores, and stays inflammations, by washing them with the water, and laying on them a green leaf or two in Summer, or dry leaves in Winter. The water gargled warm in the mouth, and drank, cures the quinsy, or scrofula in the throat.

The HYSSOP-LEAVED PURPLE LOOSESTRIFE, is much like the former, and its virtues are about the same.

LOOSESTRIFE OR WILLOWHERB.

DESCRIPTION—There are three kinds of Loosestrife; the yellow, the Hyssop-leaved, and the purple speckled. The common *yellow* Loosestrife, *Lysimachia Vulgaris*, grows about five feet high, with great round stalks, a little crested, diversely branched from the middle of them to the tops into great and long branches, on which, at the joints, grow long and narrow leaves, but broader below, and usually two at a joint, yet sometimes three or four, somewhat like willow leaves, smooth on the edges, and a fair green colour from the upper joints of the branches, at the tops stand many beautiful yellow flowers, with yellow threads in the middle, which turn into small round heads containing small cornered seeds, the root creeps under ground almost like couch-grass. It grows in moist meadows, and by water-sides. It flowers from June to August.

MEDICINAL VIRTUES.—This herb cures bleeding at the mouth, nose, or wounds, and the bloody flux, given either to drink, or taken by clysters; it restrains profuse menstruation, and is a very good wound-herb; the young leaves bruised and bound about a fresh wound, stay the bleeding, and quickly close together the lips of the wound. It has demulcent and astringent virtues, which render it useful in inveterate diarrhœa.—Dose of the powdered herb, 1 drachm three times a day; of the decoction 1 ounce of the herb boiled in a pint of water; take 2 ounces at a time. It is often used in gargling for sore mouths, The smoke of the herb burned, drives away flies and gnats, which in the night-time molest people dwelling near marshes, and in fenny countries.

LOVAGE.

DESCRIPTION.—*Ligusticum Officinale.*—It is a salad plant, having a strong and peculiar odour. The stalk is round, thick, and hollow, and deeply striated or channelled. The leaves are very large, each being composed of a number of smaller; these are set on a divided stalk, and are short, broad and indented at the edges. The flowers are small and yellow; the seeds are flat and brown. The root is thick, large and brown, having many fibres.

MEDICINAL VIRTUES.—The roots and fruit are aromatic, stimulant, and diaphoretic, and may be used as remedies for flatulency, and hysterical disorders arising from uterine obstructions. The fresh roots provoke urine, and are good in jaundice. As they are sudorific, they are good in fevers. Half a drachm at a time of the dried root in powder taken in wine, wonderfully warms a cold stomach, and promotes digestion. It relieves inward gripings and pains. The decoction of the herb is good for the ague, and to ease pains in the bowels caused by cold. The seed is still more effectual. The distilled water or a strong decoction, as a gargle, relieves quinsy. The decoction drank three or four times a day is effectual in pleurisy. The juice applied to the eyes takes away inflammation. The leaves bruised, and fried with a little hog's lard, and laid hot to any blotch or boil, will quickly break it.

LUNGWORT.

Description.—*Pulmonaria Officinalis.*—It is found in gardens. The stalk is about a foot high. The flowers branch out at the tops of the stalk; they are generally red before they expand; afterwards they are of a blue colour.

Medicinal Virtues.—It derives its name from its supposed efficacy in diseases of the lungs. It is mucilaginous and rather astringent, and is regarded as emolient and pectoral. It is good therefore for coughs, wheezing, and shortness of breath. Haller says that its viscous juice, possessing some acidity, is very useful for dryness of the throat, for cough accompanied with spitting of blood. An infusion is the best way of taking it.

MADDER.

Description.—*Rubia Silvestris.* It has many long weak four-square, reddish stalks, trailing on the ground, rough and hairy, and full of joints: at every one of these joints come forth divers long and narrow leaves, standing like a star about the stalks, rough and hairy, at the tops come forth many small pale yellow flowers and then small round heads, green at first and reddish, but black when they are ripe, wherein is contained the seed. The root is long, and deep in the ground, red and very clear while fresh. It grows in cornfields, and flowers at the end of summer.

Medicinal Virtues. It has an opening quality, and afterwards binds and strengthens. It is a sure remedy for the yellow jaundice, by removing obstructions of the liver and gall, and cleansing those parts; and also obstructions of the spleen. It is good for palsy and sciatica, and for inward and outward bruises, and is much used in vulnerary drinks. The root may be boiled in wine or water, as the cause requires, and some honey and sugar added. The seed taken in vinegar and honey, reduces the swelling and hardness of the spleen. The leaves and roots beaten and applied to any part that is discoloured with freckles, or any such deformity of the skin, takes them away.

THE DYE MADDER, *Rubia Tinctora*, is chiefly valued for the excellent dye which it furnishes. This plant has been said to possess the same properties, to be diuretic and an emmenagogue, and was formerly much used in dropsy, jaundice, and female complaints.

MAIDEN HAIR,—GOLDEN.

DESCRIPTION.—*Adiantum Aureum.*—It has many small, brownish, red hairs to make up the form of leaves growing about the ground from the root; and in the middle of them, in Summer, rise small stalks of the same colour, set with very fine yellowish green hairs on them, and bearing a small gold, yellow head, less than a wheat corn, standing in a large husk. The root is very small and thready. It grows in bogs and on moors, and in dry shady places.

Its *Medicinal Virtues* are much the same as those of the White Maiden Hair. It makes an excellent wash for the hair, cleansing it, and promoting the growth.

There is also a BLACK MAIDEN HAIR, *Adiantum Nigrum.* It is like the Common Fern of the divided kind, only very small. It grows nearly ten inches high. The stalks are thick and glossy, and black. The leaves are beautifully divided into many parts, of a short bright green, and notched at the edges. The seeds lie on the edges of the under part of the leaves in form of a brown dust.

Its *Medicinal Virtues* are similar to the other Maiden Hairs. A decoction of it works powerfully by urine. It relieves a troublesome cough.

MAIDEN HAIR,—WHITE.

DESCRIPTION.—*Adiantum Album.*—It is also called *Wall Rue.* It is gathered by children under the name of Ladies'

Hair. It has very fine, pale green stalks, almost as fine as hairs, set confusedly with several pale green leaves on very short foot-stalks, somewhat in form, but more diversely cut in on the edges, and thicker, smooth on the upper part, and spotted finely underneath. It grows on old walls, near ruins, and dry places. It is green in winter as well as in summer.

MEDICINAL VIRTUES.—A decoction of the herb is a good remedy for coughs, difficulty of breathing, yellow jaundice, and obstructions of the spleen, and urine. It is very effectual in removing stones from the kidneys, and in obstructed menses. It restrains internal bleedings and fluxes. A decoction of the green leaves is aperient, removing bad bile, and tough phlegm, from the lungs and the liver. It purifies the blood, so as to give to the body a good colour. The herb boiled in oil of cammomile, removes knots, swellings, and dries up moist ulcers. A ley made thereof cleanses the head from scurf, and from dry and running sores; it prevents the hair from falling off, and causes it to grow. For this purpose some boil it in wine, adding a little Smallage, and a little wine.

MALLOW, - COMMON.

DESCRIPTION.—*Malva Sylvestris.* A wild plant growing about hedges, in fields, and gardens. It grows three or four feet high. The stalk is round, thick, and strong. The leaves are roundish, indented, and divided, at the edges. The flowers are numerous, round, and red. The root is long and white, tough and firm.

MEDICINAL VIRTUES.—The root has most virtue. The leaves are used in decoction for clysters. The decoction made strong is excellent to promote urine, and to cure strangury and gravel, and for removing sharp humours from the bowels.

The **VERVAIN MALLOW** is common in pastures. It grows two feet high; the stalks are round, thick, erect, and a little hairy. The lower leaves are rounded and slightly divided at the edges; those on the stalks are beautifully cut into very small parts. The flowers are of a very bright red, three times the size of the Common Mallow. The root is white. The root is used. It has the same virtues as the Common Mallow, though not quite as strong. The leaves have the same effect.

MANDRAKE.

Description.—*Atropa Mandagora.*—It is an exotic; but began to be cultivated in England, 1560. Superstition has said much about it. Its root sometimes dividing into two below and shooting on each side, give a resemblance to a man, and aided by art, this resemblance became so complete as to deceive the multitude. It was said to be death to dig up the root; that screams were heard when these became wounded; and that they were to be drawn out by a dog, which perished; and in this way only could they be extracted.—As an amulet, it was once placed on Mantel-pieces to avert misfortune, and to bring prosperity and happiness.

The Mandrake has no stalk; the large leaves rise immediately from the root, a foot long, four inches broad, of a dusky green colour, and disagreeable smell. The flowers stand upon foot-stalks four inches high, slender and hairy, and rise immediately from the root; these flowers are large, of a dingy purplish colour, and of a bad smell. The fruit is of the size of a small apple, like a small pear, yellow when ripe. The root has been described. By designing people the roots are taken up, shaped like a man, and then put back to grow, and thus people are deceived.

Medicinal Virtues.—It is narcotic, and soporific. Some say that even the smell of the plant produces sleep. It was employed by the ancients in maniacal cases, and Pallas mentions its frequent use in dreadful chronic disorders which require alleviation by some powerful drug. In scrofulous or glandular affections, the leaves boiled with milk are reported by Boerhaave as beneficial. The root finely scraped into a pulp, and mixed with brandy, has been found efficacious in chronic rheumatism. The berries eaten, above two or three, are dangerous; five have been known to produce syncope, and other dangerous symptoms.

MANNA.

Manna a concrete juice, is the production of the flowering Ash, *Ornus*, vel *Fraxinus*. Sometimes the juice flows spontaneously, or is obtained by tapping the tree. It has a sweet and slightly bitter taste, and is a gentle purgative, so mild in its operation that it may be given with safety to children, persons of very weak habits, and in pregnancy. In some constitutions, however, it produces flatulency, and therefore requires the addition of a suitable aromatic, especially when given to an adult. As it is a very mild purgative, it may be combined with a decoction of senna, or rhubarb, and an aromatic, say, a small portion of Cayenne pepper.

MARIGOLDS.

Calendula Officinalis.—They need no description, they are so common, nearly in every garden.

MEDICINAL VIRTUES.—They strengthen the heart exceedingly, and are very expulsive and little less effectual in bringing out the small-pox and measles than saffron. The juice of Marigold leaves mixed with vinegar, and any hot swelling bathed with it, instantly gives ease. The flowers, either green or dried, are much used in possets, broths, and drink, as a comforter of the heart and spirits. A plaister made with the dry flowers in powder, lard, turpentine, and rosin, applied to the breast strengthens and succours the heart in fevers.

MARJORAM SWEET.

DESCRIPTION.—*Amaracus.*—Sweet Marjoram is so well known, as an inhabitant in every garden, that it is needless to write any description of it, nor of the Winter Sweet Marjoram or Pot Marjoram.

MEDICINAL VIRTUES.—Sweet Marjoram is aromatic, and warming in the cold diseases of the head and stomach, and other parts, taken inwardly, or outwardly applied. The decoction is good for diseases of the chest which obstruct breathing, and it removes obstructions of the liver and spleen. It neutralizes cold griefs of the womb, and the windiness thereof. The decoction thereof made with some pellitory of Spain, and long pepper, is good for the first stages of dropsy, for those that cannot make water, and against pains in the belly. The powder mixed with honey, it obliterates the black marks of blows and bruises; it is good for inflammation and watering of the eyes, mixed with fine flour, and laid upon them. The juice dropped into the ears, eases pains and a singing noise. It is profitably put into ointments and salves that are warm, and comfort the outward parts, as the joints and sinews; and for swellings. The powder snuffed provokes sneezing, and purges the brain, and chewed in the mouth, it promotes expectoration of phlegm. The oil is very warm and comfortable to stiff joints, to mollify and supple them. It is the principal compound of the various *rubbing bottles*, sold for outward application, "I have known," says Dr. Roberts, "the dried herb put into a bag and immersed in hot water, prove a capital fomentation for tumours and swellings. A strong infusion for a foot-bath is very effectual in relieving violent pains.

MARJORAM,—WILD.

DESCRIPTION.—*Origanum Vulgare.*—Called also Origanum, Eastward, Marjoram, and Grove Marjoram. Wild or Field Marjoram root which creeps much under ground, and continues a long time sending up sundry brownish, hard square stalks, with small dark green leaves, very like those of Sweet Marjoram, but harder, and broader; at the top of the stalks stand tufts of flowers, of a deep purplish red colour. The seed is small and blacker than that of Sweet Majoram. It grows abundantly in the borders of corn-fields, and in some copses.

MEDICINAL VIRTUES.—It strengthens the stomach and head much, there being scarcely a better remedy growing for such as are troubled with acidity of the stomach; it is a stomachic, and restores the appetite, relieves cough and consumption of the lungs; it cleanses the body of choler, expels poison, and helps the infirmities of the spleen; It is an antidote to Hemlock, henbane, or opium. It provokes urine, and the terms in women, relieves dropsy and scurvy, scabs, itch, and yellow jaundice. The juice being dropped into the ears, relieves deafness, pain and noise in the ears. It is generally taken as an infusion, which is very serviceable to nervous habits. The volatile Oil, called *Originum*, has been highly extolled as a cure for toothache.

MARSHMALLOWS.

DESCRIPTION.—*Althœa Officinalis.*—A plant of the natural order *Malvaceœ.* Marshmallows have soft hairy white stalks, rising three or four feet high, with many branches, the leaves are hairy, less than the other Mallow leaves, but longer pointed, cut into some few divisions, but deep. The flowers are many, but smaller than the other Mallows, and white, sometimes with a reddish taint; after which come long round cases and seeds, as in the other Mallows. The roots are many and long, shooting from one head, of the size of a thumb or finger, very pliant, tough, and like liquorice, of a whitish yellow colour on the outside, and whiter within.

MEDICINAL VIRTUES.—The root is most used. It has emollient and demulcent properties, which render it useful in inflammations and irritations of the alimentary canal, and of the urinary and respiratory organs. The dry roots boiled in water give out half their weight of a gummy matter like starch. Decoctions of this plant have been very useful where the natural mucus has been abraded from the coats of the intestines; in catarrhs from a thin rheum; in nephritic and calculous disorders; in cases where the lochia have been too thin and sharp after child-birth. The decoction ought not to be made too thick and viscid. It is excellent to promote urine, and bring away gravel and small stones. It cures strangury, and is good in coughs. It is a gentle aperient, easing pains in the bowels. Boiled in wine or milk it relieves diseases of the chest and lungs, if taken frequently. Pliny says that whosoever shall take a spoonful of the juice shall that day be free from all diseases, and that it is specially good for the falling-sickness. The syrup and conserve made of the flowers, are effectual for the same diseases, and to open the body when costive. The leaves bruised, and laid to the eyes with a little honey, take away imposthumes, and to persons stung with bees, wasps, &c., it presently takes away pains, redness, and swellings caused by them. A poultice made of the leaves, boiled and bruised, with some bean or barley flour, and oil of roses, is a special remedy against hard tumours, inflammations, imposthumes, or swellings of the privates and other parts, and against hardness of the liver or spleen, being applied to the places. The juice of the Mallows boiled in oil takes away scurf, roughness of the skin, dandriff, or dry scabs in the head, if they be anointed with it, or washed with the decoction; it preserves the hair from falling off. It is also effectual against scaldings, burnings, St. Anthony's fire, and other hot and painful swellings. The flowers boiled in oil or water, with a little honey and alum, is an excellent gargle to cleanse, or heal a sore mouth or throat. The green leaves, (says Pliny) beaten with nitre, and applied, draw out thorns or prickles in the flesh. The decoction is first rate for clysters to ease all pains of the body, opening the urinary passages, making them slippery that the stone may descend easily, and without pain, out of the kidneys and bladder, and to ease the torturing pains. But the roots are the most powerful for coughs, shortness of breath, hoarseness. The roots and seeds boiled in wine and water, are successfully used by those who have inflammation of the intestines, or the bloody-flux. Boiled in wine, it is a good wash for scrofulous sores, imposthumes of the throat; the dried roots boiled in milk, is good for the Hooping-cough. Hippocrates gave the decoction of the roots or the juice to those who were wounded, and faint through loss of blood, and he applied the same, mixed with honey and rosin to the wounds. It is healing to bruises, falls or blows, or bones out of joint, or any swelling, pain, or ache in the muscles, sinews or arteries. The mucilage of the roots, and of linseed and fenugreek mixed, is much used in poultices, ointment, and plaisters, to soften and remove hard inflamed swellings, and to ease pains in any part of the body.

My son had the bloody-flux with great excoriation of the bowels. I was in the country at the time but was sent for. I gave him nothing but bruised Mallows and in two days he was cured.

About 4 or 5 ounces of the dried root, 2 ounces of raisons, freed from their seeds, put into 5 pints of water, and boiled down to 3 pints, and then strained, is a good form of administration. Half a wine-glass to be taken frequently to allay cough and irritation. The addition of liquorice, coltsfoot, and horehound, would make it still more pectoral.

The syrup of Marshmallows is made by boiling 8 ounces of the fresh root sliced, in 4 pints of water; adding 2½ lbs. of lump sugar; dose half an ounce to 1 ounce. The ointment of Marshmallows is a very healing application. The lozenges are also very useful in hoarseness, coughs, &c. They may be made of the syrup by adding a little more Sugar, and Mucilage of Gum Tragacanth.

MASTERWORT.

Description.—It grows two feet high, the stalks are round, striated, hollowed, erect, not very strong. The leaves are composed of three smaller ones; they are of a dark green colour, blunt at the points, and edges indented. The flowers are small and white, standing in little umbels at the tops of the branches. The roots are long, brown, divided, of a strong smell, and a sharp aromatic taste.

Medicinal Virtues.—The root greatly promotes perspiration, it warms a cold stomach. Haller says, that it is beneficial in diseases of the chest, arising from a load of mucus, and in the pituitous asthma, and in those diseases arising from defective circulation, as chlorosis and dropsy, and it has succeeded in a quartan ague even after cinchona had failed. Employed as a clyster it facilitates parturition; and the same when taken inwardly. It expels worms. It is good in gravel, promoting urine, and expelling stone. It is good for dropsy and cramps. The juice dropped on lint, and applied to green wounds or ulcers, cures them.—A drachm of the root in substance, and a drachm in infusion to be taken four times a day.

MATICO.

Arbanthe Elongata.—It is a native of South America, and belongs to the Pepper tribe. It is now used in British Medical practice as an astringent styptic. It is used in chronic bloody flux, or dysentery, and diarrhoea, given as an infusion. The undersides of the leaves, or powdered, will, when applied, arrest the flow of blood from cuts, bruises, or obstinate leech-bites. The Tincture mixed with water, is a good astringent lotion for the mouth. Dose of the Powder, from 10 to 30 grains. The infusion, made by pouring two pints of water on two ounces of leaves; it may be taken in agreeable doses 3 or 4 times a day. The Tincture is made thus. Leaves, 2 ounces; Proof Spirit, 1 pint. Take from 1 to 2 drachms.

MEADOW SAFFRON.

Description.—*Colchicum Autumnale.*—It is a perennial bulbous-rooted plant which grows in wet meadows. It flowers in September. They rise with long slender tubes about four inches high. The green leaves appear in March, about four to a full-grown root. It is a native of most parts of Europe, and it grows in many parts of this land. It is poisonous to animals of all classes; but their instinct, implanted in them by the All-wise and Beneficent Creator, leads them to avoid the foliage in the field.

Medicinal Virtues. Stoerck, Collin, and Pleuk have praised its virtues as a diuretic in hydrothorax, and other dropsies. Some use the juice to destroy vermin in the hair. In Germany and France it is very popular amongst practitioners, who employed oxymel colchici in the afore-mentioned complaints very effectually. In England, of late years, Colchicum, or Meadow Saffron, has been extensively used in the form of Tincture, and powder, for the cure of gout and rheumatism; in both of which it is a specific. It has been recommended in gonorrhœa with Tincture of Opium, low diet, and warm baths. On the continent it is used for humeral asthma.

Dr. Graham says, "it operates chiefly on the duodenum, or

first intestine; and its action is that of a purgative, diuretic, and narcotic. It stimulates the excretory ducts of the liver and pancreas, and the mucous membrane of the intestines, producing copious bilious stools, and diminishing febrile action. It is sometimes of great service in diseases of the heart, gout, rheumatism, and inflammatory complaints; but in order to its being of much permanent benefit in these maladies, it requires to be administered with caution and judgment; otherwise it may prove detrimental, instead of being useful."

When it is properly prepared, it is a safe and powerful medicine. In gouty and rheumatic affections, it allays the pains of those cruel disorders sooner and more completely than any other remedy. Its principal forms of administration are *Vinegar of Colchicum*, which is made by merely steeping the bulb in vinegar for two or three days, *dose*, from 25 to 90 drops: *Oxymel and Syrup* 1 to 2 drachms; Extract, ½ a grain to 2 grains; Tincture ½ a drachm to 1 drachm. The Tincture is made by putting 2 ounces of Colchicum seeds, 1 pint of proof spirit, and macerate for twelve days.

MEADOW SWEET.

Description.—*Spiræa Ulmaria.*—A wild plant growing by river sides. It has divided leaves, and beautiful tufts of white flowers. The stalk is round, striated, erect, firm, pale green, sometimes purple. The leaves are each composed of about three pairs of smaller, set on a thick rib, with an odd leaf at the end; of a fine green on the upper side, whitish underneath.

The flowers are small and white, but they stand so close that the whole cluster looks like one large flower. The seeds are set in a twisted order.

Medicinal Virtues.—An infusion of the fresh tops produces perspiration. It is rather astringent. The root has been a specific remedy in fevers. Decoct the root in white wine, and take one or two table-spoonfuls at a time. An infusion of the flowers, drank as a common beverage, is good for cutaneous eruptions, greatly improving the skin, and tending to remove scrofulous affection. Let the body be bathed and well-rubbed at the same time, and the system will be greatly invigorated.

THE MEDLAR.

Description.—*Mespilus Germanica.*—It grows nearly to the size of the Quince Tree, spreading branches moderately large, with longer and narrower leaves than either the apple or quince, not dented at the edges. At the end of the sprigs stand the flowers, made of five white, broad pointed leaves, nicked in the middle with some white threads also; the fruit is of a brown green colour, bearing a crown on the top, which, having fallen away, the head is hollow. The fruit is very harsh before it is mellowed. It is cultivated in gardens.

Medicinal Virtues.—A strong decoction of unripe medlars arrests diarrhœa. A plaster made of the fruit dried before they are rotten, and other convenient things, and applied to the kidneys prevents abortion. They are powerful to stay fluxes of blood or humours; the leaves have the same quality. The fruit prevents unnatural longings in females. The decoction is good to gargle and wash the mouth, throat and teeth, when affected with pains and swellings. It is a good bath to sit over for the bleeding piles. If a poultice or plaster be made with dried Medlars, with the juice of red roses, and a little clove and nutmeg, and applied to an unsettled and foul stomach, it gives relief. The dried leaves in powder strewed on fresh bleeding wounds heals them quickly. The Medlar-stones powdered, and put into wine in which parsley roots have been boiled a little, is effectual in removing stones from the kidneys.

MELLILOT.

Description.—*Melilotus Officinalis.*—It grows wild in the English hedges, in corn fields, and in field borders. It is also called King's Clover. It has three leaves at a joint, and long straggling spikes of yellow flowers. It is about eighteen inches high. The stalk is weak, slender, and striated. The leaves are oblong, and blunt at the ends. The flowers are small, shaped like those of tares by a rough roundish green pod. The plant has a singular, but not unpleasant smell. The plant is prolific of honey, and makes excellent pasturage for bees; hence the Latin name is derived from *Mel.*

Medicinal Virtues.—Mellilot boiled in wine, and applied, softens hard tumours, and inflammation of the eyes, fundament, or privities; sometimes the yolk of a roasted egg, or fine flour, or poppy-seed, is added. A ley made of it is a good wash for ulcers in the head, especially if affected by mania. It relieves pains of the stomach, applied fresh, or boiled with any of the afore-named things; also pains in the ears, being dropped into them; and steeped in vinegar, or rose-water, it eases the head-ache. The flowers of Mellilot and Camomile form a good clyster to expel wind and ease pains; and poultices for the same purpose, and to assuage swelling tumours in any part of the body. The juice dropped into the eyes, is a singular good medicine to take away the film which dims the sight. Boiled with lard, it makes an excellent ointment for sores, and for dressing blisters.

MERCURY,—DOG.

Description.—This is also of two kinds, male and female, having many stalks, slender and lower than French Mercury, without any branches, the root is set with two leaves at every joint, larger than the female, but more pointed and full of veins, and harder in handling; of a dark green colour, and less dented at the edges. At the joints come forth longer stalks than the former, with two hairy round seeds upon them, twice as large as those of the former Mercury; the smell is strong and virulent. The female has harder leaves upon longer foot-stalks, and the stalks are longer; from the joints come forth spikes of flowers like the French Female Mercury. The roots are full of small fibres, which run under ground, and mat very much, abiding the Winter, and shooting forth new branches every year.

☞ This is a highly poisonous plant, and must be guarded against. There is not a more fatal plant than this, and it has been described more to prevent mischief. Its medical properties have not been accurately made known. The qualities attributed to it by Culpeper are absurd in the extreme, quoted from some of the old astrological botanical writers. The virtues given to it by Culpeper must apply to some other plant; for those of Dog Mercury have not yet been discovered, except the poisonous.

MERCURY.—ENGLISH.

DESCRIPTION.—*Chenopodium.*—Called also *Good King Henry*—and English Mercury, to distinguish it from French Mercury. It grows a foot high; stalk round, thick, seldom erect; is greenish and purplish, and is covered with a kind of grey powder unctuous to the touch. Leaves large, broad, the shape of an arrow-head, stand on long stalks, pale green above, greenish underneath, covered with a grey powder. Flowers small, greenish yellow, in long spikes at the tops of the branches. The plant is common in farm-yards.

The young shoots are eaten as spinach. The juice of the whole plant works gently and well by urine; and the dried herb is used in decoctions for clysters.

MERCURY,—FRENCH.

DESCRIPTION.—*Mercurialis mas et fœmina.*—It grows ten inches high. The stalks are angular, green, thick, but not firm, and rather erect. The leaves are oblong, broadest in the middle, sharp-pointed, serrated at the edges, and of a deep green colour. The female plants produce two seeds growing together at the top of a little spike. The male plants produce only one spike of dusty flowers, without any seeds. People mistake, calling the female the male.

MEDICINAL VIRTUES.—A decoction of the fresh gathered plant is gently aperient, and diuretic, promoting urine; it is cooling, and good for hot constitutions and over-fulness. The dried herb is used in decoction for clysters.

MEZEREON.

Description.—*Daphne Mezereum.*—This shrub is a kind of Spurge Laurel. It is cultivated in gardens on account of the beautiful early flowers, in February and March. The flowers come before the leaves. It grows four feet high, and sends off several branches. The leaves are few, tender, and lance-shaped. The flowers are in thick clusters, each composed of a single petal, cut into four oval segments, of a bright red colour. They produce numerous red berries, which are black when ripe. They are very inviting, but poisonous, and they should be kept beyond the reach of children.

Medicinal Virtues.—It has been used with success in syphylis. Dr. Home not only found the decoction to cure scirrhous tumours, which remain after lues venerea, and after the use of mercury; but it healed also some scirrhous tumours from other causes; he found it useful in cutaneous eruptions. In difficult swallowing caused by paralytic affections, Dr Withering tested its efficacy. The patient was directed to chew a thin slice of the root as often as she could bear it, and in about a month she recovered the power to swallow. For three years she had been able to swallow liquids and solids only very imperfectly.

The Russian peasantry take 30 or 40 of the blossoms as a purgative, and give them as an emetic to children with hooping cough; in this country 8 or 10 of them will cause purging. The bark, both of the root and the stem, is used medicinally. Internally taken, it is stimulant, having a tendency towards the side and kidneys. It is of considerable efficacy in chronic *rheumatism*, and *scrofula*; and also in *syphilis*, combined with Sarsaparilla, as a decoction. Boil 2 drachms of the bark, and half an ounce of liquorice root in three pints of water down to two. The dose is 3 to 6 ounces, two or three times a day.

It has been used instead of a perpetual blister with much less pain and inconvenience. A square piece of the bark, an inch long, and an inch broad, macerated in a little vinegar, is applied to the skin, over which is bound a leaf of Ivy or Plantain; renewed till it cauterizes the part, and brings on a serious discharge. As a plaster it may be applied behind the ears to relieve the eyes. An *ointment* of the juice of the leaves, flowers, and bark, is valuable for dressing issues, &c.; it is superior to Savine or any other ointment for this purpose.

MINT,—HORSE.

Monarda Punctata.—This plant is much used in American practice. Like all the Mints it is aromatic and carminative, and yields a volatile oil, very stimulant, and having a powerful odour. It grows besides ditches, and in America it is cultivated.

"I have known," says an American Doctor, "its efficacy in removing flatulency, colic, and difficult breathing. It is a great purifier of the breath.—It is excellent for earache, and snuffed up the nose, for headache. The oil is given as a carminative in doses of two or three drops, on a lump of sugar. Outwardly, it is a good rubefacient. The leaves and twigs are made into an infusion, which is excellent in flatulent colic. This plant is also an emmenagogue.

MINT,—PEPPERMINT.

DESCRIPTION.—*Mentha Piperata.*—It is a garden plant, much like the Wild Mint. It grows two feet and a half high. The stalk is square, firm, and upright, of a pale green. The leaves stand two at each joint; broad, not very long, dark green, deeply serrated at the edges. The flowers grow in thick spikes, not long, yet large and pale red. The smell is fragrant and agreeable, the taste hot, like pepper.

MEDICINAL VIRTUES.—The whole plant is used fresh or dried; but the distilled water is the best. It cures the colic, often almost instantaneously, and is good against the gravel. Peppermint Water should be distilled from the fresh plant. To 1 gallon of water, and 8 ounces of Proof Spirit, put 2½ lbs. of fresh Peppermint. Distil one gallon. But Peppermint Water is now generally made by rubbing down the oil with a little lump sugar, and a few drops of spirits of wine, and then filtering it. The oil is peculiarly pungent, very carminative and stimulant, which render it very useful in indigestion, flatulence, and diarrhœa. The dose of this oil is from 1 to 3 or 4 drops. It may be taken in water or any other vehicle. It has the same virtues as the other Mints, but more powerful. The infusion of the leaves is very useful in bowel complaints, as laxity especially, and flatulency.

MINT,—SPEARMINT.

DESCRIPTION.—*Mentha Viridis.*—Spear Mint has several round stalks, and long narrowish leaves set thereon, of a dark green colour. The flowers stand in spiked heads at the tops of the branches, being of a pale blue colour. The plant has a fragrant smell, and a pleasant aromatic taste. It is cultivated in gardens. Its roots are abundant.

MEDICINAL VIRTUES.—It is valuable for its carminative and aromatic properties which reside in its volatile oil, of a pungent and peculiar odour. Dioscorides says it has a heating, binding and drying quality, and therefore the juice taken in vinegar, stays bleeding. It dissolves imposthumes being applied with barley-meal. The application of the juice mixed with honey relieves pains in the ears, and roughness of the tongue. Applied to the forehead and temples, it relieves pains in the head, and the heads of children, against breakings-out, sores or scabs. The whole plant is used fresh or dried, and is excellent for flatulency, sickness, vomiting and weakness of the stomach. It generally stops vomiting and creates an appetite. Some apply the fresh herb bruised to the stomach for the removal of its complaints. Bruised and mixed with salt it is said to cure the bite of a mad dog. Given as an infusion it has relived diarrhœa. The decoction gargled in the mouth, cures sore gums and mouth. I have frequently cured young ladies of relaxed and consumptive habits by ordering them to go with the maid a milking for a few mornings, and take with them a new laid egg beaten up with a table-spoonful of Rum, and a little Spear-Mint cut small, to which add a tea-cup full of new milk from the cow. This drank in the field, and the morning air have done wonders.

MINT,—WATER MINT.

DESCRIPTION.—*Mentha Aquatica.*—It grows wild by ditch sides. It grows a foot and a half high. The stalks are square, erect, firm, and strong, generally of a brown colour; leaves broad and short, they stand two at a joint, and are of a brownish or dark green colour, rather hairy, and serrated about the edges. The flowers are larger than those of common mint, and are of a pale red colour; they stand in round thick clusters, at the tops of the stalks and round the upper joints, The smell is rather agreeable, mixed as if Mint and Pennyroyal.

MEDICINAL VIRTUES. The distilled water is a remedy for colic, pains in the stomach and bowels, and it promotes menstruation. A single dose frequently cures the colic. Its virtues are great, and it ought to be better known, and more used. It may be given in infusion. It removes obstructions, and strengthens the system.

MISLETOE.

DESCRIPTION.—*Viscum Album.*—This parasite rises up from the branch of the tree, on which it grows, with a woody stem, putting itself into sundry branches, and again divided into many other smaller twigs, interlacing themselves, and covered with a greyish green bark, having two leaves set at every joint, and at the end likewise, which are somewhat long and narrow, small at the bottom, but broader towards the end. At the joints of the branches grow small yellow flowers, which run into small, white, transparent berries, three or four together, full of a glutinous juice, with a blackish seed in each of them, which was never known to spring, when put into the ground. It grows on various trees in woods and groves, and sometimes on fruit trees.

MEDICINAL VIRTUES.—The leaves dried and powdered are a wonderful remedy for the falling sickness. They are good in all nervous disorders, and have been known to perform great cures by perseverance in taking an infusion. Instances of the efficacy of Mistletoe, are to be found in the writings of Paracelsus, Pliny, &c. The late Drs. Fothergill. Willan, Gilbert, Thompson, and Fraser, employed this medicine with great success for the cure of epilepsy. The juice, or bird-lime, softens imposthumes, ripens and heals them. Mixed with rosin and wax, it cures ulcers and sores.

MONEYWORT.

Description.—*Lysimachia Nummaria.*—It is called also *Herb Twopence.* From a small thready root, come forth several long, weak, and slender branches, running on the ground two or three feet long, set with leaves two at a joint one against another at equal distances, which are almost round, but pointed at the ends, smooth, and of a good green colour. At the joints with the leaves from the middle forward come forth at every point sometimes one yellow flower, sometimes, two, standing on a small foot-stalk, consisting of five leaves, narrow-pointed at the end, with yellow threads in the middle. It grows plentifully in moist grounds by hedge-sides and in grass-fields.

Medicinal Virtues.—The juice is a well-known remedy for profuse menstruation. The leaves powdered are excellent against scurvy, loss of blood, fluxes, weakness of the stomach, and vomiting. Take 8 or 10 grains at a time, as the disease may demand. It is good for ulcerated lungs. Made into an ointment with lard, it is healing to wounds, either fresh or old. The decoction is a good wash for inveterate sores, &c.

MOONWORT.

Description.—*Lunaria.*—It rises up with one dark green, thick, and flat leaf, upon a short foot-stalk; when it flowers it bears a small slender stalk about four inches high, having but one leaf, much divided on both sides, into five or seven parts on a side, each of which is small like the middle rib, but broad forwards, pointed and round, resembling a half moon, the uppermost parts being larger than the lowest. The stalks rise above this leaf two or three inches, bearing many branches of small long tongues, each like the spiky head of the adder's tongue, of a brownish colour, which at last resolve into a mealy dust. The root is small and fibrous. It grows on hills and heaths, where there is much grass. It is to be found only in April and May.

MEDICINAL VIRTUES. Moonwort is cold and drying more than adder's tongue, and therefore more available for all wounds both inward and outward. The leaves boiled in red wine, stay profuse menstruation and the whites, also bleeding, vomiting and other fluxes. It heals blows and bruises, and is good for ruptures; but it is chiefly used with other herbs to make oils or balsams to heal fresh or green wounds, inward or outward.

MOSSES.

I shall speak only of two kinds, viz. Ground Moss and Tree Moss, both of which are very well khown.

The Ground Moss *Muscus Clavatum*, grows in moist woods, and in the bottom of hills in boggy grounds, and in shadowy ditches. The Tree Moss grows only on trees.

MEDICINAL VIRTUES. The Ground Moss is said to be good to break the stone, and to expel it by urine, boiled in wine and drank. The herb being bruised, boiled in water and applied, eases inflammations and pains arising from a hot cause, as the pains of the gout.

The Tree Mosses, *Lichen Plicatus*, are cooling and binding, and have a digesting and mollifying quality. But each Moss partakes of the nature of the tree from whence it it is taken; therefore that of the oak is more binding, and is of good effect to stay fluxes, vomiting, or bleeding, the powder being taken in wine. The powder taken in drink for some time is good against the dropsy. The oil that has had fresh Moss steeped therein for a time, and then boiled and applied to the temples and forehead, eases the headache coming of a hot cause. The powder of this Moss is a good astringent. It is good against the whites, and spitting of blood. It deserves to be much more regarded. The dose is half a drachm.

MOTHER OF THYME.

Description.—*Serpyllun.*—A common wild plant, very pretty and fragrant. It grows in little tufts by waysides, and on dry hillocks ; the stalks are round, slender, reddish, six or eight inches long. Leaves, very small, of an oval figure ; they grow two at each joint, are smooth, and of a bright green. The flowers are of a pale red, in little tufts at the top of the stalks ; the plant has a fragrant smell, and an aromatic and agreeable taste.

Medicinal Virtues.—In nervous cases, it is a better medicine than most that are used. An infusion of the fresh plant may be used ; the taste is agreeable, and if there be perseverance in the use, nervous disorders will be cured. The infusion drank before going to bed will effectually prevent nightmare.

MOTHERWORT.

Description.—*Cardiaca.*—A tall and pretty plant. It grows wild in farm-yards, and dry places. It is a yard high ; the stalk is square, thick, and erect. The leaves stand on long foot-stalks, two at each joint. They are divided into three parts, and are much indented at the edges ; colour, dark green, smell, bad ; flowers, pale red ; they grow in a kind of prickly cups.

Medicinal Virtues.—There is no better herb for strengthening and gladdening the heart ; therefore it is called Cardiaca by the Latins. It is exhilarating in travail, and therefore callèd Motherwort. It may be made into a Syrup, which, when taken, will allay inward tremors, faintings, &c. It is good against hysteric complaints, and especially for curing palpitation of the heart, arising from hysteric causes.

MOUSE-EAR.

Description.—*Pilosella.*—This is a small herb possessing great virtues.

Mouse-Ear is a low herb creeping upon the ground by small

strings, like the Strawberry plant, by which it shoots forth small roots, and many short leaves, set in a round form together, very hairy, which being broken, give a whitish milk: from among these leaves spring up two or three small hoary stalks about a span high, with a few smaller leaves thereon; at the tops but one flower appears, consisting of many pale yellow leaves, broad at the point, and a little dented in three or four rows, very like a dandelion flower, and reddish underneath the edges. The seeds are winged with down. It grows on ditch banks, and in dry ditches, and in sandy grounds. It flowers about June or July, and is green all Winter.

Medicinal Virtues.—The juice taken in wine, or the decoction drank, is good in jaundice, even of a chronic character, to be taken in the morning and evening, and abstain from other drink three hours after. It is a special remedy against the stone, and the tormenting pains thereof, and griping pains of the bowels. The decoction with succory and centaury is very effectual in dropsy, and the diseases of the spleen. It restrains fluxes of blood, either at the mouth or nose, and inward bleeding also. It is a specific for wounds both inward and outward. There is a syrup made of the juice and sugar by the apothecaries of Italy, and other places, which they deem a remedy for cough and consumption. The green herb bruised, and bound on a cut or wound, quickly heals it. The distilled water is a good wash for wounds and sores.

MUGWORT.

Description.—*Artemisia Vulgaris.*—It has various leaves lying upon the ground, much divided, or cut deeply in about the brims, like wormwood, but larger, of a dark green colour on the upper side, and hoary white underneath. The stalk rises four or five feet high, having on it such leaves as those below, but rather smaller, branching forth towards the top, on which small pale yellowish flowers, like buttons appear in tufts. The root is long and hard, with many small fibres. It grows plentifully by water sides, and by small water-courses.

Medicinal Virtues.—Mugwort removes obstructions of urine caused by stone. A decoction is said to cure the ague.

The Chinese use it to heal wounds, applying the fresh plant bruised. A drachm of the leaves powdered was given four times a day, by Dr. Home to a woman who had been affected with hysteric fits for many years. The fits ceased in a few days. All other medicines had failed. Being made up with lard into an ointment, it takes away wens and kernels that grow about the neck and throat; it is more effectual by adding a few field daisies. Three drachms of the powder of the dried leaves taken in wine, is a speedy and certain remedy for sciatica. A decoction of it with camomile and agrimony, and the place bathed, while it is warm, takes away the pains of the sinews, and the cramp.

MULBERRY TREE.

Morus Nigra. This is so well known where it grows that it needs no description.

Medicinal Virtues.—The Mulberry is of different parts; the ripe berries, by reason of their sweetness and slippery moisture, open the body, and the unripe bind it especially when they are dried; they are good to stay fluxes, and profuse menstruation. The bark of the root kills worms called tænia or tape-worm. A syrup made of the juice of the berries, cures inflammations or sores in the mouth, throat, and palate of the mouth when it is fallen down. The leaves beaten with vinegar are good for burns. A decoction made of the bark and leaves is good to wash the mouth and teeth when they ache. The leaves of Mulberries applied are said to stay bleeding at the mouth or nose, or the bleeding of the piles, or of a wound. The Syrup may be made by boiling the juice of the ripe fruit with twice the quantity of sugar.

MULLEIN.

Description.—*Verbascum Album.*—This from the texture of the leaves, is also called Poor Man's Flannel. Common White Mullein has many fair, large, woolly white leaves, lying next the ground, longer than broad, pointed at the end, and dented about the edges. The stalk rises four or five feet high, covered over with similar leaves, but less ; so that no stalk can be seen for the multitude of leaves. The flowers come forth on all sides of the stalk in great numbers upon a long spike, of a yellow colour, consisting of five round pointed leaves. The root is long, white, and woody. It grows by way-sides, lanes, and on ditch banks.

Medicinal Virtues.—Catarrhs and diarrhœas are said to be arrested by this plant. Dr. Home tried it in these diseases, but allows its virtue only in the latter disorder. He relates four cases in which it was given ; and he says, "that it is useful in diminishing or stopping diarrhœas of an old standing, and in easing pains in the bowels. This arises from the emolient and gently astringent qualities of the plant. The decoction is made by boiling two ounces of the leaves in a quart of water for twenty minutes—two or three ounces to be given every three hours. A strong decoction eases the toothache, A decoction of the leaves, and of sage, marjoram, and cammomile flowers, and the places bathed therewith, eases cramp in the sinews, and joints. Three ounces of the distilled water of the flowers, drank morning and evening for some days together, is an excellent remedy for the gout. The juice of the leaves and flowers laid upon rough warts, or the powder of the dried roots rubbed on takes them away. The decoction is of great effect to dissolve the tumours, swellings, or inflammations of the throat. The leaves bruised and wrapped in double papers, and covered with hot ashes to bake a while, and then taken and laid warm on any blotch or boil happening in the groin or share, soon heals them.

MUSTARD.

Sinapis Nigra.—This requires no description. The seeds are used ; ground, the powder called mustard is used as a condiment. They contain an acrid principle, and a fixed oil, which give them a pungent smell and taste, and stimulant, diuretic, and aperient properties. They are also anti-flatulent. The seeds of the black mustard are more pungent then those of the white. It is to be regretted that this valuable article is so frequently adulterated. Mustard seeds excite the stomach, and stimulate the nervous energy, and act as a laxative. In costiveness and indigestion they are really useful. They act very mildly, yet effectually as an aperient.

Dr. Graham says, "they exert a considerable alterative effect on the constitution when perserved in, owing to their containing sulphur, and also to their regular laxative operation. *For whatever substance acts regularly and mildly as an aperient, is at the same time alterative; a fact which demands attention.* This depends no doubt, on the marked influence which a regular healthy action of the bowels has on the whole system." Dose, a table-spoonful, or less, twice a day. They have also been given with advantage in dropsy, and torpid state of the bowels which accompanies palsy, for weakness of stomach, and impurity of blood. The seeds are good for all cold diseases.

Mustard is frequently used externally, and is generally beneficial when applied over the seat of inward inflammation, as the chest, belly, or throat. A Mustard Cataplasm, or poultice, is made by mixing good *fresh* mustard with water, (some use with it flour or linseed-meal, to moderate it,) as for the table, and spreading it thickly on a piece of linen or calico; put a thin piece of muslin over it, and then apply it to the part affected for 15 to 20 minutes so that it may redden the skin, without producing a blister; if it should burn much when taken off, sprinkle the part with flour. Should a mustard plaster be applied to one in a state of insensibility, it should not remain above half an hour; otherwise, it might produce ulceration. Never apply a mustard-plaster where you are assured a hot bran, or a hot oat-meal poultice would be more soothing and useful.

Mustard is a safe and effectual *emetic*, in doses of one, two, or three tea-spoonfuls in water. It is thus used in paralytic cases; and it is often effectual when other emetics fail. Mustard lotions and ointments are sometimes used for local friction in hœmoptysis, or spitting of blood, applied to the chest or extremities, as the legs, &c.—and for chilblains and other indolent swellings. In cases of poisoning, torpor, or paralysis, a Mustard foot-bath may be employed to rouse the system.

MUSTARD,—TREACLE.

DESCRIPTION.—*Theriaca Sinapis.*—It is known also by the name of Treacle Mustard. It has a hard round stalk a foot high, parted into branches, having soft green leaves, long and narrow, and waved, but not indented. The flowers which grow at the tops of the branches, are white, in spikes one above another; each flower produces a blackish brown seed on each side of a pouch parted in the middle. The roots are small and thready.

MUSTARD.—MITHRIDATE.

DESCRIPTION.—*Sinapis Mithridaticum.*—It grows higher than Treacle Mustard, having more and larger branches; its leaves are smaller and narrower, unevenly indented at the edges. The flowers are small and white, growing on long branches; the seeds are formed in the same way, yet smaller, and sharper in taste. They grow under walls and hedges.

MEDICINAL VIRTUES.—Both these Mustards are purgative, cleansing the body both upwards and downwards. They promote menstruation, break inward imposthumes, taken inwardly and used as clysters, and outwardly applied they are good for sciatica. The seed is very effectual. They are tonic and antiseptic.

MUSTARD,—HEDGE MUSTARD.

DESCRIPTION.—*Sepes Sinapis.*—It is a different plant from the garden Mustard. It has one blackish green stalk, slender, but tough, branched into several parts, and sometimes with several stalks, full of branches, on which grow long, rugged leaves, much cut on the edges in many parts, some larger and some less; of a dirty green colour. The flowers are small and yellow, at the tops of the branches in long spikes, flowering by degrees. The seeds are yellow, of an acrid taste, and so is the herb. It grows by the way and hedge-sides, and in the open fields. It flowers in July.

MEDICINAL VIRTUES.—It is good in all the diseases of the chest and lungs, hoarseness, for loss of voice, and lowness of spirits. The juice made into syrup, with honey or sugar, is no less effectual for the same purpose, and for all coughs, wheezing, and shortness of breath. It is a remedy for the jaundice, pleurisy, pains in the back and loins, and for colic, being also used in clysters. The seed is a special remedy for sciatica, joint-aches, ulcers and cankers in the mouth; throat, or behind the ears, and for hardness and swelling of the testicles, or women's breasts.

MYRRH.

DESCRIPTION.—This is a resinous gum which exudes from a small tree belonging to the natural order *Terebinthaceæ.* Its classical name is *Balsamodendron Myrrhæ.* Though mentioned in Scripture, Gen. xxxvii. 25, so early, yet very little is yet known of the production. At that early period it was probably known as an antiseptic, and was used in enbalming. The tree from which it is thought to exude is a native of Arabia, Abyssinia, and the countries on the shores of the Red Sea.

MEDICINAL VIRTUES.—It is antiseptic, and possesses tonic, antispasmodic, and stimulant, and expectorant properties. It acts upon the mucous membrane as a balsamic, checking excessive secretions. It is advantageously administered in *indigestion, old coughs*, in *green sickness*, *chronic asthma*, and the latter stages of *consumption;* and it should be given in *small* doses in the *incipient* stages. The gum, with a *small* quantity of aloes, and a *minute* portion of ginger, should be made into pills, and taken occasionally. Where the bowels are relaxed, the aloes and ginger must be omitted. It has been found very beneficial for coughs peculiar to pregnancy, or coughs after abortion, and in bronchitis. On account of its antiseptic properties, it is excellent for ulcerated lungs; dose, from eight to fifteen grains twice or thrice a day. If hectic fever prevails, combine with the gum Myrrh a little nitre or cream of tartar. The Tincture of Myrrh is one of the most agreeable washes in affections of the mouth. Half an ounce of Tincture to half a pint of water, and a few drops upon the tooth-brush, is a most excellent mode of cleansing the teeth, especially if the gums are weak or spongy. It is still more efficacious if combined with Tincture of Catechu; this is also a first-rate gargle for sore throat and elongated uvula, or soft part of the palate. The Tincture of Myrrh, Tincture of Catechu, to which is added, Calcined Alum, is a cure and a preventive of toothache. It may be diluted with water.

NAILWORT, OR WHITLOWGRASS.

Description.—*Paronychia Rutula Foliosa.*—It derives its name from its virtues. This small and common herb has no roots, but a few strings; it grows about four inches high, leaves very small, rather long, not unlike those of chickweed, among which rise up several slender stalks, bearing many very small white flowers one above another, after which come small flat pouches containing very small seed, of a sharp taste. It grows upon old stone and brick walls, and in dry gravelly grounds, if there be grass or moss to protect it. It flowers in February; for before the end of April it is not to be found.

Medicinal Virtues. It is held to be exceeding good for those imposthumes in the joints, and under the nails, which they call whitlows, felons, and nail-wheals.

NETTLE.

Urtica Dioica.—It is common everywhere. Every one knows it.

Medicinal Virtues.—This is a valuable plant. The young shoots in spring, form a wholesome vegetable, boiled, like other greens. Nettle broth is good against the scurvy. It is a great purifier of the blood, and removes the phlegmatic superfluities left in the body by winter. A table-spoonful of the expressed juice given four times a day stops spitting of blood; and lint dipped in it, and put up the nostrils, has stopped bleeding at the nose, when every other remedy has failed. Cancers have been said to yield to the juice of nettles, rubbing with the juice mixed with oil and laudanum, and the juice taken inwardly very freely. Paralytic parts, being stung with nettles have regained their vigour, and the use of limbs, lost by rheumatism, has been restored. Excessive corpulency may be reduced by taking a few of the seeds only. Fourteen or fifteen of these seeds powdered, and taken night and morning, will cure goitre, or enlargement of the thoroid gland, causing frightful swelling of the throat, without injuring the stomach or the health. It is a good gargle for it, and a poultice of the leaves should be applied. Nettle is anti-asthmatic; the juice of the roots or leaves made into an electuary with honey and sugar opens the bronchial tubes of the lungs, the stoppage of which causes wheezing, shortness of breath, &c. It stimulates expectoration of phlegm very freely. It is a good deobstruent for suppressed menstruation, used as a decoction, and for the retention of urine, for the gravel and stone. For this purpose the flowers and seed should be made into a conserve. The decoction kills worms in children.

Some say that a leaf put upon the tongue, and pressed against the roof of the mouth, will restrain bleeding of the nose. "The fresh juice of the Nettle has been highly recommended," says Dr. Spencer Thompson, "in cases of internal hœmorrhage, particularly from the lungs and womb. Dose one tea-spoonful three times a day. Nettle is now coming into use as a material for the manufacture of paper. The seeds serve to fatten fowls, and are said to infuse life and spirit into horses.

NIGHTSHADE,—DEADLY.

DESCRIPTION—*Atropa Belladonna.*—A wild plant of a gloomy aspect. It grows five feet high; stalks angulated, dark green; leaves large, broad, and flat, of a dull dead green. The bell-shaped flowers stand thickly on long foot-stalks, rising from the bosom of the leaves; they are large, hollow, and hang down. Externally the colour is dusky between brown and green; and within of a deep purple. They are succeeded by berries about the size of cherries, violet black, glossy, sweet, and pleasant to the taste; hence they have been eaten by children ignorant of their very poisonious qualities, with fatal results. In 1793, some orphans, at the Hospice de la Pete, at Paris, were employed in weeding a botanical garden. They were attracted by the tempting looking fruit of a Belladonna plant, of which they ate a large quantity. Fourteen of them died a few hours afterwards in consequence. This lamentable catastrophe justifies the generic name *Atropa*, from one of the fates, who was supposed to cut the thread of life. *Belladonna*, signifies *beautiful lady*, because the Italian ladies used the distilled water of this plant as a *cosmetic*.

MEDICINAL VIRTUES.—It is a valuable medicine in proper hands. The leaves were first used externally to discuss scrofulous and cancerous tumours, and as an application to ill-conditioned ulcers. Some physicians began to employ them internally for the same disorders, on account of their external efficacy. This plant alleviates pain, nervous excitement, and spasm; it is useful in neuralgia, convulsive affections and rheumatism. The vapour of the decoction is sometimes inhaled to relieve asthma.

Belladonna is said to be efficacious in protecting against the infection of scarlet fever, when given in repeated small doses, during the prevalence of the disease, to those who are exposed to it. Eight grains of the extract are to be rubbed up with 1 fluid ounce of water, and from 5 to 20 drops, according to age, given twice a day. After all, its use ought to be in skilful hands.

NIGHTSHADE,—WOODY.

Its Latin name is Dulcamara (*dulcis*, sweet; *amarus*, bitter.) In various countries it has different names; as, Mortal, Bitter Sweet, and Felon Wort.

DESCRIPTION.—It is a climbing plant, and is common in moist hedges; its stems often reach to the height of five or six feet. The branch has a whitish bark, and a pith in the middle of it. The main stem divides into many small ones with claspers, laying hold on what is next to them. It bears many leaves, rather long and broad, and pointed at the ends; some of them have one or two little leaves growing at the end of their footstalks. The colour of the leaves is pale green; the flowers are purple with a yellow centre, and they stand together in knots. The berries, when ripe, are red, approaching to scarlet, and they stand together in knots. They taste sweet at first, and then bitter. This plant is nearly allied to the potato, which it very closely resembles in the odour of its root. The berries are poisonous, but not so much so as the twigs of the plant which are very acrid and narcotic. This plant flowers in July, and the seeds are ripe at the end of July.

MEDICINAL VIRTUES.—To make the decoction, the twigs should be gathered early in spring, as thick as a goose-quill. One ounce of them to be chopped up, and boiled in a pint and a half of water, till reduced to half the quantity. It has been regarded as a powerful medicine, increasing all the secretions and excretions, to excite the heart and arteries; and in *large* doses to produce nausea, vomiting, and convulsions. The plant may be regarded as alterative, diuretic, sudorific, and mildly narcotic. It has been recommended in cutaneous affections, in rheumatic and cathartic swellings, in bad ulcers, scrofula, jaundice, obstructed menstruation, and syphillis. The dose of the powder is from 1 to 3 scruples; of the decoction about a wineglassful; of the Extract, from 5 to 10 grains; of the Syrup, half an ounce to an ounce. The berries both purge and vomit, and are extremely dangerous for children. Take a pound of the wood and leaves bruised, and infuse in three pints of white wine over a gentle fire about 4 or 5 hours; and strain. This removes obstructions of the liver and spleen, and relieves difficulty of breathing. It forms a gentle purgative.

NIGHTSHADE,—COMMON.

DESCRIPTION.—*Solanum Vulgare.*—This is a different plant from the Deadly Nightshade, which is so poisonous. It has an erect, round, green hollow stalk, two feet high, having many branches, with many leaves, rather broad, and pointed, soft and full of juice, and unevenly indented at the edges. The flowers grow in little clusters, from six to a dozen in a bunch; they are white, with a yellowish centre, and succeeded by round black berries. It grows wild under walls, among rubbish, the sides of edges and fields, and in gardens, which it soon over runs, if not stopped.

MEDICINAL VIRTUES.—The common Nightshade is wholly used to cool inflammations outwardly. It must be used carefully, as most of the Nightshades are dangerous. The juice mingled with vinegar, is good to wash an inflamed mouth and throat. The juice, as an outward application is good for ringworms, and foul ulcers. The bruised leaves applied to inflammations, scalds, burns, and eruptions on skin, are very good. A cloth saturated with the juice is a good application for gout, inflamed privities. The juice dropped into the ears, relieves pains.

NUTMEG TREE.

DESCRIPTION.—*Nux moschata.*—A tall, spreading tree, native only of the warm climates; the trunk is large, and the branches are numerous and irregular; the bark is of a greyish colour, and the wood light and soft. The leaves are large, long, and somewhat broad: they are not unlike those of the bay tree, but larger and are of a beautiful green on the upper side, and whitish underneath. They stand irregularly, but often so nearly opposite, that they seem in pairs, as we see in the leaves of some of our willows. The blossom is of the shape and size of our cherry tree, but its colour is yellow. The fruit which succeeds this, is of the size of a small peach, and not unlike it in the general form; when cut open there appears first the fleshy coat, which is a finger thick, and of a rough taste, then the mace spread over a woody shell, in which is the nutmeg. We often have the whole fruit sent over preserved.

MEDICINAL VIRTUES.—The nutmeg is an excellent spice, it strengthens the stomach, and assists digestion. It will stop vomitings, and is good against the cholic. When roasted before the fire, and mixed with a small quantity of rhubarb, it is the best of all remedies against purgings.

OAK.

Quercus Robur.—This noble tree, the king of the forest, needs no description.

MEDICINAL VIRTUES.—The bark is a powerful astringent. The decoction is very useful in bloody flux, and spitting of blood. It is diuretic, causing the flow of urine. It has been given with advantage in intermittent fevers. Boil 10 drachms of the bruised bark in two pints of water until reduced to one pint; it may be used also as an injection, gargle, or lotion. This is very useful in chronic sore throat, with relaxed uvula. Galen applied the bruised leaves to heal wounds. It removes obstructions of the liver, and is useful in gravel. The water found in the hollow places in old Oaks, is effectual in curing scabs, itch, &c. The distilled water of the leaves is a sovereign remedy for the whites. The decoction makes a first-rate wash for a rupture, if used early.

OATS.

Medicinal Virtues.—As an article of diet, when ground into meal, it is excellent. A notion prevails that it is diet fit only for the inferior animals, but it is a very erroneous one. Since Oatmeal fell into disuetude, people have degenerated in muscular strength and form. The Scottish Highlanders and the Lowland peasantry live almost entirely on oatmeal, proving its nutrition by their well-knit, muscular and bony frames, and their clear and vigorous intellects. Oats fried with bay-salt, and applied to the sides, removes pains, stitches, and wind. A poultice made of oatmeal and oil of bays, cures the itch and leprosy, fistula, and dissolves hard imposthumes. Oatmeal poultices are more stimulating, and draw more rapidly than those made of Linseed Meal.

ONE BLADE.

Description.—*Unicaulis.*—So called because it never bears more than one leaf; though sometimes it has a stalk, and in that case it has two leaves; but this seldom occurs. The leaf is of a bluish green colour, pointed with many ribs or veins, like plantain. At the top of the stalk grow many small white flowers, star-fashion, smelling rather sweet; after which come small red berries. The root is small, creeping under the crust of the earth. It grows on moist, shadowy and grassy places of woods. It flowers about May, and the berries are ripe in June.

MEDICINAL VIRTUES. It is a precious herb. Half a drachm, or a drachm in powder of the roots taken in wine and vinegar, of each equal parts, and the person laid to sweat thereupon, is held to be a sovereign remedy for those who have a sore upon them, by expelling the poison and infection. It is a very good wound herb, and is used in many compound balms for curing wounds, whether fresh or green.

ONIONS.

MEDICINAL VIRTUES.—*Allium Cepa.*—They are more an article of diet. As to medical properties, they are the same as garlic, yet much milder. They act as a stimulant, promoting appetite, easing the bowels, and disposing to sleep. A roasted onion cut in two, is a domestic remedy for boils, as it hastens their breaking. They kill worms in children, if they drink the water fasting in which they have been steeped all night. Roasted and eaten with honey, or sugar and oil, they relieve an inveterate cough, and expectorate tough phlegm. The juice snuffed up the nostrils purges the head, and removes lethargy. It has been regarded as a preservative against infection, to eat onions fasting with bread and salt. An onion made hollow, filled with treacle, and then roasted, and beaten together, is a sovereign salve for sores, or a putrifying ulcer. The juice of onions is good for scalds and burns, and used with vinegar, takes away blemishes, spots, and marks in the skin. Figs and onions beaten together, ripen and break imposthumes and other sores.

OPIUM.

Papaver Somniferum, of the natural order *Papaveraceæ.* Opium is the dried juice of white or Eastern Poppy. Perhaps it is the most useful drug in the entire list of medical agents used by man, and has probably yielded more relief to human suffering than any other physical means. Applied externally, it acts as a sedative, easing pain; given internally, in moderate doses, its first effect is that of an excitant; it quickens the pulse, and increases the heat of the skin, and induces a temdency to sleep; pain is abated or removed, irritation subdued; and the muscular system relaxed; the secretion of the bowels is lessened by it, but that of the skin is increased, and thus it acts as a sudorific. If small doses are continually taken, it intoxicates; if over-doses, it is a narcotic poison; causing intense sleep, with contraction of the pupil of the eye, which results in coma and death.

Opium should never be given to a person in a state of high fever, or inflammation; a parched tongue and a dry skin should generally forbid its use. But if the fever is only moderate, and the skin moist, with no cerebral disorder, it may safely be given to alleviate pain and subdue irritation. It is given with effect in Bronchitis combined with Camphor and Ipecacuanha; in cancer, delirium tremens, and all neuralgic disorders; in convulsive disorders it is given as a antispasmodic; in some cases as a diaphoretic; and in dysentery and diarrhœa alone, or combined with astringents, there is no medicine so good as this. It is given advantageously also in typhus fever and gangrene, as it then supports the action of the system, also in rheumatism, and small-pox, and for the relief of coughs. In typhus, it should be combined with a tonic and wine; but, as aforesaid, it should not be given where the fever is high, the skin dry, &c. It is injurious where there is a disposition to local inflammation, especially of the chest, and where there is much determination of blood to the head. Combined with bark it has often cured the ague. It is of the greatest use in tetanus, St. Vitus's dance, hysterics, and cholera morbus.

Applied outwardly opium subdues pain and spasmodic action. Applied by friction, it relieves cramp, tetanus; when rubbed over the abdomen it is good for spasmodic pain of the stomach and bowels, and for hooping-cough.

The dose of opium for an adult is from ½ a grain to 3 grains; it is not safe to give it to children, except by skilful hands: Extract ¼ grain to 3 grains; tincture of laudanum 10 to 30 drops. The remedies for an over-dose of opium, are evacuation from the stomach. Acid of lemons taken immediately neutralises the narcotic influence; or half a drachm of sulphate of zinc (white vitriol) dissolved in water, or mustard, or salt, if nothing else be at hand, and even very strong coffee, mustard plasters between the shoulders, and the person constantly roused from lethargy.

ORANGE.

Citrus Aurantium.—The orange tree belongs to the natural order *Aurantaceæ.* It is a beautiful plant which gives a refreshing shade in hot climates, and perfumes the air for miles. It is extensively cultivated in every place where there is sufficient heat to bring it to perfection. The supply to this country comes principally from Spain, Portugal, the Azores, and the islands of the Mediterranean. There are several varieties of this species; but they all may be referred to the bitter or Seville Orange. The St. Michael's perhaps, is the most delicious, and this variety is grown largely in Malta and Provence. The juice of the sweet Orange, which consists principally of mucilage, sugar, and citric acid, is one of the most wholesome vegetable juices known. It is very grateful to invalids, especially when fever and thirst prevail. The flowers of the Orange-tree are highly odoriferous, and have been long in great esteem as a perfume. They yield their flavour by infusion to rectified sprits, and in distillation both to spirit and water: the bitter matter is dissolved by water, and on evaporating, the decoction remains entire in the extract. On the continent the distilled water is used as an antispasmodic and anodyne; it is extremely useful in hysteria, in doses of one or two ounces.

The chief direct medicinal use of the Orange is derived from the rind, and the best for the purpose is the Seville Orange, which yields an agreeable aromatic, stimulant, astringent, and tonic bitter. The rind of the sweet orange may be used, but it is less bitter. A confection, infusion, syrup, and a tincture of orange peel, are all used. It is very often prescribed in combination with stronger bitters, such as Gentian and Quinine, and it forms a good vehicle for disagreeable and nauseous purgatives.

A very good infusion may be made thus: 1 ounce of the dry bitter orange-peel, nearly one pint of boiling water poured over, the whole to stand for an hour, and then strained. A little lump sugar and lemon juice will make it more pleasant.

It is a stomachic ; dose, a wineglass full twice a day. Orange Marmalade upon bread is a good breakfast diet for dyspeptic patients. Syrup of Orange is made by infusing 2½ ounces of the dried peel in a pint of boiling water for 20 minutes, strain, and add 2 pounds of lump sugar ; boil for 10 minutes. This mixed with water, and a little lemon juice, forms Orangeade. It is nice also to mix with punch.

ORCHIS.

DESCRIPTION.—*Orchis Masculata.*—It is called dog-stones, goat-stones, foal-stones, fox-stones, satiricon, culbeans, together with many other too tedious to rehearse. It is a beautiful plant, found in moist pastures in June, with a stem like that of the tulip, crowned at the top with a spike of beautiful purple flowers, curious in shape. The corolla is formed of three petals, and terminating behind in a spur. The leaves are long, pointed, and grow from the root. The root is a double tuber.

MEDICINAL VIRTUES.—From the root the Salep of commerce is obtained, a nutritious and wholesome farina. When carefully prepared, it is one of the best articles of diet for a weakly person, and for invalids. They are only to be washed in hot water, the brown skin scraped off with a coarse cloth, and then placed in a hot oven for about 10 minutes, and then dried for use as a powder. It is very valuable.

ORPINE.

DESCRIPTION.—*Sedum Telephium.* Common Orpine has several round brittle stalks, thick set with flat and fleshy leaves without any order, and little dented about the edges, of a green colour. The flowers are white and beautiful, growing in tufts, after which come small chaffy husks, with seeds like dust in them. The roots are thick, round, white tuberous clogs. It grows in hedges, and in woods. It flowers in July.

MEDICINAL VIRTUES.—Tragus says, that the distilled water is profitable for gnawings in the stomach and bowels, or for ulcers in the lungs, liver, and the matrix, being drank as a decoction for days together. It stays the bloody flux, and other fluxes in the body, or in wounds. The root has the like effect. It is used outwardly to cool inflamed wounds, and to ease the pain. The juice of the leaves mixed with oil is good for burns and scalds. The leaf bruised and laid to any green wound, heals it quickly; and being bound to the throat relieves the quinsy; the juice made into syrup is good for sore throat and quinsy.

PARSLEY.

MEDICINAL VIRTUES.—*Apium Petroselinon.*—The roots are the part generally used in medicine. A strong decoction of them is good against jaundice. It operates powerfully by urine, and it expels wind. It gently opens the body, and removes obstructions of the liver and spleen. Galen recommended it in falling sickness, and in obstructed menstruation. The seeds are also powerful. The distilled water of Parsley is a good medicine to give children troubled with wind in the stomach or bowels. The leaves of Parsley mixed with meal and applied to inflamed eyes greatly relieves them, and fried with butter and applied to hard breasts, greatly relieves and mollifies them. Tragus gives the following medicine for jaundice, falling sickness, dropsy, and stone in the kidneys; seed of Parsley, Fennel Annise, and Carraways, of each an ounce; roots of Parsley, Burnet, Saxifrage and Carraways, of each an ounce and a half; bruise the seeds, wash the roots and cut small; all night steep in a bottle of white wine, and in the morning boil in a close earthen vessel, until a third part be wasted; which being strained, take four ounces morning and evening, abstaining from drink after it for three hours.

PARSLEY PIERT.

DESCRIPTION.—*Percicier.*—This is also called Parsley Break-stone, from its efficacy in dissolving stone in the bladder.

The root, though it is very small and thready, continues many years, from whence arise many leaves lying on the ground, each standing upon a long small foot-stalk, the leaves are as broad as a man's nail, much indented at the edges, like a parsley leaf, but of a very dusky green colour. The stalks are very weak and slender, three or four fingers in length, set so full of leaves that they can hardly be seen, either having no foot-stalk at all, or but very short ones. The flowers are very small. The seed is small and round. It grows among corn, and in barren sandy, moist places.

MEDICINAL VIRTUES.—The whole plant is used. An infusion of it is very powerful against the gravel. It operates violently, but safely, by urine, and it removes obstructions of the liver, and is therefore useful in jaundice. Some suppose that it has the power of dissolving stone in the bladder. The powder should be taken in wine.

PARSLEY,—MACEDONIAN.

DESCRIPTION.—*Petroselinon Macedonicum.* It is also called Alisander, Horse Parsley, and Black Pot Herb. It grows wild on the cliffs of the sea-coast, and is cultivated in gardens. It is two feet high. The stalk is slender, branched, and hairy. The leaves are composed of many parts, small, and rounded; those on the upper part of the stalk are more finely divided. The flowers are small and white, like Common Parsley, and stand in clusters at the top of the stalks. The seeds are small, rather hairy, and of a dusky colour.

MEDICINAL VIRTUES.—The seed is used; it is given in powder. It operates powerfully by urine, and relieves colic and gravel arising from obstructions. It is also good against the dropsy and jaundice. It has almost the same virtues as the common Parsley.

PARSNIP,—WILD.

DESCRIPTION.—*Pastanaca Sativa.*—It is a wild plant, common on our road-sides, and in marshy places. The wild Parsnip differs little from the garden; but it has not so many leaves, and the root is shorter. It flowers in July, the seed is ripe early in August.

MEDICINAL VIRTUES.—The garden Parsnip is good and wholesome, but it has a tendency to produce flatulency. It is a very nutritious and wholesome food, easy of digestion, and as a vegetable, it ought to be more frequently eaten. It removes obstructions of the urine. The wild Parsnip has a cutting, attenuating, cleansing, and opening quality therein. It relieves pains and stitches in the sides, and dissolves wind, both in the stomach and bowels, which is the colic, and provokes urine. The root is often used, but the seed much more.

PARSNIP,—COW.

DESCRIPTION.—*Vaccæ Pastanaca.*—It is a very different plant from the former. It grows with three or four large spread-winged, rough leaves, lying often on the ground, or raised a little from it, with long, round hairy foot-stalks under them, in five divisions, the two couple standing each against the other; and one at the end, and each being almost round, yet much indented at the edges in some leaves, but not so deep in others, of a whitish green colour, smelling strongly; from which springs a round, crusted, hairy stalk, two or three feet high, with a few joints and leaves thereon, and branched at the top, where stand large umbels of white, sometimes reddish flowers, and after them whitish winged seeds, two always joined together. The root is long and white, with two or three long strings growing down into the ground, smelling unpleasant. It grows in moist meadows, near ditches, and field corners.

MEDICINAL VIRTUES.—The seed, Galen says, is of a sharp and cutting quality, a fit medicine for a cough and shortness of breath, the falling-sickness and jaundice. The root is available to all these purposes, and of great use to take away the hard skin that grows on a fistula, if it be but scraped upon it. The decoction of the seed cleanses the chest from tough phlegm, eases them that are liver-grown. The seed and root boiled in oil, and the head rubbed therewith, cures those who have fallen into a frenzy, legthargy, and drowsiness. It relieves the head ache, if it be used with rue. It helps also the running scab and the shingles. The juice of the flowers dropped into the ears that run and are full of matter, cleanses and heals them.

PEACH TREE.

DESCRIPTION.—*Persica malus vel Amygdalis.* It is very nearly allied to the Almond, and generally included in the same family. They are nursed in gardens and orchards, and need no further description.

MEDICINAL VIRTUES. · The flowers are to be made into a syrup by pouring a pint of boiling water on a pound of peach blossoms, to stand 24 hours, and then strained, and dissolve in it 2 pounds of sugar over the fire. It is a good syrup for children, and adults who have become debilitated. It is good against the jaundice, and worms. It is mildly aperient, and taken largely, it is a safe emetic. The powder strewed on fresh wounds arrests bleeding, and closes them up. The flowers made into a conserve, have the same effect. The liquor that drops from the tree, being wounded, is given in the decoction of Coltsfoot, for cough or shortness of breath, adding some sweet wine and saffron. It is good for hoarseness and loss of voice; it clears and strengthens the lungs, and relieves those who vomit and spit blood. The kernels of the stones effectually relieve both colic and the stone. Take fifty kernels of peach stones, and one hundred of the kernels of cherry stones, a handful of elder flowers, and three pints of muscadel; infuse for six days near the fire, after which distil, and take a wineglassful occasionally. The oil drawn from the kernels, applied to the temples, procures sleep for the sick. The oil applied to the belly removes pains caused by colic. An infusion of the dried leaves of peach has been used for the expulsion of worms.

PEAR-TREE.

MEDICINAL VIRTUES.—*Pyrus Communis.*—All the sweet and luscious sorts are gently aperient, and cooling. Pears boiled with a little honey, relieve an oppressed stomach. The pulp is excellent to bind on green wounds, to cool and stay the blood, and heal the wound without inflammation; Galen says, he found it so by experience. The wild Pears sooner close the lips of green wounds than others.

PELLITORY OF THE WALL.

Description.—*Parietaria Officinalis.*—This plant is generally known where there are any old walls or ancient ruins. It rises with brownish, tender, weak, and almost transparent stalks, two feet high, upon which grow at the joints two leaves rather broad and long, of a dark green colour, rough and hairy, as the stalks are also. At the joints from the middle of the stalk upwards, where it spreads into branches, stand many small, pale purplish flowers, in hairy rough heads, after which come small, black, rough seed, which will stick to any garment that shall touch it. The root is rather long, with small fibres of a dark reddish colour.

Medicinal Virtues.—The dried herb Pellitory made into an electuary with honey, or the juice of the herb, or a decoction made with sugar or honey, is a singular remedy for an old or dry cough, shortness of breath, and wheezing. Three ounces of the juice taken at a time promotes urine, and cures gravelly affections. It is combined with other herbs used in clysters to mitigate pains in the back, sides, or bowels, produced by wind. If the bruised herb, sprinkled with some muscadel, be heated, and applied to the belly, it has the same effect. A decoction with a little honey, is good to gargle a sore throat. The juice held a while in the mouth, cures the toothache. The juice dropped into the ears takes away pricking and shooting pains. The distilled water reduces hot and swelling imposthumes, burns and scalds; being bathed often with cloth dipped therein. The powdered herb mixed with lard, and applied to the fundament, is a remedy for the piles. The juice is very effectual to cleanse fistulas, and to heal them, or the herb bruised, and applied with a little salt. It is curative of green wounds, if applied for three days. A poultice made of it, bran, beanmeal, wine, and oil, and applied warm to any bruise, soon removes the pains, and effects a cure.

PELLITORY OF SPAIN.

The juice of Pellitory of the Wall boiled to syrup with honey, and a spoonful of it drank every morning; and continuing to do so for a week, is a safe and certain cure for dropsy.

PELLITORY OF SPAIN.

DESCRIPTION.—The root of the *Anacyclus Pyrethrum.*—It is a foreign plant, but it is grown in some gardens in England. It requires care and attention. The root goes down into the ground, bearing leaves, similar to, but larger than the leaves of camomile. At the top it bears one single large flower at a place, having a border of many leaves, white on the upper side, and reddish underneath, with a yellow thrumb in the middle, not standing so close as that of camomile.

The common Pellitory which grows here, has a root of a biting taste, scarcely discernible by the taste from that just described. It has several brittle stalks, a yard high and more, with narrow long leaves finely dented at the edges, standing one above another up to the tops. The flowers are many and white, in tufts like those of yarrow, with a small yellowish thrum in the middle. The seed is very small. The last grows in fields, under hedges, and other places. It flowers in June and July.

MEDICINAL VIRTUES.—I am persuaded it is one of the best purgers of the brain that grows. An ounce of the juice taken in a draught of light wine an hour before the fit of ague comes, it will drive it away at the second or third time taking. Either the herb or root dried and chewed in the mouth, purges the head of phlegmatic humours, by which headache will be removed, and coughs, falling sickness, and lethargy relieved. The powder of the herb or root snuffed up the nostrils, causes sneezing, and eases head-ache; being made into an ointment with lard, it takes away black and blue spots occasioned by blows or falls, and cures gout and sciatica. The root chewed is a sovereign remedy for tooth-ache. It is sold by the Druggists. It has been very useful in dropsy. It has cured the effects of salivation, has stimulated the palsy tongue and throat, and given relief to diseased uvula.

PENNYROYAL.

Pennyroyal, or Fleamint, the *Mentha Pulegium* of botanists, of the order *Labiatæ*, is perennial. It flowers in September. It is a well-known plant. There is a larger kind than the ordinary sort found wild with us, now cultivated in gardens, and differs from it in the largeness of the leaves and stalks, in rising higher, and not creeping upon the ground so much. The flowers are purple, growing in rundles about the stalks like the other. The wild species grows in marshy places.

Medicinal Virtues.—Dioscorides says, that Pennyroyal makes tough phlegm thin, warms the coldness of any part to which it is applied, and digests raw or corrupt matter. The herb is warm, pungent, and aromatic; somewhat similar to spearmint, but less agreeable. It is used as a popular remedy with much confidence in obstructions of the courses, especially if attended with pain and hysteria. The oil is pungent and peculiar, differing from the other mints, which it resembles in its properties. A strong decoction of the whole herb is a good application for the gout, the place being rubbed with it till it is red, and if some salt be added, it is a rubefacient for the side in liver complaints, and for the itch. It is very warming and strengthening to stiff and cold joints, and removes cramps. The green herb bruised and put into vinegar, cleanses foul ulcers, and takes away marks, bruises, or blows about the eyes. The oil is a remedy for tooth-ache. Pliny says that Pennyroyal and Mint together, help faintings, being put into vinegar, and smelled, or put into the nostrils or mouth. It eases headache, pains of the breast and belly, and gnawing of the stomach. Boiled in milk and drank, it is effectual for coughs, and for ulcers and sores in the mouth. Matthiolus says the decoction cures the jaundice and dropsy, all pains of the head and sinews that come of a cold cause, and it clears the eye-sight.

PEONY.

Description.—*Pæonia Corolina.*—The plant is distinguished by Male and Female.

Male Peony rises up with brownish stalks, whereon grow

green and reddish leaves, upon a stalk without any particular division in the leaf. The flowers stand at the top of the stalks, consisting of five or six broad leaves, of a purplish red colour, with many yellow threads in the middle standing about the head, which become seed vessels, divided into three, or four crooked pods like horns, which contain round, black, shining seeds, with crimson grains, intermixed with black. The plant is beautiful. The roots are thick and long.

The ordinary Female Peony has many stalks, and more leaves than the male; the leaves are not so large, but of a dead green, smaller, and of a more purple colour than the Male, with yellow thrums at the head. The seed vessels are like those of the Male. They are culivated in gardens.

MEDICINAL VIRTUES. Male Peony roots are the best; the roots have more virtue than the seed; next the flowers, and then the leaves. The roots fresh gathered, cure the falling sickness. The roots powdered is excellent for hysterical and nervous complaints. The root chopped small and infused in white wine 24 hours, and strained, is excellent for nervous complaints, taking a wine-glassful occasionally. A decoction of Betony should be drank between. A decoction of the root is very cleansing immediately after child-birth, and so is the black seed infused in wine; it also drives away melancholy and nightmare. The Female is often used for the purposes aforesaid, because the Male is scarce.

PEPPER.

Black and White Pepper are the fruit of the *Piper Nigrum*, belonging to the natural order *Piperaceæ*. It is a shrubby, creeping plant, growing wild in the East Indies, but chiefly in Java, Sumatra, Borneo, Malacca, &c. The berries are gathered before they are ripe, and are dried in the sun; their taste is hot and fiery, and their smell is slightly aromatic. White Pepper is the fruit of the same plant, gathered after it is fully ripe, and freed of its external coat by maceration in water. It is smooth on the surface, and less pungent than the Black Pepper.

Pepper is mostly used as a corrective of the coldness and flatulence of a vegetable diet, and is much adapted for warm climates, where the food is naturally aqueous, and of a cold nature. Hence we use it with most vegetables, especially cucumbers and peas, and as a condiment to fish.

Medicinally, it is aromatic, carminative, and stimulant. It assists digestion, and gives tone to the stomach, if taken moderately. In gout, dropsy, rheumatism, cold phlegmatic habits, the use of Pepper is advisable, and taken in a large dose, it is said to cure intermittents. In incipient quinsies, before the tumour has broken, a basin of gruel well-seasoned with Pepper, taken at bed-time, will resolve it. *Ward's Paste*, so celebrated for the cure of chronic piles, is chiefly composed of Pepper, which has been given in gonnorhœa, and applied as ointment to ringworms. As an antiflatulent it is mixed with other medicines, Mixed with bread, as a poultice, it has proved beneficial in tic doloreux, and other neuralgic pains. It is much recommended in palsy.

Ward's Paste for Piles.—1 ounce of Black Pepper, finely powdered, 1 ounce of Elecampane Root, 3 ounces of Fennel Seed, well mixed. Melt together 2 ounces of Sugar, and 2 ounces of clarified Honey, for a Syrup, which add to the mixed powder, triturate them well. Take the size of a nutmeg twice a day; wash well down with a glass of cold water or white wine.

PEPPERWORT, OR DITTANDER.

Description.—*Lepidium Campestre.*—It derives its name from the biting taste of its leaves and root. Pepperwort puts forth somewhat long and broad leaves, of a light bluish greenish colour, finely dented about the edges, and pointed at the ends, standing upon round hard stalks, three or four feet high, spreading many branches on all sides, and having many small white flowers at the tops of them, after which follow small seeds in small heads. The root is slender, running much under ground, and shooting up again in many places. It is common in corn-fields, and sometimes it is cultivated in gardens. It flowers in June and July.

MEDICINAL VIRTUES.—Pliny and Paulus Ægineta say, that Pepperwort is very successful for sciatica, for gout or pain in the joints; the leaves to be bruised, and mixed with lard and applied to the place for four hours in men, and two hours in women, the place being afterwards bathed with wine and oil mixed together, and then wrapped up with wool or skins, after they have sweat a little. It also mends the deformities or discolourings of the skin. The seeds are very effectual in warming cold phlegmatic constitutions.

PERIWINKLE.

DESCRIPTION.—*Vinca Minor.*—There are two kinds, the Garden and the common. The common has many branches running upon the ground, shooting out small fibres at the joints as it runs, rooting thereby in the ground. At the joints of these branches stand two small dark green shining leaves, somewhat like bay leaves but smaller, and with them come forth the flowers, (one at a joint) standing upon a tender footstalk, somewhat long and hollow, parted at the brims, into four or five leaves. The common sorts are of a pale blue colour: some are pure white, and some of a dark reddish purple colour. The root creeps, and spreads rapidly. Those with pale blue, and those with white flowers, grow in woods and orchards, by the hedge-sides, but the purple-flowered in gardens only. They flower in March and April.

MEDICINAL VIRTUES.— The Periwinkle is a great binder, stays bleeding at the mouth and nose, if some of the leaves be chewed. The French use it to stay women's courses. Dioscorides, Galen and Ægineta commend it against fluxes, to be drank in wine. It is a remedy for bleeding piles, the leaves bruised and made into an ointment, with lard.

ST. PETER'S WORT

DESCRIPTION.—*Petræ Herba.*—It rises up with square upright stalks, some larger and higher than St. John's Wort; brown, having two leaves at every joint, like, but larger than

St. John's Wort, a little round pointed, with few or no holes in the leaves, and having some smaller leaves rising from the bosom of the greater, and a little hairy. At the tops of two stalks stand many star-like flowers, with yellow threads in the middle, very like those of St. John's Wort, differing only in size and height. The seed is the same in both. It grows in many small low woods, and near water-courses. It flowers in June and July, and the seed is ripe in August.

Medicinal Virtues. They are nearly the same as those of St. John's Wort, yet rather weaker. Two drachms of the seeds taken at a time in honey-water, purges choleric humours, (as say Dioscorides, Pliny and Galen) and therefore it relieves the sciatica. The leaves are used as St. John's Wort, to cure burns and scalds.

PIMPERNEL.

Description.—*Anagallis Arvensis.*—This is a pretty ornament to meadows and corn-fields. Common Pimpernel has several weak square stalks lying on the ground, having two small and almost round leaves at every joint, one against another, very like Chickweed, but without foot-stalks; for the leaves compass the stalk. The flowers stand singly on tender foot-stalks; they consist of five small round-pointed leaves, of a scarlet colour, with threads in the middle. It grows almost every where, and flowers from May until August.

Pimpernel is known as the *Poor Man's Weather Glass*, the flowers opening at about 7 in the morning, and closing about 2 in the afternoon; and also the *Shepherd's Barometer* closing on the approach of rain.

Medicinal Virtues.—Galen says, they have a drying faculty, whereby they are good to close the lips of wounds, and to cleanse foul ulcers. The distilled water or juice is much esteemed by French dames to cleanse the skin from any roughness, deformity, or discolouring thereof; being boiled in wine, and given to drink. It is a good remedy against pestilential fevers, if the party after taking it be warm in bed, and sweat for two hours after, and use the same twice at least. It cures stings and bites of bees, wasps, and even mad dogs, used inwardly and applied outwardly. It removes obstructions of the liver and kidneys, provokes urine and expels gravel, and relieves inward pains and ulcers. The decoction or distilled water is effectual to be applied to all fresh wounds and to old ulcers. A little honey mixed with the juice, and dropped into the eyes, removes cloudy mists, or thick films which grow over them. Ray states that the distilled water is effectual in consumption, being mixed with milk.

PAREIRA BRAVA.

The root of the *Cissampelos Pareira*, a plant growing in the West Indies, and in South America. It has a bitterish sweet taste, and is tonic, diuretic, and aperient. It is highly valued by the inhabitants of Brazil, &c. They use a decoction of it for pains and weakness of the stomach arising from general debility. It is of great service in urinary disorders, on account of its tonic influence upon the bladder. It has been found very serviceable in ulceration of the kidneys and bladder. Dr. Graham in his "Domestic Medicine," says, "One of the most prominent symptoms of chronic inflammation of the bladder is an abundant discharge of a ropy adhesive alkaline mucus, and we have Sir B. Brodie's testimony to the fact that the use of the decoction of the root of the *Pareira Brava* is here frequently productive of excellent effects."

"The decoction is prepared by simmering 4 ounces of the root in 3 pints of water, until it is reduced to 2 pints, and then strain. The dose is a small tea-cupful, (about 4 ounces) twice or thrice a day. A little tincture of Henbane may sometimes be advantageously combined with it."

PINK,—INDIAN.

Spigelia Marilandica.—This grows in North America. It is anthelmintic, and noted for its expulsion of lumbrici worms from the alimentary canal. Some order it in doses of 10 or 15 grains, others in drachm doses, alleging that the nervous affections it sometimes produces, more readily happen from small doses; while the larger doses purge or vomit. Some give an infusion of Indian Pink and Senna for worms of all kinds. Infused in wine, it has been found useful in intermittent fevers. Dr. Barton recommends it in the insidious remittent fever of children, which often lays the foundation of water in the head.

PLANTAIN.

Plantago Major.—It grows in meadows and fields, and by pathsides. It is also called Way-bread, and Way Broad Leaf.

MEDICINAL VIRTUES.—The leaves are bitter and astringent, and have been long held in popular esteem as a wound herb. They are used as an external application to ulcers, and indolent scrofulous tumours. The root has been found useful in intermittents. A mucilage prepared from the seeds has been found beneficial in the catarrhal and mild inflammatory form of diarrhœa. The juice is excellent for pains in the bowels; it restrains fluxes, spitting of blood, bloody urine, proceeding from an ulcerated bladder, and bleeding wounds. A decoction of the roots sweetened with honey or sugar is excellent in consumption, allaying cough, &c. It is also good in ague. The herb (but especially the seed) is effectual against dropsy, falling sickness, yellow jaundice, and obstructions of the liver and reins. The roots of Plaintain and Pellitory of Spain, beaten into powder and put into the hollow teeth, take away pain. The clarified juice, or distilled water, dropped into the eyes, cools inflammation, and clears the sight, and dropped into the ears, eases pain and removes the heat. The bruised leaves form a good application for burns and scalds. The juice mixed with lard is a good application for the piles. The juice mixed with oil of roses, and the temples and forehead bathed with it, eases pains of the head arising from heat, and is very applicable to lunatic and frantic persons; to hot gouts in the feet or hands, especially in the beginning. It is good to be applied where bone is out of joint, to hinder inflammations, swellings, and pains. The powder of the dried leaves taken in drink destroys worms One part of plaintain in decoction, and two parts of the brine of beef, boiled together and clarified, is a sure remedy to heal spreading scabs, or itch in the head and body, also ringworms, the shingles, &c. It is remarkable that it is the chief remedy for the cure of the rattlesnake, for which discovery an Indian received a great reward from the assembly of South Carolina.

There is another species of Plantain, called Hoary Plantain, *Plantago Media.* The leaves are small, and less blunt than in the last, hoary, lying close to the ground. Its *Medicinal Virtues* are much the same. The seeds boiled in milk are laxative and demulcent. Boyle recommends an electuary, made of fresh Comfrey roots, juice of Plantain, and sugar, as very efficacious in spitting of blood. Plantain juice mixed with lemon juice, is an excellent diuretic.

POLYPODY OF THE OAK.

Description.—*Polypodium Vulgare.*—This is a perennial herb of the fern tribe. It is a small herb consisting of nothing but roots and leaves, bearing neither stalk, flower, nor seed. It has three or four leaves rising from the root, each one single by itself, of about a hand length, are winged, consisting of many small' narrow leaves, cut into the middle rib, standing on each side of the stalk large below and smaller up to the top, not dented at the edges as the male fern is, of a sad green colour, and smooth on the upper side, but on the other side rough, by reason of some yellowish spots set thereon. The root is smaller than one's little finger, creeping under the upper crust of the earth, of a sweetish harsh taste, set with rough knags on each side, having much mossiness or yellow hairiness upon it and some fibres underneath. It grows also upon old rotten stumps, or trunks of trees, as oak, beech, hazel, willow, or any other, as in the woods under them, and upon old mud walls, and in mossy, stony, and gravelly places near unto wood. That which grows upon oak is accounted the best.

Medicinal Virtues.—The fresh root is used; it is a safe and gentle purge, used as a decoction it promotes the flow of urine. It is efficacious in jaundice, dropsy, and scurvy. It is an expectorant removing phlegm copiously. Combined with mallows it drives away melancholy, removes hardness of the spleen, stitches in the sides, and colic. Combined with a little ginger it is a safe and gentle medicine, fit for all persons. A drachm or two of dried roots powdered, taken fasting in a cup of honey water, works gently, and for the purposes aforesaid. The distilled water both of roots and leaves, is much commended for the quartan ague, to be taken for days together, and with some sugar-candy dissolved therein, is good against cough, shortness of breath, wheezings, and those distillations of thin rheum upon the lungs, which cause consumption. The fresh roots beaten small, or the powder of the dried roots mixed with honey, and applied to the nose, cures the disease called Polypus, which is a piece of flesh growing therein, which in time obstructs the passage of breathing through the nostrils.

POMEGRANATE.

Punica Granatum.—It belongs to the natural order of *Myrtaceæ.* This tree grows in Asia and Africa, and in warm countries generally. It yields a pleasantly acid and sweetish fruit, which is used for the same purpose as the orange. The flowers, the rind of the fruit, and the bark of the root, have been used in medicine, as astringents. The bark is powerfully astringent, and is employed, in decoction, as a gargle for sore throats. It is also given in diarrhœa, and as an injection in leucorrhœa, and the powder in intermittent fever; dose 20 grains. The natives of India give it as a vermifuge. The bark of the root is reckoned a powerful remedy for tape-worm. Dr. Christian says, "It seems scarcely ever to fail, if properly used."—Steep 2 ounces of the fresh bark in 2 pints of water for 12 hours; then boil down to 1 pint, strain, and give a wine-glassful every two hours till the whole is taken. Sometimes joints of the worm come in less than an hour after the last dose; but often the doses must be repeated several successive mornings before the effect is complete; and it is right to repeat occasionally for 4 or 5 days after joints have ceased to come away. Laxatives should be administered from time to time.

PONDWEED.

Description.—*Potamogiton Natans.* Called also Crab's Claw, Water Houseleek, &c. It grows plentifully in the Lincolnshire fens. It has long narrow leaves, with sharp prickles on the edges. The stalks have a forked head, like a crab's claw, out of which comes a white flower of three leaves with yellowish hairy threads in the middle. It roots in the mud in the bottom of the water.

Medicinal Virtues.—It is a great strengthener of the kidneys; it is beneficial in Erysipelas, and reduces swellings, inflammations, &c. An ointment made of the leaves with Hog's Lard is very healing. It is one of the most valuable remedies for diseased kidneys.

POPLAR TREE.

Description.—*Populus Nigra.*—There are two kinds of Poplars, viz. Black and White. The White Poplar grows large and high, covered with thick, smooth, white bark, especially the branches, having long leaves cut into divisions almost like a vine leaf; they are a glossy shining green. The catkins which come before the leaves, are long and of a reddish colour; which fall away, seldom bearing good seed with them.

The Black Poplar grows higher and straighter than the White, with a greyish bark, bearing broad green leaves, somewhat like ivy leaves, not indented on the edges like the White, ending in a point, and not white underneath, hanging by slender long foot-stalks, which continually shake like the aspen leaves. The catkins hereof are greater than those of the White, composed of many round green berries, in a long cluster, containing much downy matter, which being ripe is blown away with the wind. The clammy buds before they spread into leaves, are gathered to make Unguenum Populneum, and are of a yellowish green colour, and small, rather sweet, but strong. On both these trees grows a sweet kind of musk, which formerly was used to put into sweat ointments.

Medicinal Virtues.—White Poplar, says Galen, is of a cleansing property: one ounce in powder of the bark being drank, says Dioscorides, is a remedy for those that are troubled with the sciatica, or the strangury. The juice of the leaves dropped warm into the ears, eases pains in them. The young clammy buds, or eyes before they break out into leaves, bruised and a little honey put to them, is a good medicine for a dull sight. The Black Poplar is held to be more cooling than the White, and therefore the leaves bruised with vinegar, and applied relieve the gout. The seed drank in vinegar is held good against falling sickness. The water that drops from the hollow places of this tree, takes away warts, wheals, and other like breakings out of the body. The young Black Poplar buds, says Matthiolus, are much used by women to beautify their hair, bruising them with fresh butter, straining them after they have been kept for some time in the sun. The ointment called Populneum, which is made of this Poplar, is good for all inflammations in any part of the body, and tempers the heat of wounds. It is much used to dry up the milk of women's breasts, when they have weaned their child.

POPPY

Description.—*Papaver Album*, has three kinds, viz. the White, Black, and the Red Poppy.

The White Poppy has at first four or five whitish green leaves lying upon the ground, which rise with the stalk, compassing it at the bottom, are very large, much cut on the edges, and dented; the stalk which is four or five feet high, sometimes no branches at the top, usually but two or three at most, each bearing one head wrapped up in a thin skin, hanging down before it blows, and then rising, the flower breaks out, consisting of four large white round leaves, with many whitish round threads in the middle, set about a small round green head, having a crown or star-like cover at the end thereof, which growing ripe becomes as large as an apple. This head contains a great number of small round seeds, in several partitions next to the shell, the middle thereof remaining hollow and empty. These plants, while they remain fresh and green, yield a milk when they are broken, of an unpleasant bitter taste, and of a strong smell, which being condensed is called Opium.

The Black Poppy, *Papaver Nigrum*, little differs from the former; but the flower, which is somewhat less, and of a black purplish colour, but without any purple spots in the bottom of the leaf. The head of the seed is much less than the former, and opens itself a little round about the top, under the crown. The seed is black.

The wild Red Poppy, or Corn Rose, *Papaver Erraticum*, has long and narrow leaves, very much cut in on the edges into many divisions, of a light green colour, sometimes hairy; the stalk is blackish and hairy also, but not so tall as the garden kind, having similar leaves thereon to grow below, parted into three or four branches, on which grow small hairy heads, on which is the flower, of a yellowish red, crimson, or scarlet colour, without any spot in the bottom of the leaves, having many black threads at the middle, compassing a small green head, which contain much black seed, smaller by half than that of the garden. The former two are cultivated in gardens, the latter grows in corn-fields, on ditch banks, &c.

Medicinal Virtues.—It is a valuable plant, for all its parts, and especially the capsule, or seed-vessel, yield a white opaque narcotic juice, called Opium. Syrup of Poppy is made from the capsule. But it should be given by the skilful hand, for it is dangerous otherwise. It is taken to procure ease, rest, and sleep for invalids; and also to ease coughs, hoarseness, and loss of voice. The Poppy heads used for fomentation, are mostly of home growth; their anodyne properties render them valuable to soothe inflammations and pain. They should be broken up, and boiled, the liquor only to be used. A flannel dipped into it, wrung out, and applied to the part affected, and renewed as it begins to cool. The decoction also taken in moderation, relieves pain, and promotes sleep.

The Extract of Poppies is not so strong as opium, and may be given in doses from 2 to 10 grains. Made thus:—Bruised Poppy heads 15 ounces; boil in 1 gallon of water down to 4 pints; strain, and evaporate to a proper consistence.

The Wild Poppy, or Corn Rose, is good to prevent the falling sickness. The Syrup made with the leaves and flower, is effectual in pleurisy, and St. Anthony's fire, or Erysipelas. The dried leaves decocted have the same effect

PRIMROSES.

Primula Veris.—The root is used. The juice snuffed up the nose causes sneezing, and is a good remedy against headache. The dried root powdered has the same effect.

PRIVET.

Description.—*Ligustrum Vulgare.*—A little wild shrub in hedges. It grows four feet high. The flowers are small and white. The fruit is a black berry. But it is well known as it frequently forms a beautiful hedge.

Medicinal Virtues.—The tops are used; and they are best when the flowers are in bud. Matthiolus says, that the oil made of the flowers of Privet infused, and set in the sun, is good for inflammations of wounds and headache coming of a hot cause. There is a sweet water also distilled from the flowers, that is good for all those diseases that need cooling or drying. A strong infusion of the tops in water, with the addition of a little honey and wine, make an excellent wash for the mouth, and throat when there are little sores in them, and when the gums are apt to bleed. It is a good wash for all sores.

PRUNES.

The dried fruit of the Plum, or *Prunus Domestica*, of the natural order *Rosaceæ.* Prunes possess much mucilaginous and saccharine matter. They abate heat, and gently open the bowels, which they perform by lubricating the passages and softening the excrement. They are of great service in costiveness, accompanied with heat and irritation, which the more active cathartics would tend to aggravate. Where prunes are not sufficiently purgative of themselves, their action is promoted by combining with them a little rhubarb, or by putting them in an infusion of Senna, adding a little ginger to prevent flatulency. They form a part of the Lenitive Electuary; and even taken alone, gently, in some constitutions, open the body. The French Prunes are the best.

PURSLANE.

DESCRIPTION.—*Portulaca Sativa.*—Garden Purslane, as a salad herb is so well known as to require no description.

MEDICINAL VIRTUES.—It is good to cool heat in the liver, blood, reins, and stomach, and in hot agues nothing better. It restrains hot and choleric fluxes, the whites and gonorrhœa, distillation from the head, and pains therein proceeding from heat, want of sleep, or the frenzy. The seed is more effectual than the herb to cool the heat and sharpness of urine. The seed bruised and boiled in wine, and given to children, destroys worms. The juice of the herb is effectual to stay vomitings, and taken with some sugar or honey, it relieves an old dry cough, shortness of breath, and immoderate thirst. The juice also is singularly good in the inflammations and ulcers of the privities and bowels. The herb bruised and applied to the forehead and temples, allays excessive heat, and applied to the eyes, it removes inflammation and St. Anthony's fire. If a little vinegar be put to it, and laid to the neck, with as much of galls and linseed together, it takes away pain. The juice is used with oil of roses for the same purposes; applied to the navels of children that project, it reduces them; it is also good for sore mouths and gums that are swollen, and to fasten loose teeth. Camerarius says, that the distilled water took away pain in the teeth, when all other remedies failed, and the thickened juice made into pills with the powder of gum tragacanth and arabic, being taken, is a remedy for bloody urine, and applied to gouty limbs, it eases pain.

QUASSIA.

Quassia Chips come from Jamaica and the Caribbean Islands. It was called after *Quassi*, a negro of Surinam, who first discovered its tonic and febrifuge properties, which he employed with great success in the cure of malignant fevers. It is a very powerful tonic, invigorating the digestive organs and the intestinal canal, with little excitement of the circulation, or increase of animal heat. Its taste is intensely bitter. It is excellent for nervous irritability, intermittent, and bilious remittent fevers, looseness, and gout. It is good for female complaints, as hysterics, the effect of debility. An infusion may be made by pouring a pint of boiling water on a drachm of the chips, as a tonic and antiseptic, in bilious fevers, united with Alkaline Salts. Dose from 1 to 2 ounces, repeated twice or thrice a day; in gout, with aromatics and ginger; in hysteria, with Camphor and Tincture of Valerian.

QUINCE TREE.

Cydonia Vulgaris.—It is now cultivated in gardens, especially in the south of England. It yields a fruit which is used for imparting a pleasant flavour to tarts and pies. Quinces are also made into marmalade; and the syrup made from them is a pleasant addition to beverages during sickness. The juice of the ripe Quince made into a syrup with sugar is excellent to stop vomiting, and to strengthen the stomach. The green fruit is astringent, and restrains flux, and diarrhœa. The syrup made of the juice is still more so. The mucilage is used externally as an emollient and sheathing application to cracked lips and nipples. *Bandoline*, used by hairdressers as a cement for dressing the hair in braids, is merely this mucilage evaporated. It apppears to have narcotic properties, for a strong decoction sweetened with honey, destroys flies. If a little vinegar be added, it promotes appetite. Some spices being added, it revives fainting spirits, and removes obstructions from the liver. If you would have them purging, put honey to them instead of sugar; and if more laxative, rhubarb; but if more forcibly to bind, use the unripe Quinces. The crude juice of Quinces, is a sure preservative against deadly poison. Some say that the very smell of a Quince hath taken away all the strength of the poison of white hellebore. The seeds when boiled in water make a good mucilaginous decoction which is useful in thrush, and other irritable conditions of the mucous membrane:—Quince seed 2 drachms in 2 pints of water, boil 10 or 15 minutes, and strain. Sweeten with sugar or honey.

QUININE.

Quinine is a chemical preparation from the Yellow Peruvian Bark, by means of Sulphuric Acid. It appears as a pure white powder, partly soluble in hot water, and wholly so in diluted Sulphuric Acid, and also in Spirits of Wine. For internal administration, it has almost superseded the bark on account of the minute dose required. Eight grains are equal to about one ounce of the bark. There is scarcely any drug so valuable as Quinine.

In cases of violent periodic headache, it is most useful. It is also a powerful tonic. In agues and intermittent fevers of all kinds, it is found to be indispensable. In neuralgic affections, and those caused by debility, its efficacy is marked and decided. It is adopted in cases of typhoid fever, and in the sinking stage, combined with Port Wine, it is very beneficial; and in recovering from low fever, and other severe diseases, very debilitating, the Quinine is often prescribed with great advantage. The simplest mode of administration, in dyspepsia, and as stomachic, is, *Quinine*, 1 grain; Elixir of Vitriol 5 drops; Water, 1 ounce; Syrup of Orange Peel, 1 drachm. Mix, and take occasionally. Combined with Valerian, it is highly recommended as a nervine and antispasmodic.

RADISH.

Raphanus Sativus.—The garden Radish is so well known that it needs no description.

Medicinal Virtues.—The juice of Radish roots, fresh gathered, with a little white wine, is an excellent remedy in the gravel. Scarcely any thing operates more speedily by urine, or brings away little stones more successfully. The Radish is fit only for those who have a good digestion, not for the dyspeptic.

RAGWORT.

Description.—*Senecio Jacobæa.*—It is also called St. James's Wort, and Stagger-Wort, and Stammer-Wort, Segrum, and Ragweed.

The greater common Ragwort has many large, long dark green leaves lying on the ground; it has very ragged leaves, from which rise sometimes one, and sometimes two or three square blackish purple stalks, three or four feet high, somtimes branched, bearing such like leaves upon them, unto the top, where it branches into many stalks bearing yellow flowers, consisting of various leaves, set as a pale or border, with a dark yellow thrum in the middle. The root is very fibrous, and the seed is downy.

There is another sort that rises not so high, the leaves are not so finely jagged, nor of so dark a green colour, but rather whitish, soft and woody, and the flowers paler. Both grow wild in pastures, and untilled grounds, and oftentimes both in one field.

Medicinal Virtues.—The decoction of the herb is good to wash the mouth or throat affected with ulcers or sores, and for swellings, hardness, or imposthumes, for it thoroughly cleanses and heals them; also the quinsy, and the king's evil. It is useful in catarrhs, thin rheums, and defluctions from the head into the eyes, nose, or lungs. The juice is good to heal green wounds, and to cleanse and heal old ulcers, inward wounds and ulcers, running cankers, and hollow fistulas. It gives relief to aches and pains either in the fleshy part, or in the nerves and sinews; as also the sciatica, or pain of the hips or huckle-bone, by fomenting with a decoction of the herb, or anointing them with an ointment made of the herb, bruised, and boiled in hog's lard, with some mastic and olibanum in powder added unto it after it is strained.

RANUNCULUS.

The various species of Ranunculus, or *Buttercup*, so common in this country, are chiefly remarkable for their acridity, proved by chewing a small portion of their leaves. Their action is emetic, and when bruised and applied to the skin, irritating, acting like a mustard-plaister, or blister. See *Crowfoot.* Their acridity arises from a volatile principle, which is destroyed by boiling, or even by drying. It is not fit to be taken inwardly, on account of its poisonous influence. The juice of most members of this genus of plants when applied to the skin acts as a rubefacient; in some cases it acts as a blister. The knowledge of this might prove very useful.

RASPBERRY.

This well-known plant is the *Rubus Idæus* of botanists. In some parts it grows wild, but is usually cultivated in gardens. Its fruit is fragrant, sub-acid, and cooling. It is very wholesome, and allays heat and thirst better than any other kind of fruit, except Strawberry, which it equals. Both of them are not liable to acetous fermentation in the stomach. *Raspberry Jam* is one of the most pleasant and wholesome of confections. In fever and feverish diseases generally, when the acid is not an objection, the well-known *Raspberry Vinegar* is an agreeable and salutary beverage. It is an excellent gargle for sore throats. When the acid is not proper, a pleasant beverage is made by mixing the preserve or jam, with water. An infusion or decoction of Raspberry leaves is a sure remedy for great laxity of the bowels. I have known this prove effectual in the severest cases.

RATTLE GRASS.

Description.—*Quassatio Gramen.*—Of this there are two kinds, viz. the red and yellow. The common Red Rattle has reddish hollow stalks, and sometimes green, mostly lying on the ground, some growing more upright, with many small reddish or green leaves set on both sides of a middle rib, finely dented at the edges; the flowers at the tops of the stalks are of a purplish red colour, like small gaping hooks, after which come blackish seed in small husks, which being loose, rattle with shaking. The root is fibrous.

The common Yellow Rattle has only one round great stalk, about half a yard or two feet high, with few branches, having two long and rather broad leaves set at a joint, indented on the edges, like the comb of a cock, broadest next to the stalk, and smaller at the end. The flowers grow at the tops of the stalks, with shorter leaves, hooded like the former, but of a fair yellow colour, or in some paler, and in some whiter. The seed and root are the same as the former. They grow in meadows and woods, and flower from Midsummer until August.

Medicinal Virtues.—The Red Rattle is good to heal fistulas and hollow ulcers, and to stay the flux or humours in them, and profuse menstruation, or any other flux of blood, being boiled in red wine and drank.

The Yellow Rattle, or Cock's-Comb, is said to be good for cough, or dimness of sight, if the herb, being boiled with some honey, be drank, or dropped into the eyes.

REST HARROW.

Description.—*Ononis Arveusis.*—A little tough and almost shrubby plant, common in dry fields, and by road sides. Some call it Cammock. It is one or two feet high. The stalks are round, reddish, tough, nearly woody. It has numerous leaves, three standing on each foot-stalk, close to the stalk. There are several short and sharp prickles about the stalks, principally at the insertions of the leaves. The flowers are small, purple, and stand among the leaves towards the tops of the stalks, shaped like pea-blossoms, but flatter, each is followed by a small pod. The root is white within, long, tough, and woody.

Medicinal Virtues.—It removes obstructions in the kidneys. The bark of the root powdered is a good remedy for the stone. It should be taken in wine. Matthiolus says that it cures the disease called Hernia Carnosa, the fleshy rupture, by taking the powder for some months constantly, and that it has cured some which seemed incurable by any other means than by cutting or burning. The decoction is an excellent diuretic; and it is very powerful to open obstructions of the liver and spleen. It is celebrated as a remedy for rheumatism, especially the chronic. Though it may not be successful in every case, it can do no harm. It has been known to cure many cases that had long resisted other means. The powder of the root made into an electuary, or lozenges, with sugar, also the bark of the fresh roots boiled tender and afterwards beaten to a conserve with sugar, has the like effect.

RHATANY ROOT.

This is the root of the *Krameria Triandria*, a native of Peru, where it is called *Ratanhia*. It is a powerful astringent, and tonic, and is very efficacious in debility and relaxation, in chronic diarrhœa, and passive hæmorrhages, or dysentery. It is much used in the manufacture of Port Wine, and in some cases with Logwood, to which it gives its rich red colour, and astringency. It may be administered in infusion; half an ounce of the root bruised to six ounces of boiling water; and by decoction, by boiling two ounces of the bruised root in a pint of distilled water; Dose of each from one to two ounces. The tincture is very useful. Take a tea-spoonful or two in water, two or three times a day.

RHODODENDRON.

This is a well-known beautiful garden shrub. It belongs to the natural order *Ericæe.* They all possess medicinal properties. The juice is acrid, and to some extent, narcotic. Hence the ancients said, that the honey obtained by the bees from the species, *Azalea Pontica*, made those mad who ate it. In Siberia, the *Rhododendron Chrysanthemum* is used as a remedy in rheumatism; an infusion of the leaves is taken, which causes a creeping or pricking sensation, which gradually subsides, and with it the rheumatic pains. It is good in palsy and syphilis. Those grown in our gardens have the same effect.

But skill, and caution are requisite in the use of their narcotic properties. Beautiful ornaments of gardens and shrubberries, they are redolent with poison.

RHUBARB,—BASTARD.

It is also called the Great Round Leaved Dock. It is the *Garden Rhubarb*, which every body knows. And what is said of the virtues of the Foreign Rhubarb, may be said of this *in degree.* Culpeper has written many absurd things about Rhubarb. I will not disfigure this book with them; but extract the best. The juice of the leaves or roots or the decoction of them in vinegar, heals scabs and running sores. A decoction of the seed eases pains in the stomach, and strengthens it, by increasing the appetite. The root strongly decocted is a good wash for scrofulous sores, &c. And taken inwardly, it removes obstructions of the liver, and cools the blood. In short Garden Rhubarb differs not from the Foreign, except the latter is more powerful.

Garden Rhubarb, used as food, has a slight aperient action upon the bowels. In some cases, this may be beneficial; but those who have tender bowels had better abstain from it. Some mix with it a little ground Ginger in puddings, pies, &c., which counteracts that tendency. It is a very wholesome and cooling diet. Its agreeable acid depends on the presence of the oxalic (slightly) and malic acids, which it abundantly contains. Persons subject to urinary irritation should take it very sparingly, or not at all.

RHUBARB,—FOREIGN.

This is sold by Druggists in the root, or the root powdered. It is one of the most useful drugs. The species of *Rheum* which produce it are thought to be *Rheum Palmatum, Undulatum, Raponiticum,* and *Australe.* It principally grows in Chinese Tartary, and is gathered in summer from plants six years old. A portion of this Rhubarb goes to China, the remainder passes through Russia, and is known in this country as Russian or Turkey Rhubarb. This is the best. It is in roundish pieces, of a yellow reddish colour on the outside, soft and easily reducible, having many streaks of a beautiful bright red colour. It has generally a hole in the middle, as it is the custom to string them when newly gotten, in order to dry the pieces. It is also cultivated in Oxfordshire; and that is the kind sold by men dressed up as Turks as the genuine Rhubarb. Some of this is very good; yet so powerful and unreasonable is prejudice, that very little of it can be sold.

Few medicines are more valuable or safer. It is a mild and effectual aperient, the action depending upon the amount of the dose. It rarely gripes; it has a beneficial tonic action upon the stomach. It is astringent, and therefore has a little tendency to constipate after its purgative effect is over. Dr. Graham says, "In the dose of one, two, or three grains, twice or thrice a day, it acts as a valuable stomachic, stimulating the stomach, increasing the appetite, and promoting a healthy flow of bile, and is of much service in *indigestion*, *low spirits*, *jaundice*, and a weakened relaxed state of the bowels. It acts chiefly on the stomach and first intestines, and in these complaints may be advantageously combined with soap, dried subcarbonate of soda, ipecacuanha, or extract of gentian. A pill of two grains of rhubarb, one of ipecacuanha powder, and one of soap, repeated three or four times a-day, is sometimes of superior benefit in indigestion, and bilious complaints, especially of elderly persons.

Rhubarb may be taken alone as an aperient, in doses from ten to thirty grains, mingled with water, or made into pills. Some persons carry the root with them, and chew it occasionally, and this is a good way of taking it. Where the bowels are sluggish, it makes an excellent dinner pill, combined with ginger and a little Castile soap. Rhubarb is very useful in a lax state of the bowels, as it expels any acrid matter that may be offending the bowels, before it acts as an astringent. It strengthens the intestinal canal, and therefore it is a safe and valuable purgative for children, "in whom," as Dr. Graham says, "that canal generally possesses a great degree of relaxation, aud morbid irritability." "When it is intended to act on the bowels, it should be given in conjunction with about fifteen grains of super-sulphate of potash, which covers its taste, and causes it to act more readily and with greater certainty."

Gregory's Powder is valuable, as a stomachic, and mild aperient, very advantageous to both adults and children. Composed thus:—Rhubarb, 2 parts, Calcined Magnesia, 4 parts, Ginger, 1 part. It may be taken in simple water, or in water and a few drops of sal-volatile, which will increase its stimulant and tonic properties. It should not be taken regularly, as the quantity of magnesia might irritate the coats of the stomach, and bring on diarrhœa.

The *Compound Rhubarb Pill*, is a safe and valuable aperient. Rhubarb, 4 drachms; Aloes in powder 3 drachms; Myrrh in powder, 2 drachms; Hard soap, scraped, ½ a drachm; Oil of carraway, ½ a drachm. Make up with treacle or mucilage.

The *Tincture of Rhubarb* is one of the best stomachics known. Made thus:—2½ ounces sliced rhubarb; saffron, 3 drachms; liquorice, bruised, 6 drachms; proof spirit, two pints; macerate for a week, and strain.

Extract of Rhubarb, dose, 10 to 20 grains. The *Infusion* is made by macerating 3 drachms of the sliced roots in 1 pint of boiling water for 2 hours. Dose, a wineglassfull. It will not keep.

Syrup of Rhubarb is made with Sugar, &c. It is excellent for young children. Dose 1 to 2 drachms—All may be obtained at the Druggists.

The powder of Rhubarb sprinkled on foul indolent ulcers excites them to a healthy action.

RHUBARB,—MONK'S.

DESCRIPTION.—*Lapathum sativum, vel patientia.*—It is also called Garden Patience. It bears the name of Rhubarb on account of its aperient properties. It has large tall stalks, set with broad and long fair green leaves, not dented. The tops of the stalks are divided into many small branches, bear reddish or purplish flowers, and seed, like dock seed. The root is long, great and yellow, like the wild docks, and if it be a little dried, showeth less store of discoloured veins than the Bastard Rhubarb when it is dry. Its virtues also are not so strong.

RICE.

Oryza Sativa.—This is a tropical plant, and it is well-known. As an article of food, Rice is very nutritious, easily digested, and therefore suitable for delicate stomachs. As it has no laxative effect, it is very suitable for those persons who have tender bowels. Rice water is good for those whose stomach and bowels are subject to irritation. It should be made in the same way as Barley-water; a little sugar and lemon-peel may be added to improve the flavour, and a little isinglass to render it more astringent. When intended to correct relaxed bowels, it should be used ground. It is not so nutritious as wheat, &c., yet it affords sustenance to about three-fourths of the inhabitants of the globe. It should always be well-cooked, otherwise it will not be so digestible. The property of Rice, intending to confine the bowels, renders it a valuable food for sick persons so requiring it. For young persons and invalids, nothing is so good as puddings made of Rice. Softened, and then boiled in milk, and sweetened, it is very agreeable.

ROCK CRESS.

Description.—*Arabis Hirsuta.*—It is also called Swine's Cress. It is a small wild plant, growing in fields and gardens. The stalks are five inches long, firm and thick, reposing on the ground, much branched, and full of leaves. The leaves direct from the root are long, and deeply divided; those on the stalks are smaller. The flowers are small and white, standing among the leaves, at the tops of the branches.

Medicinal Virtues.—A decoction of the plant is a good diuretic, powerful, but very safe. The juice may be expressed and taken as a remedy for the scurvy, the jaundice, and all inward obstructions. It is a good Salad herb, and some persons cultivate it in the garden for that purpose.

ROCKET.

DESCRIPTION.—*Reseda Sativa*.—The Garden-Rocket being rather used as a salad herb than for any medicinal purpose, I shall speak of the common wild Rocket only. The common wild Rocket has longer and narrower leaves, more divided into slender cuts and jags on both sides the middle rib than the garden kinds have; of a sad green colour, from which rise divers stalks two or three feet high, sometimes set with the like leaves, but smaller upwards, branched from the middle into several stiff stalks, bearing yellow flowers, of four leaves each, as the others are, which afterwards yield small reddish seed, in small long pods, of a more bitter and hot biting taste than the garden kinds, as the leaves are also.

MEDICINAL VIRTUES.—The Garden rocket works by urine, and is good against the scurvy. The wild Rockets should not be used alone. A decoction sweetened promotes digestion, and relieves cough, and destroys worms in children. An infusion of the leaves made into a syrup causes expectoration, and relieves cough and difficult breathing, The seed mixed with honey, and used on the face, cleanses the skin from morphew, and used with vinegar, takes away freckles and redness in the face, or other parts.

WINTER ROCKET, OR CRESSES.

DESCRIPTION.—*Reseda Luteola*.—The winter rocket is a different plant from the former. It has rather large sad green leaves lying upon the ground, torn or cut in various parts, like Rocket or turnip leaves, with smaller pieces next the bottom, and broad at the ends, which abide all Winter, from which rise up several small round stalks, full of branches, bearing many small yellow flowers of four leaves a-piece, after which come small pods, with reddish seed in them. The root is rather stringy. It grows in gardens and fields, and by the way-sides.

MEDICINAL VIRTUES. It provokes urine, helps strangury, and expels gravel and the stone. It is good for the scurvy, and found by experience to be a singular good wound herb to cleanse inward wounds; the juice or decoction being drank, or outwardly applied to wash them, will prevent dead flesh from growing, and heal them by astringency.

ROSA SOLIS, OR SUN-DEW.

DESCRIPTION.—*Drosera Anglica.*— It is also called Red-rot, and Youth wort. It has various small, round, hollow leaves, rather greenish, but full of certain red hairs, which make them seem red, each standing upon its own foot-stalk, reddish and hairy. The leaves are moist in the hottest day. Among these leaves rise up slender stalks, reddish also, three or four fingers high, bearing small white knobs or flowers one above another, after which in the heads are contained small seeds. The root is a few small hairs. It grows in bogs and wet places, and sometimes in moist woods.

MEDICINAL VIRTUES. Rosa Solis is good for those that have a salt rheum distilling on the lungs, which induces consumption, and therefore the distilled water in wine, is fit for such to drink. The same water is held to be good for all diseases of the lungs, as phthisic, wheezings, shortness of breath, or cough; and also to heal ulcers in the lungs; and it is good for nervous fainting spirits. The leaves outwardly applied to the skin, will raise blisters, which has caused some to think it dangerous to be taken inwardly; but many things will draw blisters, yet are not dangerous to be taken inwardly. It is reckoned a great cordial, good against convulsions, hysteric disorders, and trembling of the limbs.

ROSEMARY.

DESCRIPTION.—*Rosmarinus.*—It is too well known to need description.

MEDICINAL VIRTUES.—The flowers and tops are used medicinally. They contain a fragrant volatile oil, which is stimulant, antispasmodic, and carminative. It is an agreeable addition to more active medicines. The dose of this oil is from 2 to 3 drops as a carminative. The oil may be added to liniments, as a fragrant stimulant. A spirit of Rosemary is made, which may be used as an antispasmodic in doses of 30 drops, in water, or on sugar. If the flowery tops of Rosemary are used as a tea, they are excellent against headache, tremblings of the limbs, and all nervous disorders. A conserve made of the same has similar power. Beat up the fresh gathered tops with three times their weight of sugar. A strong decoction applied to the temples removes fainting, and taken inwardly, it expels wind, and strengthens the stomach. It tends to enliven the whole frame. It removes obstructions of the liver, and promotes digestion. It is very good against the jaundice. The leaves and flowers burnt are a good disinfectant. Both the flowers and leaves are good against the whites, if they be daily taken. Smoking the dried leaves shred, like tobacco, is a remedy for cough, phthisic, or consumption, by warming and drying the thin distillations which cause those diseases. The leaves make a good fomentation, made into ointment, or oil, for cold benumbed joints, sinews, or members, which are much relieved thereby.

ROSES.

The Rose is esteemed the Queen of flowers. Its botanical name is *Rosa*, of the natural order *Rosaceæ*. The varieties of this plant are very numerous. Three kinds are used medicinally, as follows:—

The Dog Rose, *Rosa Canina*. It grows wild in hedges, and is well known as the Wild Rose. The fruit is chiefly used. The *Hips* are made into a confection, which is used as a vehicle for other remedies. It is pleasant and acidulous, and allays thirst caused by fever. The confection is thus made, The pulp is separated from the skins and seeds, and beat up into a conserve with sugar. Rub them well together. It is astringent, and very useful in diarrhœa, dysentery, and coughs. The flowers gathered in the bud and dried are more astringent than the Red Roses. A tea made strong of these dried buds and some of them taken in powder, checks profuse menstruation. The seeds dried and powdered, work by urine gently, and are good against gravel.

The CABBAGE, or *Hundred-leaved Rose*, *Rosa Centifolia*. Of this species Rose Water is made by distilling the leaves, or by mixing with water the volatile oil. It is a useful vehicle, a good eye-water, and much used in lotions. The petals make an excellent laxative Syrup.

The DAMASCUS ROSE, *Rosa Damascena*. The flowers are used. From them is obtained the delicious perfume Otto, or Attar of Roses, of great celebrity throughout Europe, and Eastern lands especially. The Syrup is an excellent purge for children. There is not a better purgative for adults than this Syrup. Rose Water is also distilled from this kind.

The RED OR FRENCH ROSE, *Rosa Gallica*. The flowers are used. Gather them when in bud; cut from the husks, without the white bottoms, and dry. The conserve of Red Roses is made of these buds; they are beaten up with three times their weight of sugar. The infusion is made thus:—Dried Rose leaves, 3 drachms, on which pour boiling water, 1 pint; then add dilute Sulphuric Acid, or Elixor of Vitriol 1½ drachms; macerate for 40 minutes in a covered vessel, strain, and add 6 drachms of lump sugar. Thoroughly mix.—The infusion is a useful beverage in fevers. It is an excellent gargle, and vehicle for many active remedies. It is given with advantage in Consumptive sweats, and fever; and with additional acid, and nitrate of Potass, in uterine and pulmonary hœmorrhages, or spitting of blood. The Infusion also strengthens the stomach, prevents vomitings, and restrains dysentery.

Some affirm that the White Roses possess equal virtures, and are rather more astringent. The leaves ground, and made into an ointment with lard, and a minute portion of Laudanum, are curative of the piles, and other inflamed parts. Rose leaves and Mint, heated and applied to the stomach, stay vomitings and strengthens a weak stomach. They form a good cooling fomentation for inflamed and pained parts.

RUE,—GARDEN.

Ruta Graveolens.—It is so common in gardens, that it requires no description. It was anciently valued for its medicinal virtues; but has of late been little esteemed. This is a mistake; for if valuable at one time, why not now? Strange if herbs are to be subjected to "the fashions." It acts as a stimulant, and antispasmodic; but in large doses it is narcotic. It is very useful in hysteria, and in flatulent colic. It has been found useful in infantile convulsions, and as a destroyer of worms, especially the thread-worms, used as an injection. In accumulations of flatulence in the bowels, *tympanitis*, a strong infusion of Rue given as an injection, is of great use. In suppressed menstruation, when stimulants are required, the Rue clyster is of great use. Boerhaave says that mixed with wine and salt, it stops gangrene, restores vitality to the part, prevents suppuration and heals the wound. Medical men sadly neglect Rue, as a medicinal agent. Why go to foreign lands when we have remedies at our doors? A decoction of it relieves the colic, and all inward pains. The leaves bruised and well rubbed on the parts, relieves pain, sciatica, inflammation of the chest. Some of the ancients believed that it arrested generation. They regarded it too as anti-pestilential, and the judges had their noses regaled with this fœtid plant; they believed that Mithridrate, in which Rue has a principal share, repelled all poisons. Rue, and honey, and the gall of a cock, they said, cured dimness of sight. An ointment, made of the juice with lard, oil of roses, and a little vinegar, cures erysipelas, running sores in the head, and ulcers. The antidote used by Mithridates, every morning fasting, to secure himself from any poison or infection was this: take twenty leaves of Rue, a little salt, two walnuts and two figs, beaten into a mess, with twenty juniper berries, the quantity appointed for every day. Another electuary is made thus: take of nitre, pepper, and cummin-seed, of each equal parts; of the leaves of Rue clean picked, as much in weight as all the rest, beat them well together, and put as much honey as will make it up into an electuary, (but you must first steep your cummin-seed in vinegar twenty-four hours, and then rather roast it in a hot oven) and it is a remedy for pains in the chest or stomach, of the spleen, belly, or side, by wind or stitches, of the liver by obstructions, of the reins and bladder by the stopping of urine, and it reduces corpulency. The fresh leaves have been applied to the temples to relieve headache. A decoction of the herb in wine, used as a gargle, is a good remedy for scurvy in the gums.

RUE,—MEADOW.

DESCRIPTION.—*Ruta Pratense.*—It is also called Spurious Rhubarb, or Rue-Weed. Meadow Rue rises from a yellow stringy root, much spreading in the ground, shooting new sprouts round about, with many green stalks, two feet high, crested all the length of them, set with joints, with many large leaves on them, above as well as below, divided into smaller leaves, dented in the forepart of them, of a red green colour on the upper side, and pale green underneath; at the top of the stalk the branches have two, three, or four small heads or buttons, which eventually shoot forth a tuft of pale greenish yellow threads, which falling away, small three-cornered pods succeed, containing small, long and round seed. The plant has a strong unpleasant scent. It grows in the borders of moist meadows, and ditch-sides, and flowers in July and August.

MEDICINAL VIRTUES.—Dioscorides says, that this herb bruised and applied, perfectly heals old sores, and so does distilled water of the herb and flowers. It is used by some among other pot herbs to open the body; but the roots washed clean, and boiled in ale and drank, purge more than the leaves, yet very gently. The root boiled in water, and the parts of the body troubled with vermin and lice, washed therewith while it is warm, destroys them utterly.

RUPTURE WORT.

DESCRIPTION.—*Herniaria Glabra.*—It spreads many thready branches upon the ground, about a span long, divided into many smaller parts, full of small joints, very thick together; the stalks lying on the ground form a kind of circular figure. The leaves are very small, nearly oval, of a pale green; they stand two at each joint, and are also of a pale green, tinged yellow. The flowers are very small, and yellow, scarcely discernible from the stalks and leaves. The root is very long and small, and deep in the ground. It grows in dry, sandy, and rocky places, and is cultivated in gardens.

MEDICINAL VIRTUES.—It has not its name in vain; for it is found by experience to cure the rupture, not only in children, but also in adults, if the disease be not too inveterate, by taking a drachm of the powder of the dried herb every day in wine, or a decoction for some days together. The juice or distilled water of the green herb, relieves fluxes, vomiting and gonorrhœa. It relieves those who have the strangury, or the stone or gravel in the bladder. It removes stitches in the sides, griping pains, obstructions of the liver. It cures yellow jaundice, and kills worms in children. The bruised herb bound on wounds, heals them. It is a very good remedy for all wounds and sores.

RYE.

Rye is one of the cereals whose cultivation has been a great blessing to man. Its botanical name is *Secale Cereale.* It produces a nutritious flour having less bran and more farina than wheat has though darker in colour. It is not so nutritious as wheat, but it is easier to digest, and it slightly promotes the action of the bowels. It makes excellent poultices for imposthumes, boils, and other swellings. Rye-meal moistened with vinegar, placed between a cloth, and well heated in an oven, and applied to the head, very much relieves its pains. *Ergot of Rye*, or the Spurred Rye, is a diseased production which grows on the ear of Rye. It is of a poisonous nature. This substance has however been employed as a child-bed remedy. Its great influence over the uterine system is undoubted. It is the only medicine now employed as an excitent of the womb, or to rouse the energies of that organ in cases of lingering labour. Dose from five to twenty-five grains in powder. It is good also for Leucorrhœa. Matthiolus says that the ashes of Rye straw steeped in water twenty-four hours, will cure chapped hands.

SAFFRON.

It is produced from the *Crocus Sativa*, or the blue autumn flowering crocus, cultivated in this country, and on the continent. Saffron is sold by the druggists either in the form of *Hay Saffron*, or of "Cake Saffron." The former is composed of the loose dried stigmata. It is used as medicine, and as colouring matter. It was at one time a favourite stimulant and antispasmodic. It is now given when scarlatina, or the measles are suspected, as an expulsive, to hasten the eruption. It is good in asthma, cough, and difficulty of breathing, and is a good remedy for the jaundice. It must be used as a decoction.

SAGE.

Salvia Officinalis.—The common garden Sage has tonic properties, as its aromatic odour and bitter taste indicate. It is often made into tea, and is tonic, astringent, and carminative; as a gargle with vinegar, or honey and alum, it is good for inflamed throats, or relaxed uvula. It removes obstructions of the kidneys, and of the menstrual flux. Orpheus says, three spoonfuls of the juice of Sage, taken fasting with a little honey, arrests spitting or vomiting of blood. These pills are much commended: take of spikenard, ginger, of each two drachms, of the seed of Sage, eight drachms, of long pepper, twelve drachms, all being powdered, add as much juice of Sage as may make them into pills, taking a drachm every morning fasting, and at night, drinking water after them. Mathiolus says, it is very good for pains in the head, coming of cold and rheumatic humours; for all pains in the joints, and for the falling sickness, lethargy, palsy, and is of much use for diseases of the chest or breast. The leaves of Sage and nettles bruised together, and laid upon imposthumes behind the ears, cures them.

The juice of Sage taken in warm water relieves hoaresness and cough. Sage taken with wormwood is good for the bloody-flux. And with other hot herbs, Sage is boiled to bathe the body and legs in the Summer time, especially to warm cold joints or sinews, troubled with cramp, and to strengthen the parts. The volatile oil is sometimes prescribed in doses of 1 or 2 drops. It is a useful ingredient in embrocations for rheumatism. An infusion is very cooling in fevers, a little lemon-juice being added. It cleanses and purifies the blood.

SAGE,—WOOD.

DESCRIPTION.—*Salvia Agrestis.*—It is also called Wood Germander. It rises up with square hoary stalks, two feet high, with two leaves at every joint, like other Sage leaves, but smaller, softer, whiter and rounder, and a little dented about the edges, and smelling rather stronger. At the tops of the stalks and branches stand the flowers, on a slender large spike, turning all one way when they blow, and are of a pale and whitish colour, smaller than Sage, but hooded and gaping like them. The seed is blackish and round; the root is long and stringy. It grows in woods and by wood sides, and in bye lanes.

MEDICINAL VIRTUES.—The decoction of Wood Sage promotes the flow of urine, and perspiration, and reduces swellings in the flesh. The decoction of the green herb, made with wine, is a safe and sure remedy for those who by falls, bruises, or blows, suspect some vein to be inwardly broken, to disperse and void the congealed blood, and consolidate the veins. The juice of the herb, or the powder dried, is good for moist ulcers and sores, to dry them and cause them to heal more speedily. It is no less effectual in green wounds.

SAGO.

Sago is prepared from the pith of several species of Palm, especially those of the genus *Sagus Lævis.* The granular form is given to it by passing it when half dry through a coarse sieve. The process of refining it, and giving it a pearly lustre, is attributed to the Chinese. Thus prepared, it is called *Pearl Sago;* this is reckoned the best, yet many aver that the browner and coarser kinds possess the most nutriment. Sago is nearly pure starch, and closely resembles Arrow-root, for which it is a cheap substitute. Sago affords very little nourishment, and is, therefore well adapted for invalids labouring under acute diseases. It has demulcent properties, which render it very useful in irritated state of the bowels and rectum. Where inflammatory action is slight, a very small portion of wheaten flour may be added for the sake of nutriment.

Sago is made into puddings, boiled in milk and cooked a variety of ways. Sago Posset is an excellent cordial, where acute diseases have left the body debilitated. Made thus:—Put 2 ounces of Sago to 1 quart of water, and boil until a mucilage is formed; then rub half an ounce of lump sugar on the rind of a lemon, and put it, and a tea-spoonful of tincture of ginger into half a pint of Sherry Wine; add this mixture to the Sago mucilage, and boil the whole five minutes. A wine-glassful may be taken every four or five hours. But during sickness Sago Gruel must be made of Sago and water only, except a little sugar and lemon juice to render it more palatable.

SAMPHIRE.

DESCRIPTION.—*Crithmum Maritimum.*—A plant common about sea coasts, very much like fennel, but not so tall; it has been called sea-fennel. It grows on rocks that are often saturated with sea-water. It has a tender green stalk about two feet high, branching forth almost from the bottom, and stored with thick and almost round leaves, of a deep green colour, sometimes more on a stalk, and sappy, and of a pleasant, hot, and spicy taste. At the top of the stalks and branches stand umbels of white flowers, which produce seed like fennel-seed, but larger. The root is large, white, and long, and of a hot, spicy taste.

MEDICINAL VIRTUES.—The leaves are used fresh, but those nearest the root are the best. It is diuretic, and tonic. The juice of the fresh leaves operate very powerfully by urine, and is good against the gravel and stone, menstrual suppression, and the jaundice. It is excellent for promoting digestion. It makes a fine pickle, which was formerly highly esteemed. The sale of it has been almost stopped by adulteration.

SANICLE.

DESCRIPTION.—*Sanicula Europæa.*—A pretty wild plant growing in woods and under shady hedges. It has many large round leaves standing upon long brownish stalks, every one deeply cut, or divided into five or six parts, and some of these also cut like the leaf of crow's-foot, or dove's-foot, and finely dented at the edges, smooth, and of a dark shining colour, and reddish about the brim; from which rise up small, round, green stalks, without any joint or leaf, except at the top, where it branches into flowers, having a leaf divided into three or four parts at that joint with the flowers, which are small and white, starting out of small round greenish yellow heads, in a tuft, in which afterwards are the seeds, which are small round burs, almost like the leaves of clevers, and stick in the same manner upon any thing they touch. The root is fibrous.

Medicinal Virtues. It heals green wounds speedily, or any ulcers, imposthumes, or inward bleeding, and it is good for tumours; for the decoction or powder taken in beer, and the juice applied outwardly, dissipates the humours; and there is not found any herb that can give such instant help, when the disease falls upon the lungs or throat. It is good for healing malignant ulcers in the mouth and throat, by gargling with the decoction of the leaves and roots made in water, and a little honey. It has been celebrated for the cure of ulcers, and ruptures.

There is another Sanicle, called *Yorkshire Sanicle*, or *Butterwort or Marsh Violet;* and there are four varieties of it. It grows wild on wet bogs on the moors in the north of England and Scotland, on the mountainous parts. This and its fellow the Bladderwort, are, on account of their beauty, cultivated in some gardens. The Butterwort is easily known by its violet-coloured flowers, and its thick plaintain-shaped leaves growing at the root. The remarkable greasy feel of the leaves, have caused it to be applied to chapped hands and sore nipples. It is applicable to all kinds of sores.

SARACEN'S CONFOUND

Description.—*Saracenica.*—It is also called Saracen's Woundwort. Sometimes it grows with brownish stalks, and also green, to a man's height, having narrow green leaves snipped about the edges, like those of the peach-tree, or willow leaves. The tops of the stalks have many yellow star-like flowers, standing in green heads. The seed is rather long and brown, downy when ripe, and is blown away. The root is fibrous. The taste is strong and unpleasant, and so is the smell. It grows in moist and wet grounds, by wood-sides, and in the moist places of shadowy groves and by the water side.

MEDICINAL VIRTUES.—Among the Germans this wound herb is preferred before all others of the same quality. Being boiled in wine and drank, it reduces inflammation of the liver, and frees the gall from obstructions; and therefore it is good for yellow jaundice, dropsy, inward ulcers of the reins, mouth, or throat, and inward wounds and bruises. Steeped in wine, and then distilled, it is good to ease gnawings in the stomach, or other pains of the body. A decoction in water is good for the ague; and it is very effectual to heal any green wound, or sore or ulcer. Briefly, the medicinal virtues of Bugle or Sanicle belong also to Saracen's Confound.

SARSAPARILLA.

Smilax Sarsaparilla.—The Sarsaparilla plant is a native of the West Indies, Mexico, and South America. It has a mild bitterish and glutinous taste, not disagreeable. The root is used. It consists of one head, from which many fibres, or small roots proceed about the thickness of a goose quill. These are the parts producing Sarsaparilla.

This drug is known to possess tonic, demulcent, and alterative properties; and sometimes diuretic and diaphoretic. It possesses the power of improving the general state of the system, and restoring the vigour of the constitution when broken down by long protracted disease. That these beneficial effects result from the use of Sarsaparilla, Dr. A. Thompson says his experience has fully demonstrated. It is necessary to give it in large doses—from half a pint to a pint, for instance, of the decoction should be taken in the course of the day, and continued for weeks. The decoction has been regarded as a cure for lues venerea. Now, strong decoctions of it, made with 3 ounces of the root to a quart of water, are much used in those disorders.

A small quantity of antimonial wine, (from 30 to 60 drops to the quart,) to these decoctions, which much increases their efficacy. These decoctions are found to be of great use in purifying the blood, and resolving obstructions in scorbutic and scrofulous cases, and in cutaneous eruptions, and many other diseases. "I have known," says Dr. Thornton, "two obstinate swellings that had resisted the effects of other remedics for twelve months, cured by drinking a quart of this decoction daily for some weeks.

Dr. Graham says, "It is given with advantage in various *obstinate internal chronic diseases, and in swellings, ulcerations*, and other local maladies, depending upon *constitutional indisposition.* I have fonnd it of inestimable value in cases of extreme irritation and debility of the mucus membrane of the digestive organs. In *nocturnal pains* in the limbs, *painful enlargements* of the knee and elbow-joints, *nodes*, and *cutaneous ulcerations*, arising from a *syphilitic* taint, it is superior to any other remedy," The Doctor instances two cases in which Sarsaparilla was the means of saving life.

The powder of Sarsaparilla, is an invaluable alterative, more efficacious than the decoction. From one to two drachms may be taken in water, twice or thrice a day. The Liquid extract, which contains a portion of spirit, will keep any length of time; dose from half a drachm to 2 drachms in water. The Compound Decoction is made thus :—5 ounces of Sarsaparilla chips in 4 pints of water; let it gently simmer for 2 hours; take out the chips, bruise and replace them in the water; boil down to two pints. While boiling add Sassafras, sliced; Guiacum wood, rasped; and Liquorice-root, bruised, of each 10 drachms; Mezereon roots 3 drachms, boil for 10 or 15 minutes, then strain. The Concentrated Essence is the most convenient and portable form for its administration, and, from the nicety and caution observed in evaporating, it will rarely disappoint the hopes of the invalid.

SASSAFRAS.

A beautiful tree, native of America, the wood of which is used in medicine. *Sassafras Officinale* belongs to the natural order *Lauraceæ.* It has a sweet aromatic taste, and an odour like that of fennel, owing to the presence of a volatile oil, in which its virtues chiefly reside, though it contains fatty matter, resin, gum, albumen, wax, &c.

It is best taken in infusion, or tea; it is a very pleasant beverage; it promotes sweat; and is a remedy for scurvy, and foulness of the blood, of which it is a great purifier. It has been found to recruit exhausted strength more rapidly than either cocoa, chocolate, or any farinaceous substances, and to sit lighter on the stomach, than either animal or vegetable jellies. It is a most nutritious beverage; "but the scandal of its being good in *Venereal cases*, is a great detriment to its credit, which prevents good being done by it; for it is a first-rate sweetener of the blood."

SAUCE ALONE.

Description.—*Erysimum Alliaria.*—It is also called Jack by the Hedge. The lower leaves are rounder thon those towards the tops of the stalks, and are set singly on the joints, being round and broad, pointed at the ends, dented at the edges a little like nettle leaves, but of a fresher green colour, hot rough or pricking: the flowers are white, growing at the tops of the stalks one above another. The seeds are in pods, round and blackish. The root is stringy and thready. The plant being bruised, smells of garlic, and tastes hot and sharp, like rocket. It grows under walls, by hedge-sides, and pathways in fields.

Medicinal Virtues.—This is eaten by many country people as sauce to their salt fish, and wonderfully warms the stomach, and promotes digestion. The juice boiled with honey is as good as hedge mustard for cough, to cut and expectorate tough phlegm. The seed bruised and boiled in wine, is a good remedy for colic, or stone, being drank warm. The leaves also or the seed boiled, is good to be used in clysters to ease the pains of the stone.

SAVINE.

Description.—*Juniperus Sabina.*—It rises two or three feet high. Its leaves are numerous, and firmly pointed. The flowers are very small, of a yellowish colour, producing a blackish purple berry. It is a native of the south of Europe, and of the Levant; but grows in English gardens.

Medicinal Virtues.—It has powerful cathartic, emmenagogue, and stimulant properties, acting especially on the uterus of the female. Those who take it for the purpose of abortion greatly endanger their lives; in many cases it has ruined the constitution, and in some produced instant death; for taking large doses for that purpose, it is an irritant poison, proving fatal. The herb powdered, and mixed with honey, makes a good dressing for all kinds of sores, carbuncles, ringworms, scrofulous runnings at the ears, neck, &c. Dr. Cullen observes, "Savine is a very acrid substance, and I have often, on that account, not employed it in the quantity to render it emmenagogue. Yet it indicates a more powerful determination to the uterus than any other plant I have employed. But it requires *a great deal of caution*. Dr. Home had great success with it; for in five cases of amenorrhœa at Edinburgh Royal Infirmary, four were cured by Savine, which he gave in powder from a scruple to a drachm twice a day. He says it is well suited to the weak, but improper in plethoric habits. It makes an excellent *drawing* ointment for issues, as under:—Fresh Savine leaves separated from the stalks, and bruised, quarter of a pound; hog's lard, 1 pound; yellow wax, quarter of a pound. Boil the leaves in the lard until they become crisp, then filter, with expression; add the wax, and melt them together.

SAVORY.

Saluria Hortensis.—There are two kinds, Winter and Summer Savory. It is well known as a kitchen garden plant.

Medicinal Virtues.—It is a sovereign remedy for the colic, and the Iliac Passion; keep it by you all the year, keep it dry, make conserves and syrups of it for your use, and take notice that the Summer kind is the best. They are both of them hot and dry, especially the Summer kind, which is sharp in taste, expelling wind from the stomach and bowels. It is very beneficial to take during pregnancy. It is a good expectorant, removing tough phlegm from the chest, and improving the breathing. The juice dropped into the eyes, removes dimness of sight, if it proceed from thin cold humours distilled from the brain. The juice heated with oil of Roses, and dropped into the ears, removes noise and singing, and deafness. Outwardly applied with wheat flour, like a poultice, it gives ease to them. It also takes away the pain that comes by stinging of bees, wasps &c.

SAXIFRAGE,—BURNET.

DESCRIPTION.—*Pimpinella Saxifraga.* It grows with long stalks of winged leaves, set directly opposite one to another on both sides, each being rather broad, and a little dented at the edges, of a sad green colour. At the top of the stalks stand umbels of white snowy flowers, after which come small blackish seed. The root is long and whitish. The lesser Burnet Saxifrage has much finer leaves than the former, and very small, set one against another, deeply jagged about the edges, and of the same colour as the former. The umbels of the flowers are white, and the seed and root very small. The taste is very hot. These grow in moist meadows, hid among the grass. They flower in July.

MEDICINAL VIRTUES.—They are hot as pepper. They have the same properties as Parsley ; but in provoking urine, easing the pains thereof, and of wind and colic, are more effectual, the roots or seed being used either in powder, or in decoction. They are diuretic, and good against gravel and stone. They assist to expectorate. • It has been used for the removal of tumours and obstructions of the glands, and in scorbutic and cutaneous diseases. The juice of the herb dropped into the most grievous wounds of the head, dries up their moisture, and heals them quickly. Some women use the distilled water to take away freckles or spots on the skin or face.

SAXIFRAGE.—WHITE.

DESCRIPTION.—*Saxifraga Alba.*—The common white Saxifrage has a few small reddish kernels of roots covered with skin, lying among small blackish fibres, which send forth round, yellow green leaves, greyish underneath, lying above the ground, unevenly dented about the edges, and hairy, each upon a little footstalk, from whence rise brownish, hairy, green stalks, two or three feet high, with round leaves, rather branched at the top, on which stand pretty large white flowers, of five leaves apiece, with yellow threads in the middle, standing in a brownish green husk. After the flowers comes a round hard head, forked at the top, containing small black seeds. The grains of the root are usually called the White Saxifrage-seed, and so used. It grows in the dry corners of meadows, and grassy sandy places. It usually flowers in May.

MEDICINAL VIRTUES.—It is said to expel stone and gravel from the bladder, to relieve strangury. The decoction of the herb or roots in wine, or the powder of the small kernal root in wine. The distilled water of the whole herb, root and flowers, is most familiar to be taken. It cleanses the stomach and lungs from thick tough phlegm. There are not many better medicines to break the stone than this.

SCABIOUS.

DESCRIPTION.—*Scabiosa Succisa.*—There are several kinds of Scabious, but those here described are the most familiar.

Common field Scabious grows up with many hairy, soft, whitish green leaves, some of which are very small, a little jagged on the edges, others much rent and torn on the sides, and have threads in them, which upon breaking may be plainly seen; from which rise hairy green stalks, three or four feet high, with hairy green leaves deeply and finely divided and branched a little; they are naked and bare of leaves for a good space, but on the tops stand round heads of flowers, of a pale blueish colour. The flowers are the size of a small walnut, and composed of many little ones. The root is large, white, and thick, growing deep into the ground, and abides many years.

There is another sort of Field Scabious different in nothing from the former, but in being smaller.

The Corn Scabious differs little from the first, but it is larger in all respects, and the flowers more inclining to purple, and the root creeps under the crust of the earth.

The first grows usually in meadows. The second in dry fields, but not so plentifully as the former. The third in standing corn, or fallow fields. They flower in July, and August.

Medicinal Virtues.—Scabious is very effectual in the cure of coughs, shortness of breath, and all other diseases of the breast and lungs, digesting and expectorating cold phlegm. *Etmuller* extols it for " Asthma and Pleurisy, and inward abscesses, ulcers, and imposthumes. The decoction purifies the blood, and taken inwardly, and used as a wash externally, it is a first-rate remedy for cutaneous eruptions. Some make the decoction in wine. The green herb bruised and applied to any carbuncle or sore, is found by certain experience to dissolve and break it in three hours. The decoction removes pains and stitches in the side. The juice or decoction drank, takes away scabs and breakings out of the itch. The juice made into an ointment is effectual for the same purpose. The dried root given in powder, promotes sweat, and is beneficial in fevers. By its astringency it tends to heal all inward wounds. A syrup made of the juice and sugar, or honey has the same effect. The decoction of the herb and roots outwardly applied, reduces hard or cold swellings, and relieves shrunk sinews or veins, and it heals green wounds and sores. The juice of Scabious, with the powder of Borax and Samphire, cleanses the skin of the face, or other parts of the body, from freckles, pimples, morphew and leprosy. The head washed with the warm decoction, cleanses it from scurf, sores, dandriff, and itch.

SCAMMONY.

This purgative substance is the concrete gum of the Convolvulus Scammonium. It is imported from Smyrna. It is a powerful drastic purge, closely allied, in its operation, to jalop, but more active and irritating, yet not so nauseous.

It is used as a smart purge for children, especially for those who have worms, on account of the smallness of the dose necessary to produce its effect, the slight taste, and the energy of its operation. It is useful as a hydragogue in dropsies. As a vermifuge it might be combined with powdered Wormwood, or Tansy, &c. It is inadmissible, however, in inflammatory conditions of the alimentary canal.—The dose of the powder for adults is, from 5 to 10 grains; for children, from 2 to 5 grains. It should always be combined with an aromatic to prevent griping. The Compound Scammony Powder of the shops is the best; dose of it, for an adult, from 10 to 20 grains; and for children from six to twelve years old, half that quantity.

SCURVYGRASS.

Description.—*Cochlearia Officinalis.*—English Scurvygrass has many thick flat oblong leaves, smooth on the edges, and sometimes a little waved; sometimes plain, smooth and pointed, of a sad green, and sometimes a bluish colour, each standing by itself upon a long foot-stalk, brownish or greenish also, from which arise many slender stalks, bearing few leaves but longer and less than those near the root. The flowers stand at the tops of the stalks in little clusters; they are white, small, and bright. They are succeeded by short roundish, seed vessels. The root is white and fibrous. It grows wild on the sea coast, and also in gardens. It flowers in April and May.

Medicinal Virtues.—The plant possesses antiscorbutic and diuretic properties. It has wonderful efficacy to cleanse the blood, liver, and spleen. The juice, for this purpose, taken in Spring, every morning fasting, will answer this purpose. The decoction has the same effect; it opens obstructions, evacuates cold, clammy and phlegmatic humours from the liver and spleen, and restores the body to a more lively colour. Scurvygrass is considered a good wash for the mouth and gums in scurvy. It may be mixed with Seville Orange juice to make it more agreeable.

SELF-HEAL.

DESCRIPTION.—*Prunella Vulgaris.*—It is also called Carpenter's Herb, Hook-heal, and Sickle-wort.

Self-heal is a small, low creeping herb, having many small, roundish-pointed leaves, like leaves of wild mints, of a dark green colour, without dents on the edges; from which rise square hairy stalks, a foot high, which spread into branches with small leaves set thereon, up to the tops. The flowers are small, and of a bluish purple; they stand in a kind of short spikes, or heads; the cups of them are often purplish. The roots consist of many fibres downward, and spreading strings. The small stalks, with the leaves creeping on the ground, shoot forth fibres taking hold on the ground, whereby it is made a great tuft in a short time. It is found in woods and fields. It flowers in May.

MEDICINAL VIRTUES.—This herb is a curative of inward and outward wounds. As a decoction, or syrup, inwardly, and the juice of the roots and leaves alone, or made into an ointment, for external application for bruises and sores. As Self-heal is like Bugle in form, so also in its medicinal virtues. If it be accompanied with Bugle, Sanicle, and other wound-herbs, it will be more effectual to wash or inject into ulcers outwardly. Where it is necessary to repress the heat and sharpness of humours flowing to any sores, inflammations, or swellings, or to staunch the flow of blood in any wound, this is used with good success. It is a special remedy for all green wounds, to close and heal them. The juice used with oil of roses to anoint the temples and forehead, cures the head-ache, and the same mixed with honey of roses, cures ulcers in the mouth and throat. And the proverb of the Germans, French, and others, is verified in this, that he needs neither physician nor surgeon who has Self-heal and Sanicle to cure himself.

SENNA.

The leaves of different species of Cassia. It is a very old medicine, having been used by the Arabians. The plant is a native of Upper Egypt. It is also cultivated in India. Alexandrian Senna is most highly esteemed.

Senna Leaves are a very useful purgative, operating mildly, and yet effectually. The only inconvenience complained of in this drug is its tendency to gripe, and its sickly nauseous flavour. This may be obviated by the addition of an aromatic, as ginger, cinnamon, &c.; and its operation may be facilitated by drinking copiously of any warm mild diluent. The best form of administering it is that of watery infusion, two drachms being infused in 4 or 5 ounces of tepid or warm water, (it should never be boiled) to which add 3 or 4 drachms of compound tincture of cardamoms, or some aromatic, as stated before, to prevent griping. Sugar or manna, covers its taste, and makes it more agreeable to children. Dose from one to three ounces. It is often given in combination with Epsom Salt, Glauber's Salt, or Soluble Tartar. It should not be administered when irritation and fever are present, nor during pregnancy.

Black Draught;—Epsom Salt, ½ ounce, infusion of Senna, 1½ ounce, Tincture of Senna, 1 drachm, Syrup of Ginger, 1 drachm, Spirit of Salvolatile, ½ a drachm. Mix. Take according to age and constitution.—

An Infusion of Senna may be taken as under:—One ounce of Senna leaves infused in a pint, or more, of tepid water; strain, and add to it one ounce of Camphor mixture, which will neutralise its griping tendency. Four table-spoonfuls of this infusion, with a tea-spoonful, or rather more of Epsom Salt, is a good purgative.

Electuary of Senna.—Senna leaves, in fine powder, 4 ounces; pulp of French Prunes, 1℔.; pulp of tamarinds, 2 ounces.—molasses, 1½ pint; essential oil of Carraway, 2 drachms; boil the pulps in the Syrup to the thickness of honey; then add the powder; and when the mixture cools the oil; lastly, mix the whole intimately.

SERPENTARIA, OR SNAKE ROOT.

Aristolochia Serpentaria. **It is a native of America. We owe the knowledge of this medicine to the American Indians,**

who give it as a remedy for the poisonous bite of the Rattlesnake. It possesses great virtues. Dr. Tennant brought it into England, and it has been regarded as a powerful remedy in pleurisy, quinsy, and all other diseases where the blood is sizey. It was said to dissolve the dangerous texture better than all other known remedies. It is a warm cordial, aromatic, tonic, and acts as a diaphoretic. It is calculated to support vitality, and promote free perspiration in low and putrid fevers. The ague yields to Peruvian bark much sooner when it is combined with Serpentaria. It is also promotive of digestion; and wonderfully arrests gangrene or mortification, combined with Opium and other cordials.

It may be given in infusion by pouring 1½ pint of water on 1 ounce of the bruised root. Strain after 12 hours. Two tablespoonfuls to be taken three or four times a day.

English *Polygala*, Snake-root, or the common blue, or white-flowered Milkwort, has the same effects. They have been given in pleurisies with great effect.

SERVICE TREE.

Pyrus Domestica.—It is so well known in the place where it grows, that it needs no description.

MEDICINAL VIRTUES.—Services when they are mellow, stay fluxes, scouring, and casting, yet less than medlars. If they be dried before they are mellow, and kept all the year, they may be used in decoctions for the said purpose, either to drink or to bathe the parts requiring it; and are used to stay the bleeding of wounds, of the mouth or nose, to be applied to the forehead, and nape of the neck.

SHEPHERD'S PURSE.

DESCRIPTION.—*Thlaspi Bursa Pastoris.*—It is also called Shepherd's Scrip, Shepherd's Pouch, Toywort, Pickpurse, and Casewort. It is a very common plant, overrunning garden-beds, farm, and court yards. The leaves spread upon the ground, are long, rather broad, a little indented at the edges. The stalks are round, erect, 9 or 10 inches high, and have few leaves. The flowers stand at the tops in little clusters, they are small and white. The seed vessels are like a bag or pouch. The seeds are small, yellowish, and the roots are white.

Medicinal Virtues.—It is very astringent and glutinous. It is good for bleeding at the nose and spitting of blood, and in diarrhœas, dysenteries, and bloody urine. It may be applied with great success to cuts and fresh wounds; and made into a poultice, and applied to the wrists, it cures the ague; apply it before the fit comes on. The same is beneficial also in Erysipelas. An ointment may be made of it for wounds.

SLOE BUSH.

Prunus Sylvestris.—It requires no description.

Medicinal Virtues.—All the parts of Sloe are astringent, and effectual to stay bleeding at the nose and mouth; or bloody flux, profuse menstruation; and it eases pains of the sides and bowels, produced by diarrhœa. The decoction of the bark or fruit to be used. The conserve also is taken for the same purpose. The distilled water relieves pains in the stomach, sides, and bowels. The leaves make a good lotion to gargle and wash the mouth and throat in which are swellings, sores, or kernels; to cool inflammations of the eyes, and to ease pains of the head, bathing the temples and forehead. The distilled water of the flowers is very effectual for the same purposes.

SMALLAGE.

Description.—*Apium Graveolens.*—A common wild plant about ditch sides, a kind of Parsley, but resembling Celery. Leaves many and large; stalks two feet and a half in height, round, smooth, striated, and branched; leaves like those from the root, broad and indented, but smaller. The flowers stand in little umbels at the division of the branches; they are small, of a yellowish white.

Medicinal Virtues.—The roots are most used. Smallage is hotter, drier, and much more medicinal than parsley. It is more effectual in opening obstructions of the liver and spleen. It provoketh urine and is good against the yellow jaundice, tertian and quartan agues, if the juice be taken, but especially if made into a syrup. The juice also put to honey of roses, and barley water, is very good to gargle the mouth and throat affected by sores and ulcers. The same lotion also heals ulcers and cankers. The seeds dried are good against the colic, worms, and they strengthen the stomach. The root is more powerful in operation than the herb, especially to open obstructions, and remove ague, if the juice be taken in wine, or the decoction in wine be used.

SOLOMON'S SEAL.

Description.—*Polygonaton.*—There are two kinds of this plant, the common and the sweet smelling. The common Solomon's Seal grows a foot and a half high. The stalk is round, striated, and of a pale green; naked half way up, and from thence to the top, it has large oval leaves of a pale green, blunt, smooth, ribbed, unindented at the edges. Small, hollow white flowers hang from the under part of the stalk; the fruit is a berry about the size of a pea, and when ripe, black. The root is white and knotted in some places, and creeps. It is a flat, round circle, representing a seal, from which it derives its name. It grows wild in many places, and it grows in gardens.

Medicinal Virtues.—The root is the part used. It is a very good application for external bruises, blows, &c. It cures a black eye sooner than any thing; first apply the bruised root mixed with a little cream, and then the bruised leaves made into a stiff ointment with lard. It is good to close the lips of green wounds, and to heal all kinds of sores. The powdered root is good against purgings attended with bloody stools; and the fresh root made into a conserve with sugar, stays the whites. The decoction of the root in wine is a suitable beverage for persons with broken-bones, as it disposes the bones to knit; also for those who have ruptures. The decoction or the distilled water of the whole plant applied to the face, or other parts of the skin, cleanses it from freckles, spots, or marks, leaving the place fresh, fair, and lovely.

SOPEWORT.

Description.—*Saponaria Officinalis.*—It is also called Bruisewort. The root creeps under ground, with many joints, of a brown colour on the outside, and yellow within, shooting forth weak and round stalks, full of joints, each set with two leaves a-piece on the contrary side, which are ribbed like the herb Plantain, and formed like the common field White Campion leaves, seldom having any branches from the sides of the stalks, but set with flowers at the top, standing in long husks like the Wild Campions, having five leaves each, round at the ends and dented in the middle, of a rose colour, almost white, sometimes deeper, sometimes paler. It grows wild in low and wet grounds, by brooks and by running waters. It flowers in July, August, and part of September.

Medicinal Virtues.—It is an old fashioned remedy for gout and skin diseases. It possesses alterative, diaphoretic, and diuretic properties; it is very mucilaginous and will make a lather like soap, instead of which it is sometimes used. It may be used in infusion or decoction. A decoction of the root removes obstructions, and promotes the flow of urine, and perspiration. It is a great purifier of the blood. It is of great service in Asthma, and in all disorders of the breast which require expectoration. The country people in some places bruise the leaves of Sopewort, and lay them upon their fingers, hands or legs, when they are cut, in order to heal them. It is very powerful to expel gravel and the stone from the kidneys or bladder, and also to expel or prevent the accumulation of water in persons disposed to dropsy. In syphillitic affections, it is more effectual than Sarsaparilla, or Guaicum. As a purifier of the blood, it is worthy of attention.

SORREL.

Rumex Acetosa.—Sorrel grows in gardens, and wild in fields. It is well known.

MEDICINAL VIRTUES.—Sorrel is useful in all hot diseases to cool inflammation of blood in agues, or sickness and fainting in fevers, and to procure an appetite in fainting, or decaying stomachs. It destroys worms, and is a cordial to the heart. The seed is most powerful and astringent, and very useful in the bloody flux. The root in decoction, or in powder, is effectual for all these purposes. The decoction of the roots is good against jaundice, and the gravel and stone in the kidneys. The decoction of the flowers made with wine cures the black jaundice, and ulcerated bowels. A syrup made with the juice of Sorrel and Fumitory, is a sovereign remedy for the itch. The juice with a little vinegar, is a cure for tetters, ring-worms, &c. It removes kernels and sores in the throat; the juice being gargled in the mouth. The leaves wrapped in a cabbage-leaf, roasted, and applied to a hard imposthume, boil or plague sore, ripen and break it.

SORREL,—WOOD.

DESCRIPTION.—*Oxalis Acetosella.*—This is a different plant from the former. It grows upon the ground, having leaves coming from the root comprising three leaves, like trefoil, broad at the ends, and cut in the middle, of a yellowish green colour, each standing on a long foot-stalk, which at first are folded together, to the stalk, till they expand; they have an acid taste. The juice turns red when it is clarified and makes a fine clear syrup. Among these leaves rise up tender, weak footstalks, with a flower at the top, comprising five small-pointed leaves, star-fashion, of a white colour, and in some with a small show of bluish, on the back side only. After the flowers follow small round heads, containing small yellow seeds. The roots are yellowish, small, and fibrous. The herb grows in woods, and wood sides. It flowers in April and May.

MEDICINAL VIRTUES.—This is more effectual than the other Sorrels in preventing putrefaction of blood, and ulcers in the mouth and body, to quench thirst, to strengthen a weak stomach, procure an appetite, stay vomiting, and to prevent contagious sickness or fevers. It operates by urine, and removes obstructions in the viscera. The syrup made of the juice and the distilled water of the herb are equally effectual. Sponges or linen cloths saturated with the juice, and applied to any hot swelling or inflammation, tends to reduce them. The juice gargled in the mouth repeatedly, is a remedy for canker or ulcers therein. It is very good to heal wounds, or to stay bleedings. *Salts of Lemon* is obtained from this plant, used to take ink-spots out of linen, and Oxalic Acid also, both rank poisons.

SOUTHERN WOOD.

Abrotonum Mas.—Every one knows this plant, especially by the name of Lad's-Love.

Medicinal Virtues.—The tops of the young branches are used. A decoction of them destroys worms. It is not very pleasant to take. They may be made into a conserve by adding sugar, cinnamon in powder, cloves, or any thing aromatic, to render it agreeable. It corrects a bad stomach, and strengthens it much. It restrains the Whites. It is a nervine, and therefore good against nervous disorders, and all hysterical complaints. It is also anti-scrofulous, and deobstruent, therefore valuable in urinary suppression. The oil applied to the backbone, before fits of ague, prevents them. Boiled with barley-meal, it takes away pimples, &c. The ashes mingled with old sallad oil, causes the hair to grow again. Daranters says that Southern Wood oil, and a little White Hellebore, is very effectual to kill lice in the head. The distilled water of the herb is said to remove the stone, and diseases of the spleen and womb.

SOW THISTLE.

Sonchus Asper. Sow Thistles are so well known that they need no description.

Medicinal Virtues.—Sow Thistles are cooling, binding, and very fit to cool a hot stomach, and ease its pains. The herb boiled in wine arrests decay in the stomach, and the milk taken

from the stalks given in drink relieves those that are short winded, and have a wheezing. Pliny says it has caused the gravel and stone to be voided by urine, and the eating of it cures a foetid breath. The decoction of the leaves and stalks causes abundance of milk in nurses, and their children to be well-coloured. The juice or distilled water is good for inflammations, eruptions, or heat in the skin, or itching of the hæmorrhoids. The juice thoroughly heated in a little oil of bitter almonds in the peel of a pomegranate, and dropped into the ears, is a sure remedy for deafness, singing, &c. Three spoonfuls of the juice warmed in white wine, causes women to have an easy and speedy delivery, so that they are able to walk presently after. It is good for women to wash their faces with, to clear the skin and give it lustre.

SPEEDWELL.

Veronica Officinalis.—This is one of the commonest and prettiest of the wild plants of Britain. It grows in dry pastures and on heaths. Its stalks are about 6 or 8 inches high. The leaves are short and oval. The stalks trail on the ground only rising at the upper parts. The leaves are of a pale green colour, a little hairy, and dented at the edges; the flowers are small and blue; they grow in slender spikes, arising from the bosoms of the leaves. The root is small and fibrous.

The whole herb is used, and it is best fresh. An infusion taken freely works by urine, and opens all obstructions; it promotes the menses. It is good against obstruction of the lungs, and is an excellent cleanser of the blood. It removes blotches, and cutaneous eruptions.

SPIGNEL.

Description.—*Athamanticum Meum.*—The roots spread deep in the ground, many fibres growing from one head, which is hairy at the top, of a blackish brown colour on the outside, and white within, fragrant, and of an aromatic taste, from whence arise long stalks of fine cut leaves, like hair, smaller than dill, set thick on both sides of the stalks, and of a good scent. From these leaves rise up round stiff stalks, with a few joints, and leaves, and at each top, an umbel of pure white flowers; the edges tinted with a reddish blue, especially before full blown. The seeds are brown. It grows wild, and is planted in gardens.

MEDICINAL VIRTUES.—Galen says the roots of Spignel provoke urine and women's courses; but if too much be taken, it causes headache. The root boiled in wine or water, cures stoppage of urine, expels wind, allays swellings and pains in the stomach, and joint-aches. If the powder of the root be mixed with honey, it breaks tough phlegm, and dries up rheum that falls on the lungs. It strengthens the stomach, creates an appetite, and removes colic.

SPLEENWORT.

DESCRIPTION.—*Asplenium Trichomanes*, vel *Ceterarch, Scholendrii.*—It is also called Hart's tongue by some. From a black thready, and bushy root, arise long single leaves, indented on each side irregularly, and covered on the under part with small seeds. As they spring from the root, they are folded inward, so that the under part only appears; they appear more like some insect than a leaf. It grows on old walls, and is green all winter.

MEDICINAL VIRTUES.—It is said to be binding and strengthening, and especially a cleanser of the spleen, removing stranguury, stone in the bladder, the yellow jaundice, and the hiccup. Matthiolus says, that if a drachm of the dust that is on the back of the leaves be mixed with half a drachm of amber in powder, and taken with the juice of purslain or plantain, it restrains the running of reins and that the decoction of the herb cures melancholy diseases. Camerarius says that the distilled water drank, is very effectual against the stone.

SQUILL.

This drug is the produce of the Scilla, or *Squilla Maritima*, the bulb being the part used. It is sold in the Shops. It is an expectorant medicine of great value. It also acts as a diuretic, and in large doses may cause sickness or purging. It is inadmissible when there is inflammatory action, or active irritation in the bronchi or air passages; in such cases, it aggravates cough instead of relieving it. As an expectorant, squill is most serviceable in chronic bronchitis especially in the aged, but in all cases when the phlegm is tough, viscid, and difficult to void. It is most advantageously combined with opium, as it does not impair the expectorant property of the squill, but modifies its tendency to irritate. From one to two drachms of paregoric, with 20 drops of Tincture of Squils in a wine-glassful of water, is a most excellent cough draught for night to which, if there is much debility, one drachm of sal-volatile may be added.

As a diuretic, Squill is generally given in dropsies in from one to three grain doses. The root is used dried, or infused in vinegar, 2½ ounces in a pint of distilled vinegar for a week. After straining, 1½ ounce of proof spirit is added to insure keeping, and then filtered. The Syrup of Squills is made by dissolving 3½ ℔s. of fine sugar in a pint of Squill vinegar by the aid of gentle heat. The dose is from one to two drachms. In dropsy of the abdomen, a liniment, composed of two parts of Soap-liniment, and one part of Tincture of Squills rubbed well into the skin, frequently, is said to be very serviceable. In asthma, the oxymel of Squill is very serviceable. The wine of Squills works by urine, and is good against the jaundice and dropsy.

STAR THISTLE.

Description. — *Calcitrapa.*—The Star Thistle has narrow leaves lying in a circular manner on the ground, indented at the edges, soft, or a little woolly, green, from which rise weak stalks parted into many branches, all lying to the ground, a pretty bush, set with divided leaves to the top, where stand small whitish green heads, with sharp white pricks (no part of the plant else being prickly) which are yellowish; out of which rise the flowers, composed of many small reddish purple threads; they resemble the flowers of thistle. The seeds are winged with down. The root is oblong. It grows on heaths, and flowers in July.

MEDICINAL VIRTUES.—The seeds made into powder, and drank in wine, provoke urine, and break the stone. The root in powder, given in wine and drank in the morning fasting, helps to cure a fistula in any part of the body. It opens obstructions, and is good against gravel.

STAVESACRE.

This is a plant of the crow-foot tribe, botanically known as *Delphinum Staphisagria.* Its seeds are violently emetic and cathartic. They are seldom given internally: though the powdered seeds have been given as a purge for dropsy, in very small quantities at first and increased till the effect is produced. Dose at first should not exceed two or three grains. The seeds are used as an external application to some cutaneous eruptions, and to destroy lice in the head. The decoction applied with a linen rag is effectual in curing the itch. The seeds are merely boiled in water.

ST. JOHN'S WORT.

DESCRIPTION.—*Hypericum Perforatum.*—It grows a foot and a half high. The stalks are round, thick, firm, upright, and at the top divided into several branches. The leaves are a little like those of the lesser Centuary, but narrow, short, and obtuse at the end, and if held up against the light, they appear full of small round holes. Large and bright yellow flowers abundantly grow at the tops of the branches, full of yellow threads, which, when rubbed upon the hand, stain it red, like blood. The seed is black, and smells like rosin. It grows in meadows, woods, and copses.

MEDICINAL VIRTUES.—A decoction of the flowers is very diuretic, promoting the flow of urine, is good for gravel, and inflammation of the ureters. It has been used as a vulnerary, both externally and internally, and has been considered useful in hysterics, intermittent fevers, dysentery, hemorrhages, chest complaints, worms, and jaundice. For wounds, the tops gathered fresh and bruised are used. Boiled in wine it is excellent for inward wounds and hurts. It is a first-rate wound herb, made into an ointment; it soon closes cuts, wounds, &c. The decoction of the plant and flowers, and especially of the seed, with the juice of Knotgrass, relieves vomiting, spitting of blood, and obstructions of urine. Two drachms of the powdered herb drank in a little broth, expels choler and congealed blood from the stomach. A warm decoction of the leaves and seeds taken before fits of ague, relieves, and, eventually, drives them away. The decoction of the seed, frequently and continuously taken, will cure sciatica, falling sickness, and palsy.

STONE-CROP.

DESCRIPTION.—*Sedum Acre.*—It is a kind of House-Leek, growing upon stone walls, mud walls, the tiles of houses, and amongst rubbish, and gravelly places. It grows with trailing branches upon the ground, set with many thick, flat, roundish, whitish green leaves, pointed at the ends. The yellow flowers stand together, rather loosely. The roots are small, and creep under the ground.

MEDICINAL VIRTUES.—It is astringent, and good to stay defluxions, especially such as fall upon the eyes. It stops bleeding, both inward and outward, tends to cure cancers, and fretting sores and ulcers. It abates the heat of the bile, and prevents diseases arising from bilious humours. It expels poison, prevents fevers, and tertian agues, the decoction of it being used. It is so harmless an herb, you can scarcely use it amiss. The leaves bruised, and applied to scrofulous sores, and the piles, is an effectual cure.

STRAWBERRY.

Fragaria Vesca.—This plant needs no description.

MEDICINAL VIRTUES.—Dr. Thompsom says, "The delicious fruit must be classed with the most wholesome of the vegetable kingdom." It is said of Fontenelle that he attributed his longevity to them, in consequence of their having regularly cooled a fever which he had every spring; and that he used to say, "If I can but reach the season of strawberries, I shall do well." Boerhaave regarded their continual use as one of the principal remedies in cases of obstruction, and viscidity, and in putrid disorders. Hoffman furnished instances of obstinate disorders cured by them, even consumption in its incipient stages; and Linnæus says, that by eating plentifully of them, he kept himself free from gout. They are good even for the teeth, and may also be used as a safe and effectual dentrifice.

They cool the stomach, the liver, and the spleen, quench thirst, and regulate the kidneys. The juice dropped into foul ulcers, tends to cure them. It is good to stay catarrhs, or defluxions of rheum in the lungs. The juice is good for inflamed eyes, if dropped into them.

Strawberries make a good wash for inflamed parts, and take away redness of the face, spots, &c.

SUCCORY, OR CHICORY.

DESCRIPTION.—*Chicorium.*—This is a species of the endive and is commonly known by the name of *Chicory*.

The wild Succory has long leaves, lying on the ground, very much cut in or torn on the edges, on both sides, even to the middle rib, ending in a point; sometimes it has a rib down the middle of the leaves. From the leaves rise a hard, round woody stalk, spreading into many branches, set with smaller and less divided leaves on them up to the tops, where stand the flowers, which are like the garden kind, and the seed is also; the root is whiter but harder and more woody than the garden kind. The whole plant is exceeding bitter. It grows in waste untilled barren fields.

MEDICINAL VIRTUES.—The plant has been celebrated as a cooler. It is of great service in all obstructions of the viscera, particularly of the liver. It has been extolled in complaints proceeding from a redundant bile; it is therefore good against jaundice, inflammation of the liver, and the gravel, as it works powerfully by urine. The decoction of the leaves has the same effect, if made strong; and is good also for dropsy and ague; for the latter a decoction of the leaves and root in wine. The distilled water of the herb and flowers is specially good for hot stomachs, and in agues; for swoonings and passions of the heart, for the heat and headache in children, and for the blood and liver. The bruised leaves applied allays swellings, inflammations. St. Anthony's fire, especially if used with a little vinegar.

SWEET FLAG.

Acorus Calamus.—A common wild plant that grows undistinguished among the flags and rushes by ditch-sides. It grows three feet high, but consists only of leaves without a stalk. They are long, narrow, and of a pale green colour. Amongst these there are three or four like the rest, but they have a cluster of flowers at one side, five or six inches from the top. It is long, brown, and thick, like the catkin of a filbert tree, but longer and thicker. The root is long, flattish, and creeping; at first the smell is unpleasant, but becomes otherwise in drying, quite fragrant and aromatic.

It is an aromatic stimulant, and never causes feverish excitement. It is a very powerful tonic, and very useful in weakness of the digestive organs, loss of appetite, and general weakness. Combined with Peruvian Bark, or Quinine, it has been of great service in the low stage of malignant fevers. The roots powdered, and infused, or decocted, has cured the colic, flatulence and ague. The dose of the root powdered is from 15 to 40 grains; of the Infusion from 1 to 2 ounces; of the tincture, from ½ a drachm to 1½ drachms. Outwardly, it is applied as a stimulating fomentation.

TAMARIND.

The tree is a native of the East and West Indies, *Tamarindus Indica*. The fruit is a flat pod. It contains a pulpy substance, and the seeds a stringy matter with them. The pulp, strings, and seeds are imported, and the pulp is separated for use. It is of a pleasant acid taste, and is an excellent gentle purge. It works by urine. It is good in the jaundice. The pulp is useful to cool the mouth, and to quench thirst in fevers. The efficacy of sweet purgatives is increased by this fruit, such as Cassia, Manna, &c. Preserved tamarinds, as an aperient are very suitable for the sick in fevers, or feverish diseases. It is used by infusion—in hot water, and allowed to cool.

THE TAMARISK TREE.

Tamarix Gallica.—A little tree which grows wild in France, and is kept in some English gardens.

MEDICINAL VIRTUES.—The roots, leaves, or bark boiled in wine, stays the bleeding of the hæmorrhoidal veins, spitting of blood, and profuse menstruation. This decoction is good against the jaundice and colic. A watery decoction externally applied hot is powerful against hardness of the spleen, tooth-ache, pains in the ears and inflamed eyes. The decoction with honey, is a good application to stay gangrenes and fretting ulcers, and to destroy lice. Alpinus and Veslingius affirm that the Egyptians give it to those who have the leprosy, scabs, ulcers, or the like. Its ashes quickly heal blisters raised by burnings or scaldings. It helps the dropsy, arising from hardness of the spleen. It is good in melancholy, and the black jaundice.

TANSY,—GARDEN.

It is a common plant, cultivated in gardens. It is the *Tanacetum Vulgare* of botanists. It is so well known as to need no description.

MEDICINAL VIRTUES.—This herb bruised and applied to the navel, prevents mis-carriage, at least ancient physicians reckoned so. It consumes the phlegmatic humours engendered by winter, and this caused Tansy to be eaten in spring. The decoction of Tansy, or the juice drank in wine, promotes urine, cures strangury, and strengthens the kidneys. It is very antiflatulent. The decoction is also good against worms. The seeds combined with Worm-seed, and made into an electuary, destroy worms effectually.

TANSY,—WILD TANSY, OR SILVER WEED.

DESCRIPTION.—*Tanacetum Argentina.* A common wild plant growing on way-sides. It rises to no height. The stalks creep upon the ground, and take root at the joints; but it is easily distinguished by its silvery leaves, and yellow flowers. The stalks are round and reddish. The leaves rise from these, like the leaves of Tansy. It flowers in June or July.

MEDICINAL VIRTUES. Wild Tansy restrains fluxes of blood in men and women, also spitting or vomiting of blood. The powder of the herb taken in some of the distilled water, arrests the terms, and the whites. It is also good for children that have a rupture. Boiled in water and salt, it eases griping pains of the bowels, and is good for the sciatica and joint-aches, as an external application. Boiled in vinegar, honey, and alum, and gargled in the mouth, it relieves tooth-ache, heals sore gums and strengthens the palate of the mouth when lax. It is given with success in bleeding piles, and, as a gargle, for an ulcerated mouth. The juice of the leaves and root made into an ointment is good to heal green wounds, and running sores in the legs. The distilled water frees the skin from sun burning, pimples, freckles, and the like. The juice dropped into the eyes, or cloths wet therein and applied, takes away inflammations in them.

TAPIOCA.

Tapioca is the pith of the roots of *Jatropa Manihot*, a shrub growing in Brazil and the West Indies, where it is called *Cassava.* It resembles Sago, but it is less coloured, and in larger grains. The juice of the root in its primitive state is highly poisonous, and with it the Indians poison their arrows. This juice is thoroughly removed by washing, and the starch or Tapioca, dried in the form of grains. Tapioca is used in sick-room cookery like Arrowroot and Sago. To make Tapioca into a proper mucilage for the sick, 1 ounce should be macerated in a pint of water, on or near a slow fire, or in a slow oven, for one hour, then boiled ten minutes, stirring well during the boiling. The mucilage may be sweetened with sugar, or flavoured with lemon-juice. It is a nutritious farina; but by the addition of a little flour it is rendered more so. Dr. Christison says, "No amylaceous substance is so much relished by infants about the time of weaning; and in them it is less apt to turn sour during digestion than any other farinaceous food, even Arrow-root not excepted."

TEA.

The dried leaves which we infuse, and call Tea, are produced by the *Thea Viridis*, of the natural order *Theaceæ*. The tea-plant is a native of China, Japan, Tonquin, and Assam, in India. The different varieties are caused by different modes of cultivation, or of preparation of the same species. Tea has slightly stimulant and astringent properties, and besides its daily use as a beverage, it is taken medicinally.

Dr. Thompson says, "Tea possesses a natural fragrance which requires no addition. The Chinese say, that only common tea requires scenting; nevertheless there are various scented teas which are in high estimation even in China....... Tea is liable to immense adulteration—much after it reaches this country, but partly in China. The Chinese annually dry many million pounds of the leaves of different plants to mingle with the genuine; and the leaves of the following species have been detected from time to time in samples of tea of British fabrication;—beech, elm, horse-chestnut, plane, bastard-plane, fancy-oak, willow, poplar, hawthorn and sloe."

"One of the most frequent adulterations of tea is its admixture with exhausted leaves which have been redried.....Catechu is a frequent addition to the exhausted and other leaves, to give them astringency. Sulphate of iron, rose-pink, logwood, plumbago, indigo, &c. are all used at times in the adulteration of tea.......Such additions are highly deleterious.....Green tea is so greatly adulterated, that, although there is certainly a genuine preparation of this kind, it seems doubtful whether any is sold pure. From authentic examinations, it appears that all the green teas imported into this country, are faced with a powder consisting either of Prussian blue, or sulphate of lime, or gypsum, or of some other colouring matters.

Tea, especially the green, exerts a very powerful influence upon the nervous system. "There are some persons upon whom green tea produces nearly the same effect as digitalis, and it has been medicinally employed in the diseases for which that herb so decidedly obtained a high reputation. Where persons have any tendency to dyspeptic affections, they are very apt to be aggravated by the use of tea.

Dr. Graham says, "Tea appears to me to exert a very injurious influence on the stomach, bowels, and nerves—a very marked and irritating effect on the nervous system, and is drank in this country far too often and too strong. It forms a refreshing and anti-spasmodic beverage, but should not be taken either strong or hot; the addition of milk renders it more wholesome, that of sugar less so. Individuals of a rigid and solid fibre are less injured by it than those of an opposite habit; but none should take more than two small tea-cupfuls morning and evening. I cannot think it equal to cocoa or thin chocolate for common use; and it is probable that some of our indigenous plants would yield a more wholesome and equally as palatable an infusion as the tea-leaf of China. With some tea does not agree; an infusion of *Agrimony* or some other native plant, should be used instead. I may state on very respectable authority, that the first leaves of *Wortleberry*, dried in the shade, cannot be distinguished from real tea. *Sage*, (the Tomentosa, or *Balsamic Sage)* and *Balm*, are valuable substitutes for tea, particularly in the case of debility in the stomach and nervous system. John Hussey, of Sydenham, in Kent, who lived to 116, took nothing for his breakfast for fifty years, but Balm tea sweetened with honey."

Tea is occasionally of service in ardent and bilious fever, cramp of the stomach, flatulency, and to relieve the sensations of oppressions accompanying indigestion and bilious complaints.

TEAZLE,—OR FULLER'S THISTLE.

Dipsacus Sylvestris.—It is well known, and needs no description.

The root is used; it is bitter, and given in infusion strengthens the stomach, and creates an appetite. It removes obstructions of the liver, and the jaundice. The juice diluted with water is said to take away freckles. The same also, or the distilled water dropped into the eyes, removes inflammation, and improves the sight. The juice is said to take away warts and wens.

THISTLE,—BLESSED.

DESCRIPTION.—*Carduus Benedictus.*—This plant is a native of the warmer countries, and is raised with us in gardens. It is two feet high; the stalk is reddish, slender, and weak; very much branched, and scarce able to keep upright under the weight of leaves and heads. The leaves are long, narrow, cut in on both sides, and of an obscure green, The flowers are yellow; they stand in a kind of green leafy heads: the little leaves composing these heads are prickly; and each of the cups of the flowers ends in a long brown spine, dented on both sides.

MEDICINAL VIRTUES.—It is bitter and stomachic. An infusion of it taken in large quantities, will excite vomiting: in smaller draughts, it is good to create an appetite, and prevents sickness and reachings. The leaves dried and powdered, are good against worms. It was at one time supposed to possess very great virtues against fevers of all kinds: but that is now disregarded.

THISTLE.—MELANCHOLY.

DESCRIPTION.—*Carduus Helenoides.*—It rises up with tender single hoary green stalks, bearing four or five green leaves, dented at the edges; the points thereof are a little prickly, and at the top it has but one head, yet sometimes from the bosom of the uppermost leaves there is another small head, scaly, and prickly, with many reddish threads in the middle, which being gathered fresh, will keep its colour, and fade not for a long time, while it perfects the seed, which is downy. The root is stringy and black. It is easily known by its long straight stem, purple flowers, and linear leaves. They grow in moist meadows, and flower about July or August.

MEDICINAL VIRTUES. Its virtues are not to be despised; for the decoction of the thistle in wine expels superfluous melancholy out of the body, and makes a man as merry as a cricket. Persons troubled with melancholy and depression of spirits may take a decoction of the root—a wine glassful two or three times a day, with the greatest advantage. Dioscorides asserts that it cures melancholy. Modern writers laugh at him. Let them laugh that win; my opinion is, that it is a good remedy against melancholy diseases.

THISTLE,—OUR LADY'S THISTLE.

DESCRIPTION.—*Carduus Mariæ.* It has several large broad leaves lying on the ground, indented and crumpled, hairy on the edges, of a white green shining colour, with many lines and streaks of a milk-white colour running all over, and set with many hard prickles, among which rise one or more strong round, prickly stalks, full of similar leaves to the top, where at the end of every branch, comes forth a great prickly Thistle-like head, strongly armed with prickles, with bright purple thrums rising out of the middle. The seed grows in the heads in soft white down, which is dispersed by the wind. The taste of the plant is bitter. It grows on ditch-banks, and by road-sides. It flowers in June and July.

MEDICINAL VIRTUES.—The roots and seeds are used. An infusion of the fresh root works by urine, and removes obstructions of the liver and spleen, and is therefore good for jaundice, It hinders the ague, expels the stone, and relieves dropsy. It relieves inward pains and gripings, pains in the sides, &c. It is often applied outwardly with cloths to the region of the liver, to cool the distemper thereof, and to the region of the heart, against swoonings. It cleanses the blood exceedingly; and in Spring, if you boil the tender plant without the prickles, it will change your blood as the season changes, and that is the way to be safe.

THISTLE,—WOOLLEN THISTLE.

DESCRIPTION.—*Carlina Vulgaris.*—It is also called Cotton Thistle. It has many large leaves lying upon the ground, indented and crumpled on the edges, of a green colour on the upper side, but covered over with long hairy wool, or cotton down, set with very sharp prickles: from the middle of whose heads of flowers come many purplish crimson threads, and sometimes white, but seldom. The seed in these white downy heads, is large and round, resembling the seed of Lady's Thistle, but paler. The root is large, thick, and spreading much. It grows on ditch-banks, and in corn-fields and highways.

MEDICINAL VIRTUES.—Dioscorides and Pliny write, that the leaves and roots taken in drink, cure stiff neck. Galen says that the roots and leaves are good for such persons that have their bodies drawn together by spasm or convulsion, or other infirmities; as the rickets in children, a disease that hinders their growth, by binding their nerves, ligaments, &c. It is good also in nervous complaints.

THORN APPLE.

DESCRIPTION.—*Datura Stramonium.*—It is a native of America; but is now cultivated in this country, on account of its beauty. It grows three feet high. The leaves are much toothed, of a light green; the flowers are white and trumpet-shaped. The fruit is of the size of a wall-nut, covered with prickles or thorns, hence its name.

The leaves, stems, fruit, and seeds are cut up together and sold for smoking to afford relief in *Spasmodic Asthma* which it certainly does. For this purpose it is used in Ceylon, and the poorer Turks use it instead of Opium. It acts as a sedative upon the mucus membrane, and promotes the secretion of the mucus; it allays the spasmodic symptoms attendant on the paroxysms of asthma and respiration proceeds in a calm and undisturbed manner. A little only should be smoked *at the first* and gradually increased.

Its internal use is very dangerous; for it is very stimulant and narcotic,—a deadly poison, exercising much the same influence as *belladonna*: It is given to quiet the mind during violent paroxysms of insanity: as a specific in severe chronic pain of the head. It is given in the form of Tincture or extract; of the former from 5 drops twice a day in water; the latter from $\frac{1}{4}$ of a grain. It ought to be administered by persons of medical skill.

THOROUGH WAX.

Description.—*Perfoliata.*—It is sometimes called Through Leaf. It is a beautiful wild plant growing among corn, distinguished by the stalk growing through the leaves, three feet high. The stalk is round, firm, erect, whitish, and branching at the top. The leaves are broad and oval; the stem runs through them toward the bottom; for they have no footstalks, and they surround it in their largest part ending in a blunt point; of a bluish green colour, unindented. The flowers are small and yellow, in clusters with a parcel of small leaves under them. The root is white, oblong, and slender. It flowers in July.

Medicinal Virtues.—Thorough-Wax is useful for bruises and wounds, either inward or outward, if the decoction of the herb with water and wine be drank, and the place washed with it, or the juice of the green herb bruised, made into an ointment. The decoction of the herb, or powder of the dried herb, taken inwardly, or the leaves bruised, and applied outwardly, is good for all ruptures, especially in children. If the navels of children project, the juice mixed with flour, and a little wax, cures them.

THYME.

Thymus.—A common plant in kitchen gardens, well known.

Medicinal Virtues.—It is a noble strengthener of the

lungs. An infusion of the fresh tops is good in asthmas, and stuffing of the lungs. It is excellent in nervous affections, and a special remedy for hooping cough. It expectorates phlegm, and relieves shortness of breath. It kills worms, and provokes the terms. It is so harmless you need not fear the use of it. An ointment made of it removes hot swellings and warts, relieves sciatica, dulness of sight, and pains and hardness of the spleen, it is good against the gout, and swelled testicles, pains in the back and loins. The herb taken any way inwardly, comforts the stomach and expels wind.

The *Wild Thyme*, (See Mother of Thyme) is preferable. For obstructed menstruation, a bath for the feet and legs in a strong infusion, or decoction, gives relief after the failure of all other remedies. An oil is made from the Wild Thyme, a drop or two of which cures the tooth-ache; apply with a little lint.

A writer in the "Lancet" says, "An infusion of *Wild Thyme* will, in many cases of Hooping Cough, and affections of the air passages, remove the complaint, when all other remedies fail."

TOBACCO

Tobacco is manufactured from the dried leaves of the *Nicotiana Tabacum*, a native of the Southern states of America. It is a deadly narcotic, especially the oil, so much of which is absorbed by the pipe in smoking. Its effect on the system is that of a narcotic and sedative, producing sickness, and depressing the action of the heart; it is slightly diuretic, and antispasmodic; in over-doses it produces convulsions, which are likely to terminate in death.

Like many other poisons, Tobacco is used medicinally. The American Indians bind the leaves on the bite of the Rattle-snake and cure it. And the bite of a mad dog has been cured by the application of a thick poultice of Tobacco. It has been given to relax the muscular system in colic, constipation, and hernia, and by enema to relieve spasmodic constriction of the bowels. But it is far too dangerous for domestic use.

I hesitate not to say that Tobacco has killed thousands. In

some it promotes rapid digestion, forcing the food down faster than it can be disposed of. In others causing "shameful spitting," gradually wasting the frame, or disposing it to those diseases which terminate in death. In some it affects the brain, and renders the person liable to apoplexy. In short, its evil influences are many and great. In others it produces disorder and extreme irritation of the digestive organs, often attended with extreme nervous irritability. The lips of smokers are very liable to cancer, and its injury to the teeth is notorious. Smokers too are very liable to diseases of the throat and air-passages, laryngeal phthisis and bronchitis.

☞ Snuff is even worse than Tobacco; for it often is a combination of the rankest poisons with the powdered leaves of Tobacco.

TORMENTIL.

Description.—*Tormentilla Erecta.*—Also called Septfoil, or Steptfoil. It has reddish slender branches rising from the root, lying on the ground, not quite upright, with many short leaves closer to the stalks than Cinquefoil, (which this is very like) with the foot-stalk compassing the branches in several places, but those that grow to the ground are set upon long foot-stalks, which leaves are like those of Cinquefoil, but long and less, dented about the edges, some divided into five, and some into seven, on account of which it is called Septfoil; yet many have six, and some eight, according to the fertility of the soil. The flowers are small, of a beautiful shining yellow; they grow on slender footstalks, in shape and colour like the crow-foot flowers, but more beautiful and less. The root is short and thick for the size of the plant, externally brown, and reddish within, of an austere taste. It grows in woods, shady places, and in borders of fields.

Medicinal Virtues.—Tormentil is most excellent to stay all kind of fluxes of blood. The juice of the herb and root, or the decoction, taken in Venice treacle, and the person laid to sweat, expels venom, poison, fever, or other contagious diseases, as the pox, measles, &c. The root taken inwardly is most effectual to relieve any flux of the belly, stomach, spleen, or blood; and the juice wonderfully opens obstructions of the liver and lungs, and thereby arrests the yellow-jaundice A plaster made of the root and vinegar is good for those who cannot retain their urine. It should be externally applied to the back, against the kidneys. The powder of the root mixed with the juice of plantain is a remedy against worms. The root made up with Pellitory of Spain and alum, and put into a hollow tooth, stops the pain. The juice or powder of the root combined with ointments and plasters, that are applied to wounds or sores, increases their power to heal. The juice of the leaves and the root bruised, and mixed with a little vinegar, is a good application for scrôfulous sores near the ears, on the neck, &c. and for any sore or eruption on the head, or elsewhere, and for the piles. A decoction strongly made is a good wash for the piles, and for inflamed eyes.

This plant is very astringent; so much so that it has been used in some places for tanning, and this astringency invests it with active remedial powers. If it were brought from a foreign country, it would be extensively used; *growing in England, it is too cheap.* The root is chiefly used. Powdered, it is given in from half a drachm to drachm doses. The decoction is made by boiling 2 ounces of the bruised root in 30 ounces of water, till it is reduced one third, and strained. Dose 1½ ounce. It may be used as an astringent gargle.

Dr. Graham says, "It is a mild yet powerful astringent, operates without producing any stimulant effect, calculated to check the diarrhœa of pulmonary consumption, and all diarrhœas, where the general excitement is considerable! For this purpose, its union with small doses of ipecacuanha powder forms a very simple medicine, recommended by that distinguished physician, Dr. George Fordyce. It is also beneficial in old ulcers, and in cases of weak bowels liable to frequent relaxations, although they may be of short duration."

Dr. Thornton says, "A poor man, fond of botanical excursions, knew the powers of this root, and by making a strong decoction of it, sweetened with honey, he cured agues which had resisted the bark; long-standing diarrhœas, ulcers of the legs turned out of hospitals as incurable, the worst scorbutic ulcers, fluxes, &c. This excited the attention of Lord William

Russel, who allowed him a piece of ground out of his park to cultivate Tormentil, which he kept as a secret. In fluxes of blood, I have found 1 drachm given four times a day, in an infusion of hops, do wonders.

TREFOIL.

Description.—A common wild plant in our meadows. It grows 8 inches high, stalk round, not very upright; the principal leaves rise immediately from the root, they stand three together on long foot-stalks, and are of an oval figure, but pointed; of a pale green colour, and a little hairy, having a white spot in the centre of each. The leaves on the stalks have the same form, but are less. The flowers stand at the tops, in short thick spikes; they are small and red, followed by little flat pods.

Medicinal Virtues.—The fresh flowers are fresh used, and given in infusion. They are good against the bleeding piles; and while they are balsamic and astringent in the bowels, they work beneficially by urine.

TRUE-LOVE, OR ONE-BERRY.

Description.—*Verus-Amor.*—It is also called Herb-Paris, and Four-leaved True-Love. It has a small creeping root, like couch-grass root, but not so white, shooting forth stalks with leaves, some bearing berries, and others not; every stalk is smooth, without joints, and blackish green, rising half a foot high, if it bears berries, otherwise seldom so high, bearing at the top four leaves one against another, like a cross or ribband tied (as in a true-lover's knot) which are each of them apart like a night-shade leaf, but rather broader, having three, five, or six leaves. In the middle of the four leaves rises up a small slender stalk, an inch high, bearing at the top one flower spread like a star, consisting of four small and long narrow-pointed leaves of a yellowish green colour, and four less lying between them; in the middle of which stands a round dark purplish button or head, compassed about with eight small yellow mealy threads with three colours, making it the more conspicuous, and lovely to behold. This button or head in the middle, becomes a blackish purple berry, full of juice, about the size of a grape, having within it many white seeds. It grows in woods and copses, and sometimes in the corners or borders of fields, and waste grounds. They spring up in April or May and flower soon after. The berries are ripe in the end of May, or in the beginning of June.

Medicinal Virtues.—The leaves or berries hereof are effectual to expel poison, especially that of the aconite. The roots in powder taken in wine relieve the colic. The leaves are very effectual for green wounds, and to cleanse and heal old sores and ulcers ; and to disperse old tumours and swellings in the private parts, the groin, and to allay inflammations. The juice of the leaves cures felons, and heals imposthumes or sores about the nails of the hands or feet. Children should not be allowed to eat the berries.

TURNSOLE, OR HELIOTROPIUM.

Description.—*Heliotropium.*—A plant celebrated for its fragrance. The blossom is very small, of a pale blue, inclining to white, and shedding an almond like-perfume. The name is derived from two Greek words, signifying the *sun*, and *to turn;* the leaves or flowers having been supposed to turn with the sun ; hence it is called Turnsole, or *Turn* Sol. Here it is cultivated in Greenhouses.

Medicinal Virtues.—It is a good herb. Dioscorides says, that a good handful of this herb, boiled in water, purges both choler and phlegm ; and boiled with cummin, removes stone in the kidneys, or bladder, provokes urine and menstruation. The leaves bruised and applied to places pained with the gout, or that have been out of joint, and newly set, and full of pain, give much ease ; the seed and juice of the leaves also being rubbed with a little salt upon warts or wens, and other kernels in the face, eye-lids, or any other part of the body, will by often using, take them away.

TURPENTINE.

Terebinthina.—It is an exudation from different species of Pines. It is a valuable remedy, either externally or internally. Sprinkled on flannel dipped in hot water, wrung out, and then locally applied, it is a powerful counter-irritant, acting like mustard, and even blistering. It is useful for local pains, for lumbago, sciatica, and for inflammatory diseases in the abdomen. As an external application to burns, turpentine has been much used.

Internally turpentine is anthelmintic, diaphoretic, diuretic, purgative and stimulant. It is also given as an astringent. As a destroyer of worms, it should be given in combination with Castor Oil, lest failing to purge it should over-stimulate the urinary organs. As a diuretic, it is prescribed in dropsy, and suppression of urine. As a purgative, it is useful in cases of tympanitic distension of the abdomen, and in acute stages of puerperal fever. As a stimulant to the nervous system, in neuralgia and epilepsy. Dose, as a stimulant and diuretic 6 to 30 drops—as a purgative and worm-expellant ½ ounce to 2 ounces.

TUTSAN, OR PARK LEAVES.

Description.—*Androsœmum.*—It deserves special notice, on account of its great virtues. It has brownish shining round stalks. It grows two feet high. The stalks are firm, and smooth, tolerably upright, not branched, except for some young shoots near the tops. The leaves stand two at each joint, opposite to one another, at no great distance, they are large, and nearly oval. Their colour is a brownish green, they are smooth, and not serrated at the edges. The flowers are not large, but of a beautiful yellow, like those of St. John's Wort, full of yellow threads, which stain the hands red. The fruit is a kind of berry, when ripe black, containing many small seeds. The plant in autumn frequently appears of a blood red colour, very singular and beautiful. The root is small, reddish, and irregular; it creeps under the surface. It grows in woods, groves, and woody grounds, parks, and forests.

Medicinal Virtues.—The leaves are an excellent cure for fresh wounds. Scarcely any thing is equal to them. The young and tender ones at the tops of the branches are to be used; they are to be bound upon the wound, and they stop the bleeding, and effect a very speedy cure. There have been very singular instances of the efficacy of this herb. Many other plants are celebrated for their curative properties; but the efficacy of this is surprising. A decoction of the tops promotes urine. Tutsan purges choleric humours. Its virtues are very similar to those of St. John's Wort

VALERIAN.

Description.—*Valeriana Officinalis.*—It has a thick, short, greyish root, partly lying above the ground, shooting forth all around small pieces of roots, which have many long green fibres under them in the ground. From the head of these roots spring up many green leaves, which at first are broad and long, without any divisions or denting on the edges; but those that rise up after are more divided on each side, some to the middle rib, being winged, the leaves on the stalk are more divided, but smaller towards the top than below; the stalk grows a yard high, it is sometimes branched at the top. The flowers stand in large tufts like umbels at the tops of the stalks, and are small and white, with a reddish blush. The root is of a whitish colour, composed of a great many fibres. The scent is strong and disagreeable. It is cultivated in gardens, and it also grows wild.

Medicinal Virtues.—Dioscorides says that Garden Valerian has a warming faculty, and that being dried and given to drink, it provokes urine, and relieves strangury. The decoction removes pains of the sides, provokes women's courses. Pliny says, that the powder of the root given in drink, or the decoction removes all obstructions and pains in the body. The root of Valerian boiled with liquorice, raisins, and aniseed, is good for those who are short-winded, and for those who are troubled with cough, causing easy expectoration of phlegm. The green herb with the root, bruised and applied to the head, takes away pain. The juice is good for the eyes, clearing them from inflammation, and dimness. It is an excellent medicine in nervous disorders. The root is one of the most useful remedies in hysteria and in spasmodic attacks generally. Its action is chiefly upon the nervous system, and is very useful for depression of mind, and for most affections of the nerves, melancholy. It may often be advantageously combined with bark. Dr. Cullen thought highly of it as a remedy for nervous disorders, and he remarks that it should be given in large doses. It is best given in substance, with a little mace, or cinnamon to disguise the flavour. The Ammoniated Tincture is very valuable. It may be bought at the shops. Dose, one to three spoonfuls thrice a day in water.

VANILLA.

It is the fruit of the *Vanilla Aromatica*, a creeping shrub of the Orchis tribe, growing on the mountains of Mexico and Peru, and South America. This fruit has a strong, peculiar, and agreeable odour, a warm aromatic, and sweetish taste; it appears to contain benzoic acid. As sold in the shops, Vanilla is a shrivelled pod of the kidney-bean shape, 6 inches long, wrinkled, feels oily, and adhesive to the fingers, has a balsamic odour, a taste like prunes, with the flavour of burning pastiles. It is used by perfumers, confectioners, and distillers, and to give a balsamic flavour to confectionary; and it is employed in small quantities as an adjunct to chocolate, to which it gives sweetness and a delicate flavour. It is valuable to the perfumer, the odour of the substance being one of the most exquisite imaginable. Medicinally it assists the digestion, and restores the impaired gastric forces; it gives tone to the stomach, strengthens the intestines and heart, gives vigour and activity to the brain and the mental powers; therefore it is valuable to dyspeptic and persons nervously low.

VERVAIN

Description.—*Verbena Offiicinalis.*—Called also Simpler's Joy. It has long broad leaves next the ground, deeply gashed about the edges, and some deeply dented, or cut all alike, of a dark green colour on the upper side, grey underneath. The stalk is square, branched into several parts, about two feet high, if you reckon the long spike of flowers at the tops, which are set on all sides one above another, sometimes two or three together, small and gaping, of a blue colour and white intermixed, after which come small round seed, in small long heads: the root is small and long, but of no use. It grows by the hedges and way-sides, and other waste grounds.

Medicinal Virtues.—It is slightly astringent. It removes obstructions of the liver, and strengthens the nerves. It cures the yellow jaundice, dropsy, and gout, and expels worms. It warms and strengthens the stomach, and cleanses, and strengthens the internal viscera. It is good in all urinary affections. It is good for coughs, asthma, and most affections of the lungs. It is a good wound herb, the leaves being ground, and made into an ointment with lard. It is good also for the piles. The juice mixed with vinegar is a remedy for the headache. This has often been tried with success. As a cosmetic, it very much improves the skin, being mixed with a little vinegar.

VINE.

Vitis Vinifera.—The leaves of the English Vine being boiled, make a good lotion for sore mouths; boiled with barley meal into a poultice, it cools inflammations of wounds. The ashes of the burnt branches will make teeth black as a coal, to be as white as snow, used every morning.

Grapes, the fruit of the Vine, are the most wholesome of fruits, containing much sugar, vegetable jelly, and mucilage, the characteristic tartaric acid in combination with potassa, gluten. on which depends its property of ready fermentation.

VIOLET.

Viola Odorata.—It needs no description. They flower from March till the end of July.

Medicinal Virtues.—All violets are cold and moist while

they are fresh and green, and are used to cool any heat of the body, either inwardly or outwardly, as inflammations of the eyes, in the fundament, in imposthumes and hot swellings. A decoction of the leaves and flowers should be made with water and wine. A poultice made of the flowers and leaves, and locally applied, has the same effect. A drachm weight of the dried leaves or flowers of Violets, purge the body of choleric humours, and heat, being taken in wine, or any other drink; the powder of the flowers dried, and drank in water is said to relieve the quinsy and the falling sickness in children. The flowers of the white violets ripen and dissolve swellings. The Violet-flowers are used medicinally on account of their demulcent and mildly laxative properties. They are good for coughs and lung affections, and pleurisy. The Syrup of Violets, to which has been added, a little lemon juice, and a few drops of the oil of vitriol is very powerful to cool the heat and quench the thirst. The green leaves are used with other herbs to make plasters and poultices for inflammations and swellings, and to ease pains arising from heat, and for the piles. The Syrup of Violet may be bought at the Shops; or a combination of it and Almond Oil. It relieves coughs and tightness of the chest. Syrup of violets mixed with Almond Oil, and Syrup of Senna, makes an excellent demulcent and aperient medicine. To make the Syrup, take a quantity of flowers, and boiling water sufficient to cover them; let it stand all night. Strain and add sugar, 2 pounds to each pint, and melt over the fire. It is a good gentle purge for children.

VIPER'S BUGLOSS.

DESCRIPTION.—*Echium Vulgare.*—It has many long rough leaves lying on the ground, from which rise up hard round stalks, very rough, as if set with prickles or hairs, on which are set similar prickly green leaves, somewhat narrow: the middle rib being white. The flowers stand at the top of the stalk, branched forth in many long spiked leaves of flowers, turning like the turnsole. The flowers are large of a beautiful blue with a red stamen in the middle. After the flowers are fallen, the seeds when ripe are blackish, shaped like the head of a viper. The root is large, blackish, and woody. It grows about pathways, on ditch-banks, and about old walls.

Medicinal Virtues.—The leaves are used; those growing from the root are the best. An infusion of them is cordial, and operates by sweat. It is good in fevers, cures the headache, and all nervous complaints. It relieves inflammatory pains, the seed being decocted in wine. This decoction comforts the heart, and drives away melancholy. It is a sweetener of the blood. It is said to be an expellant of poison, and venom, and to cure the bite of a viper; hence its name.

WALL-FLOWER.

Leucoion.—It needs no description.

Medicinal Virtues.—Galen says, that yellow Wall-Flower works more powerfully than any of the other kind. It cleanses the blood, and the liver and reins from obstructions, promotes menstruation, removes the hardness of the spleen, reduces inflammations and swellings, comforts and strengthens any weak part. It cleanses the eyes from mistiness and films, and ulcers in the mouth, or any other part, and is a singular remedy for the gout, and aches and pains in the joints and sinews.

WALNUT TREE.

Juglans Regia.—It requires no description.

Medicinal Virtues.—The bark and leaves of the tree are very astringent. The husk and shell, and peal of the kernels, are sudorific, especially if used while the walnuts are green. It is said to expel the broad worms, or tape-worm. No insect eats the leaves of this tree. The leaves have the same property. The juice of the green husks, boiled with honey, is an excellent gargle for a sore mouth, and inflammation in the throat and stomach. The kernels when they grow old, are more oily, and therefore not fit to be eaten, but are then used to heal wounds, gangrenes, and carbuncles. The kernels burned are very astringent, and will stay women's courses, being taken in red wine. The green husks have the same effect. The kernels beaten with rue and wine, and applied, relieves the quinsy; and bruised with some honey, and applied to the ears, eases the pains and inflammation of them. The oil pressed out of the kernels, taken inwardly, is good for the colic, and to expel wind; half an ounce may be taken at any time. The young green nuts taken before they are half ripe, preserved with sugar, are good to strengthen weak stomachs. The distilled water of the green husks, before half ripe, cools the heat of agues; dose an ounce or two at a time. It is a very cooling application to green wounds, quickly healing them. The distilled water of the green husks being ripe, is very good against the quinsy, gargling, and bathing the throat with it.

WATER PLANTAIN.

Description.—*Plantago Aquatica.*—A very common tall plant in ditches, and having not the least resemblance of any kind of plantain, except in the leaves; from which, however, it has received its name. The root is composed of a great quantity of fibres. From this, there rise in spring a number of leaves, oblong, broad, smooth, and of a beautiful green colour, and having in shape, though not at all in colour or consistence, some slight resemblance of plantain: they are perfectly smooth, of a glossy surface, and brittle. These stand for many months without the stalk; and doubtless in this state it got the name. The stalk is two feet or more in height; round, firm, and upright; and at the top it sends out a vast number of branches, which send out other smaller; and even these last are again divided. On the tops of the last divisions stand the flowers with their buds, and the seed-vessels; so that the whole has the appearance of a cone. The flowers are little and white, and consist of three leaves each; they stand but a little time, and only a few are seen together.

Medicinal Virtues.—The seed is the part used: the plant is to be suffered to stand, till this is thoroughly ripe, and then cut up gently, and laid to dry two or three days upon a table: a smart stroke or two, will dislodge a great quantity of the seeds; they are very good against the overflowing of the menses, and all other bleedings; and are given in powder, in electuaries, small doses to be taken at a time and often repeated.

WHEAT.

Medicinal Virtues.—*Triticum.*—Pliny says, that the corns of Wheat roasted in an iron pan and eaten, are a speedy remedy for those who are chilled with cold. The oil pressed from wheat, heals tetters and ring-worms; and Galen says, he has known many cures performed by it. Matthiolus recommends the same to be put into hollow ulcers to heal them. It is good for chilblains in the hands and feet, and to make the skin smooth. Slices of Wheat bread soaked in warm water, and applied to the eyes that are red and inflamed, or blood-shot, cures them. The flower of Wheat boiled in vinegar cures the shrinking of the sinews, says Pliny; and mixed with vinegar, and boiled, it heals freckles, pimples, and spots on the face. Wheat flour mixed with the yolk of an egg, honey and turpentine, draws, cleanses, and heals any boil, sore, or foul ulcer. The bran of Wheat meal steeped in vinegar and bound in a linen cloth and rubbed on the places that have scurf, scabs, &c, it will take them away. Wheat bran boiled in good vinegar, and applied to swollen breasts, reduces them, and all inflammations. Boiled in water into a thick jelly, it checks spitting of blood; and boiled with mint and butter, it relieves the hoarseness of the throat.

WILLOW TREE.

Medicinal Virtues.—*Salix.*—Both the leaves, bark, and the seed, are used to staunch bleeding of wounds, spitting of blood, and other fluxes, and to stay vomiting, if a decoction of them in wine be drank. It helps also to stay thin, salty distillations from the head upon the lungs, causing consumption. The leaves bruised with pepper, and drank in wine, relieves the colic. The seed has the same effect. Water gathered from the Willow, when it flowers, the bark being slit, is very good for redness of the eyes, and dimness of sight; to provoke urine, if it be drank; to clear the face and skin from spots and discolourings. Galen says, the flowers have an admirable faculty in drying up humours, as it is a medicine without any sharpness or corrosion; you may boil them in white wine, and drink freely of the liquor. The bark has the same effect, if used in the same manner; the burnt ashes being mixed with vinegar take away warts, and corns. The decoction of the leaves or bark in wine, takes away scurf and dandriff by washing the place with it.

WINTER-GREEN.

Description.—*Ganetharia Procumbeus.*—This plant is little known. It sends forth seven or eight leaves, from a small, brown, creeping root, upon a long foot-stalk. The leaves are hard, resembling the leaf of a Pear-tree. From them arises a slender, erect stalk, bearing at the top many small white smelling flowers, spread open like a star, with yellowish threads in the middle surrounding a green head. The seed is as small as dust. It grows in fields and woods, especially in the north. It flowers in July.

Medicinal Virtues.—It is a good wound herb, the green leaves, or the juice of them being applied. A salve made of the green herb bruised, or the juice boiled with lard, or salad oil, and wax, with a little turpentine, is a sovereign salve. The Germans use it for all kinds of wounds and sores. A decoction of the herb relieves ulcers in the kidneys, or neck of the bladder. As an astringent it arrests dysentery, immoderate courses, and bleeding of wounds. It is good for diseases of the heart.

WOAD.

Description.—*Insatis Tinctoria.*—A plant cultivated in fields, for the use of dyers.

Medicinal Virtues.—The herb is so astringent that it is not fit to be given inwardly. An ointment made thereof staunches bleeding. A plaster made of it, and applied to the region of the spleen which lies on the left side, takes away its hardness and pains. The ointment is good in such ulcers as abound with moisture, for it takes away corroding and fretting humours. It cools inflammations, quenches St. Anthony's fire, and stays defluction of the blood to any part of the body.

WOLD, WELD, OR DYER'S WEED.

DESCRIPTION.—*Genista Luteola.*—The common kind grows bushy with many leaves, long, narrow, and flat upon the ground; of a dark bluish green colour, a little like Woad, but not so large, a little crumpled, and pointed, which so abide the first year; and the next year rise up from their round stalks, two or three feet high, beset with many such like leaves, but smaller, and shooting forth small branches, which bear many small yellow flowers, in a long spike at the top of them. The seed is small and black. The root is long, white, and thick. It flowers in June.

MEDICINAL VIRTUES.—It is said to be a good expectorant of phlegm; and to be a deobstruent in affections of the liver, &c. The bruised leaves are a good application to cuts, bruises; and mixed with lard to be a specific for scrofulous sores.

WORMSEED PLANT.

DESCRIPTION.—*Erysimum Cheroides.*—A kind of Wormwood, native of the East, and not known so much as in our gardens. The plant is two feet high. The leaves are very finely divided, like those of the true Roman Wormwood, and of a pale green on the upper side, and a silvery white below. The stalks are stiff, firm, woody, and branched; they are of a whitish colour, and have a loose downy skin upon them: the flowers are small and brownish; they resemble those of wormwood, and stand in a kind of loose spikes at the tops of the stalks.

MEDICINAL VIRTUES.—The seeds are used: our druggists keep them; and very often the unripe buds of the flowers in their place are mixed with them. They are good against worms in children; the good women give them mixed with treacle: and few medicines for this purpose have better effect. For people of nicer palates, they may be powdered, and made into boluses.

WORMWOOD.

Culpeper has written a great deal of trash about this Herb; viz. the conference of Jupiter, Mars, Saturn, the Moon, &c. about its virtues. To an intelligent mind, such trash is *utterly disgusting*. I verily believe that the vain old fellow was three-fourths drunk when he wrote such rubbish; and it is very strange that persons are still found to print, and credit his astrological foolery.

There are three kinds of wormwood. The *common* is mostly in use.

WORMWOOD,—COMMON.

DESCRIPTION.—*Artemisia Absinthium.*—A wild plant growing by way-sides, and on ditch banks. It is a yard high. The stalks are round, striated, white, firm, and branched. The leaves are large, but they are divided into a great number of small parts. They are of a pale whitish green, and stand irregularly on the stalks; many larger, but of the same kind rise from the root. The flowers stand in a kind of loose spikes at the tops of the stalks; they are small and brown. The whole plant is of a very bitter taste.

MEDICINAL VIRTUES.—Its smell is strong and disagreeable, taste intensely bitter, so as to become the foundation of a proverb. The tops of the plants are to be used fresh gathered; a very slight infusion of them is excellent for all disorders of the stomach, and will prevent sickness after meals, and create an appetite. Dr. Graham says, "It is a bitter tonic of considerable service in indigestion, and low spirits, and it has also been used with great advantage in ague, gout, and scurvy. It has been reported to have been of great service in epilepsy. Its powers in expelling worms are well ascertained. It will frequently bring away the smaller sorts of worms in great quantities. The dose in powder is from one to two scruples twice or thrice a day. The Infusion is made by pouring a pint of boiling water on an ounce of the plant; of which from an ounce to an ounce and a half may be taken twice or thrice a day."

The juice of the large leaves of wormwood, which grow from the root before the stalk appears, is good against the dropsy, and jaundice, for it removes obstructions, and works powerfully by urine. Another eminent physician says, "It is used in stomach complaints and is of great service to persons labouring under hypochondria. It is most useful in intermittent fevers, (ague); I have frequently found it so, in cachectic and hydropic affections, and in jaundice. The extract is a pure and simple bitter. The essential oil is of a dark green colour, and contains the whole flavour of the plant. It is stimulating, and a powerful antispasmodic, and anthelmintic. Wormwood was formerly much used for the preparation of medicated wine and ales. It forms *purl* when used with the last, which hard drinkers are in the habit of taking in the morning, to go through their hard day's labours." Haller says that Charles V. used this plant for the gout; and for the same purpose Dr. Thornton employed a decoction of Wormwood with success upon himself, so that he had no return for many years.

SALT OF WORMWOOD, formerly much used medicinally is pure Carbonate of Potass, obtained from the ashes of this and other plants. In small doses, say 8 or 10 grains, dissolved in a little rose-water, and taken twice or thrice a day, is very useful in indigestion and billious complaints, attended with acidity in the stomach. It is rendered effervescent by mixing with a little lemon juice.

WORMWOOD,—SEA.

DESCRIPTION.—*Absinthium Seriphium.*—A plant common in our salt-marshes, and about ditches, where salt water comes. It has somewhat the aspect of wormwood, but the leaves are much narrower in the divisions, and the whole plant is smaller. The stalks are woody, firm, upright, very much branched, and a foot and a half high. The leaves are whitish and small.

The flowers stand in loose spikes at the tops of the stalks; they are little and brown; and they very much resemble those of the common wormwood, except for the size. The whole plant has a bitter taste, but not disagreeable, and it has a pleasant aromatic smell.

MEDICINAL VIRTUES.—The tops fresh gathered, and the whole plant dry, are used. They call it Roman wormwood at the markets and in the shops; and it is used for the other: it has the same general virtues. All the three kinds indeed possess them in common; but the common wormwood is the most disagreeable to the taste, and sits worst upon the stomach; this is better than that; but it is much more disagreeable than the true Roman wormwood. It is very strengthening to the stomach; it assists digestion, and prevents wind. It is commonly an ingredient in the bitter infusions, and tinctures of the shops, but it does very well alone; boiling water poured upon it, and suffered to stand till it is cold, then strained off, is an excellent medicine to cause an appetite. Put into white wine, it also gives a pleasant bitter flavour, with the same virtues.

WORMWOOD,—ROMAN.

DESCRIPTION.—*Artemisia Romanum.*—A delicate plant of the Wormwood kind, kept in our gardens. It is two feet and a half high; the stalk is round, smooth, hard, upright, of a brownish colour, and somewhat woody. The leaves stand irregularly on it, and they are small and divided into very fine segments: they are more like the leaves of the common southern wood in figure, than those of either of the other wormwoods. The flowers are little and brown, like those of common wormwood, but vastly smaller; they are very numerous, and stand at the tops of the stalks in a kind of long and thick spikes. The root is creeping and spreading, and composed of fibres. The whole plant has a bitter taste, but not at all like that of wormwood, extremely aromatic and pleasing. The flowers are very bitter, and have little of an aromatic flavour.

MEDICINAL VIRTUES.—The fresh tops are used, and the whole plant dried. It is excellent to strengthen the stomach;

but that is not all its virtue. The juice of the fresh tops is good against obstructions of the liver and spleen, and has been known singly to cure the jaundice.

YARROW.

DESCRIPTION.—*Millefolium.*—It has many long leaves spread upon the ground, finely cut, and divided into many small parts; its flowers are white, but not all of a whiteness, and stayed in knots upon divers green stalks which rise from among the leaves. It is frequent in pastures.

MEDICINAL VIRTUES.—The whole plant is used fresh gathered; but the tops of the shoots are the best. These are to be boiled in water gently a short time, and the decoction sweetened with fine sugar. It is good against the bleeding piles, bloody flux, and profuse menstruation. An ointment made of it cures green wounds and other sores. It arrests the falling off of the hair by washing the head with a decoction of it. It cures diseases of the kidneys, and the whites, and relieves those who cannot retain their water. The leaves chewed ease the tooth-ache. Yarrow tea is a good remedy for severe colds. It is also a good substitute for Tobacco. For colds, the best way is to sweeten the tea with sugar, or honey, or treacle, adding a little Cayenne Pepper.

ADDITIONAL HERBS.

BEHEN,—WHITE.

Description.—*Behen Album.*—A common wild plant in our corn fields. It is two feet high; the stalks are weak and often crooked; but they are thick enough, round, and of a whitish green colour. The leaves are oblong, broad, and of a fine blue green colour, not dented at all at the edges, and they grow two at every joint; the joints of the stalks where they grow are swelled and large, and the leaves have no stalks. The flowers are white, moderately large, and prickly. They stand upon a husk which seems blown up with wind.

Medicinal Virtues.—This is one of those plants of our own growth, that have more virtue than people imagine. The root, which is long, white, and woody, is to be gathered before the stalks rise, and dried. An infusion is one of the best remedies known for nervous complaints: it will not take effect against a violent present disorder; but is an excellent preservative, taken cautiously.

BEHEN,—RED.

Description.—*Limonium majus.*—A common wild plant about our sea-coasts, and a very pretty one. It grows to a foot in height; the stalks are naked, and the flowers red; and in their disposition, they somewhat resemble lavender, whence the plant is also called by some Sea Lavender. About the bottoms of the stalks stand clusters of large and broad leaves, rounded at the ends, of a deep green colour, and fattish substance; these rise immediately from the root, and the stalks grow up among them. The stalks are very tough and strong, and branched, and of a paler green; the root is long and reddish.

MEDICINAL VIRTUES.—The people in Essex cure themselves of purgings, and of overflowings of the menses, with an infusion of this root; and it is a very great medicine, though little known. It is to be gathered, as soon as the young leaves appear, cleaned and dried; it may be taken in powder, half a drachm for a dose. These are not the white and red Behen roots of the old writers on physic, but they are better.

WART CRESSES, OR SWINE'S CRESSES.

DESCRIPTION.—*Coronopus Ruellii.*—A little wild plant very common about our fields and gardens. It spreads upon the ground. The stalks are five or six inches long; firm, and thick, but usually flat on the earth; very much branched, and full of leaves. The leaves that rise immediately from the root are long, and deeply divided: and those on the stalks resemble them, only they are smaller: they are of a deep glossy green colour, and not at all hairy. The flowers are small and white; they stand at the tops of the branches, and among the leaves; the seed-vessels are small and rough.

MEDICINAL VIRTUES.—This is an excellent diuretic, safe and yet very powerful. It is an ingredient in Mrs. Stephens' medicine: the juice may be taken; and it is good for the jaundice, and against all inward obstructions, and against the scurvy; the leaves may also be eaten as sallad, or dried and given in decoction.

CUP MOSS.

DESCRIPTION.—*Muscus Pyxidatus.*—A common little plant on ditch banks, by wood sides, and in dry barren places. It consists of a thin coat of a leafy matter, spread upon the surface of the ground, and of a kind of little cups rising from it. The leafy part is dry and without juice, divided into several portions, and these irregularly notched; it is grey or greenish on the upper side, and whitish underneath. The cups are half an inch high. They have each a thick stem, and an open mouth, and rather resemble a clumsy drinking glass, than a cup. They are of a grey colour, often with some odd mixture of green, of a dusty surface; sometimes they grow one from the edge of another, up to the third or fourth stage: they have also many other accidental varieties; and sometimes they bear little brown lumps, which are supposed to contain the seeds.

MEDICINAL VIRTUES.—The whole plant is to be used; it is to be taken fresh from the ground, shook clean, and boiled in water, till the decoction be very strong; then there is to be added as much milk as there is of the liquor, and it is to be sweetened with honey. It is an excellent medicine for children's coughs: it is recommended particularly in that called the Hooping Cough.

CYPERUS,—LONG.

DESCRIPTION.—*Cyperus Longus.*—A wild plant in our marshes, fens, and other damp places. It is a foot and a half high. The leaves are a foot long or more, narrow, grassy, and of a bright green colour, flat and sharp at the ends. The stalk is triangular and green; there are no leaves on it, except two or three small ones at the top, from which rise a number of small tufts or spikes of flowers. These are brown, light, chaffy, and in all respects like those of the other water grasses.

MEDICINAL VIRTUES.—The root is used. It is long and brown, and, when dried, is of a pleasant smell, and aromatic warm taste. It should be taken up in spring. It is good against pains in the head, and it promotes urine.

GLASSWORT.

DESCRIPTION.—*Kali.*—A common wild plant on the sea coasts of many parts of Europe, but not a native of our country. It is called cochleated kali, from the form of its seed-vessels, which are twisted in the manner of a snail's shell. It grows to a foot and a half in height. The stalk is round, thick, fleshy, and brittle. The leaves are few, and they stand irregularly; they are oblong, and blunted at the ends, and of a bluish green colour. The flowers are small, inconsiderable, and yellow.

MEDICINAL VIRTUES.—The juice of the fresh plant is said to be an excellent diuretic; but we have no opportunities of knowing its virtues here. Some say the seed vessels have the same virtue, and give them in infusion, but we have better remedies of the same kind, of our own growth. The whole plant is burnt for its fixed salt, which is used in making glass.

HARTWORT.

DESCRIPTION.—*Seseli.*—A tall, robust, and handsome plant, a native of the Alps, but kept in our gardens. It grows five or six feet in height: the stalk is round, thick, striated, and hollow, very firm and upright, and but little branched. The leaves are very large, and they are divided into a great number of parts, by fives and by threes; they are of a yellowish green. The flowers are small and white, but they stand in great tufts or umbels at the tops of the stalks: the seeds follow, two after each flower, and they are oblong, broad, and edged with a leafy border; they are of a dark colour, a strong smell, and acrid taste.

MEDICINAL VIRTUES.—The seeds are the only part used; they promote the menses, and the necessary discharges after delivery, and are an excellent warm and cordial medicine; they work also gently by urine, and cure colicy pains; they are to be given in powder or infusion.

LEOPARD'S-BANE.

Its botanical name is *Arnica Montana;* natural order, *Asteraceæ.* It is a very common perennial plant in the Alpine parts of Germany, in Sweden, Lapland, and Switzerland, where it has long been medicinally used. The flowers are yellow, compound, consisting entirely of tubular florets and are distinguished from other similar flowers, (with which they are often mixed, from ignorance or fraud,) by the common calyx, which is shorter than the florets, and consists entirely of lancet-shaped scales, lying parallel and close to each other, of a green colour, with purple points. These flowers have a slightly bitter taste, combined with a degree of acrimony, and when rubbed with the fingers, have a somewhat aromatic smell. They contain a great deal of resin, and a portion of essential oil.

As a medicine, it has not been much used in England, although it has been employed with the greatest advantage in Germany. The plant possesses very great virtues. It is diuretic, diaphoretic, emmenagogue, and vulnerary. It is given in amaurosis, paralysis, and other nervous affections. It has been recommended for hydrocephalous, and typhous fevers, especially in the latter stages. Dose of the powdered flowers, 4 to 15 grains; powdered root, 10 to 30 grains; infusion, half an ounce; extract, 1 to 10 grains; tincture 20 or 30 drops; essential oil, 1 or 2 drops.

"The flowers," says an eminent physician," are stimulating and discutient. In small doses, and properly administered, they produce very beneficial effects, in raising the pulse, in exciting the action of the whole sanguinerous system, in checking diarrhœas, in promoting expectoration, and especially in removing paralytic affections of the voluntary muscles; but they are frequently attended with no sensible operation, except that in some cases of paralysis, the cure is said to be preceded by a peculiar prickling, and by shooting pains in the affected parts. When given improperly, or in over-doses, they excite an insupportable degree of anxiety, shooting and burning pains, and even dangerous hæmorrhages, vomiting, vertigo, and coma. For these dangerous symptoms, vinegar is said to be the best remedy."

Haller says, "that even gutta serena, or loss of sight, has yielded to the powers of this medicine." It is also recommended in chronic rheumatism; in retention of the urine, from paralysis of the bladder; in intermittent fevers, when combined with Peruvian bark, where it has been very efficacious; in putrid diseases; to promote the uterine discharge: and in internal pains and congestions, from bruises.

"In the countries where the plants are indigenous, the flowers have long been a popular remedy in these cases. They are best given in infusion, one or two scruples may be infused with half a pound of water, and drank at proper intervals. The flowers should be wrapped up in a piece of linen, to prevent the diffusion of the down in the liquid, which would cause violent irritation of the throat.

Dr. Spencer Thompson says. "It is seldom prescribed internally in this country. But as an external application, it is much and beneficially used in the treatment of wounds and contusions. From 1 to 2 drachms of the tincture in half a pint of water forms a convenient lotion. The homœopathic practitioners claim Arnica, or Leopard's Bane, as one of their own remedies, and chemists ask for their tincture an extravagant price. But the tincture may be procured equally good, and much cheaper, at many respectable chemists. Like every thing else, there is much spurious tincture sold. When the pure tincture is dropped into water, it gives a milky or opalescent appearance."

The Homœopathists recommend it as possessing very great virtues, and that justly, in contusions, wounds, produced by falls, crushes, where the skin is lacerated and bruised; for bedsores, when the skin is not much broken; for pain in any part, produced by severe physical exertions, and in muscular weakness, sore or blistered feet, and hands. The body to be sponged with the aforesaid lotion as stated by Dr. S. Thompson. "I have found it," says one, "of the greatest use in whitlows, or painful gatherings in the fingers, chilblains, where the skin is not broken, and black eyes, chapped hands and lips, in gouty pains. For this purpose the *Cerate* of Arnica is a good application. The lotion takes away the soreness and pain of any diseased part, and it is remarkably beneficial for sore gums, especially after the extraction of teeth, or the straining of any part by surgical operations. The Monthly *Homœopathic Review* gives many instances of remarkable cures by Arnica, as cataract of the eyes, inflammation of the eyes, chronic rheumatism, fractures, and even blindness, &c. The application of *Arnica* in some cases was alternated with *Aconite*, an old-fashioned, but most valuable remedy. The lotion must be applied by saturating a piece of linen or cotton with it, and covering it with a bandage, repeating as the cloth dries. Some sores, or aching parts may be washed with the lotion. Should the skin be broken, the lotion should be reduced to half its strength. Should a careless administration produce eruption, it may be neutralized by diluted laudanum, say 30 or 40 drops to 4 ounces of water, frequently bathing the part. A weak solution of Coculus Indicus is also recommended.

MARIGOLDS.

See page 168. This plant, *Calendula Officinalis*, has been used in France as a vulnerary. The tincture is useful for curing warts. It may be used as a lotion, by adding 10 drops of the tincture, to 2 ounces of soft water. It is of special service in severe cuts, and lacerations; they are speedily relieved by it, and pain and bleeding arrested by its external application. It heals wounds so completely, when properly applied, as to leave no cicatrix or scar; if there should be any, it is scarcely perceptible. It has a wonderful power to heal without producing suppuration, or the formation of matter; it contracts the mouth of the small arteries which may have been cut across longitudinally. Where the cut cannot be closed, it may be washed with the lotion; it may be diluted as above, or be used in a pure state with perfect safety. It may also be applied by cloths and bandages as in the case of Leopard's-Bane.

SPIKENARD,—INDIAN.

Nardus Indica.—An East Indian plant, of the grass kind, with triangular stalks, and yellow flowers. It is like the yellow tufted grass, frequent in our meadows in spring. Breynius calls the Spikenard plant, a kind of Cyperus grass.

The tuft of fibres at the tops of the root, is what we call Indian Spikenard; they are brown, flattish, matted together, and of a pleasant fragrant smell; they are good in the disorders of the nerves; but we have better remedies.

DIRECTIONS
FOR GATHERING HERBS.

THE LEAVES OF HERBS OR TREES.

Of leaves, choose only such as are green, and full of juice; pick them carefully, and reject decaying ones, for they will putrify the rest, observe the places in which they grow best, and gather them there; for Betony in the shade is far better than that which grows in the sun, because it delights in the shade; also such herbs as grow well near water, should be gathered near it, though you may find some of them upon dry ground.

The leaves of such herbs as run up to seed, are not so good when in flower as before; (some few excepted,) if through negligence you have gathered them when in flower, take the tops and the flowers, rather than the leaf.

Dry them well in the sun and not in the shade; for if the sun draws away the virtues of the herb, it must do the like by hay, which every farmer would regard as nonsense.

Having well dried them, secure them in brown paper, and press them not too hard together and keep them in a dry place near the fire.

THE FLOWERS OF HERBS.

The flower, which is the beauty of the plant, and often medicinal, is to be gathered when it is in its prime.

As for the time of the day to gather them, let it be when the sun shines upon them so that they may be dry · for if you gather either flowers or herbs when they are wet or dewy, they will not keep.

Dry them well in the sun, and keep them in papers near the fire. So long as they retain the colour and smell, they are good; either being gone, so are their virtues also.

SEEDS.

The seed is that part of the plant which is endowed with the vital faculty to bring forth its like, and it contains potentially the whole plant in it. Gather them in the place where they delight to grow. Let them be full ripe when they are gathered. Dry them a little, and but a little, in the sun before you lay them up. Keep them in a dry place, they will keep many years ; yet they are best the first year ; for they will grow soonest the first year after being gathered, if sown ; therefore being in their prime, they must have more power.

ROOTS.

Do not choose such as are rotten or worm-eaten, but proper in their taste, colour and smell, such as exceed neither in softness nor hardness.

The drier the time in which you gather the roots, the better they are, having less tendency to decay. Dry soft roots in the sun, or near the fire. The hard roots you can dry anywhere. Large roots will keep longer than the small, yet all will keep a year.

BARKS.

The barks of fruit are to be taken when the fruit is full ripe, as Oranges, Lemons, &c. The barks of trees are best gathered in the Spring, if of oaks, &c. for then they come easier off; but the best way is to gather barks only for present use.

As for the bark of roots, take the roots of such herbs as have a pith in them, as parsley, fennel, &c. slit them in the middle, and when you have taken out the pith, that which remains is called the bark, and is only to be used.

JUICES, SYRUPS, PRESERVES, &c.

JUICES.

Juices are to be pressed out of herbs when they are young and tender, out of stalks, and tender tops of herbs and plants, and out of flowers. Bruise them well in a stone mortar with a wooden pestle, put it into a canvass bag, press it hard in a press, then take the juice and clarify it thus:—Put it into a pipkin or skillet, and set it over the fire; take off the scum; keep on the fire till no more scum arises.

When almost cold, put it into a glass, and put so much oil on it as will cover to the thickness of two fingers; the oil will swim at the top, and so keep the air from putrifying it. When you intend to use it, pour it into a porringer, and if any oil come out with it, you may easily scum it off with a spoon, and put the juice you use not, into the glass again, it will quickly sink under the oil. Or, when you have clarified it, boil it over the fire, till (being cold) it be of the thickness of honey: this is most commonly used for diseases of the mouth.

SYRUPS.

Syrups made by infusion, are usually made of such flowers as soon lose their colour and strength by boiling, as roses, violets, peach-flowers, &c. They are thus made:—Having picked your flowers clean, to every pound of them add three pounds, or three pints of spring water, boiling hot; first put your flowers into a pewter pot, with a cover, and pour the water on them; then shutting the pot, let it stand by the fire twelve hours and strain it out; (in such syrups as purge, as damask rose, peach-flowers, &c. the best way, is to repeat this infusion, adding fresh flowers to the same liquor, several times, that it may be the stronger) having strained it, put the infusion into a pewter bason, or an earthen one well glazed, and to every pint add two pounds of sugar, which being melted over the fire, without boiling, and scummed, will produce the syrup.

Syrups made by decoction are usually made of compounds, yet may any simple herb be thus converted into syrup: Take the herb, root, or flowers, and bruise a little, then boil it in a convenient quantity of spring water; the more water you boil it in, the weaker it will be: a handful of the herb or root is a convenient quantity for a pint of water; boil it till half the water be evaporated, then let it stand till almost cold, and strain it through woollen cloth, letting it run at leisure, without pressing. To every pint of this decoction add one pound of sugar, and boil it over the fire till it comes to a syrup, which you may know, if you now and then cool a little of it with a spoon: scum it while it boils, and when it is sufficiently boiled, whilst it is hot, strain it again through a woollen cloth, but press it not.

Syrups made of juice, are usually made of such herbs as are full of juice, and the juice makes the best syrup. Having beaten the herb in a stone mortar, with a wooden pestle, press out the juice and clarify it, as before; then let the juice boil away till about a quarter of it be consumed: to a pint of this add a pound of sugar, and boil it to a syrup, always scumming it, and when it is boiled enough, strain it through a woollen cloth.

If you make a syrup of roots that are hard, as Parsley, Fennel, and Grass roots, &c. When you have bruised them, lay them to steep some time in that water in which you intend to boil them, hot, so will the virtue the better come out.

Keep your syrups either in glasses or stone pots, and stop them not with cork or bladder, only bind paper about the mouth. All syrups, if well made, continue good a year; yet such as are made by infusion, keep shortest.

PRESERVES.

Flowers are very seldom preserved; I never saw but cowslip flowers. It is thus done: Take a flat glass, we call them jar-glasses; put in a layer of fine sugar, on that a layer of fine flowers, on that another layer of sugar, on that another layer of flowers, till your glass be full; then tie it over with paper, this will make an excellent and pleasant conserve.

Fruits, as quinces, and the like, are preserved two ways.

Boil them well in water, and then pulp them through a sieve; then with the like quantity of sugar, boil the water they were boiled in into a syrup, viz. a pound of sugar to a pint of liquor; to every pound of this syrup add four ounces of the pulp; then boil it with a very gentle fire to their right consistence, which you may easily know, if you drop a little of it upon a plate; if enough, it will not stick to your fingers when it is cold.

Another way to preserve fruits is this: pare off the rind; then cut them in halves, and take out the core, then boil them in water till they are soft; then boil the water with its like weight of sugar into a syrup; put the syrup into a pot, and put the boiled fruit, as whole as you left it when you cut it, into it, and let it remain till you use it.

Roots are thus preserved. First, scrape them very clean, and cleanse them from the pith, if they have any, for some roots have not, as Eringo and the like, boil them in water till they are soft; then boil the water in which you boiled the root into a syrup; then keep the roots whole in the syrup till you use them.

As for barks, few come to our hands which can be done, oranges, lemons, citrons, and the outer barks of walnuts; if there be any more, put them into the number. The way of preserving such as are bitter is to soak them in warm water, often changing it till their bitter taste be fled: but I like not this way, because when their bitterness is gone, so is their virtue also. It is best first to boil them whole till they are soft, then make a syrup with sugar and the liquor in which you boiled them, and keep the barks in the syrup. They are kept in glasses, or in glazed pots. The preserved flowers will keep a year; the root and barks much longer.

Thus medicines are made pleasant for sick and delicate stomachs, which otherwise would loath them.

OILS.

Olive Oil, commonly known by the name of Sallad Oil, because it is usually eaten with sallads, if it be pressed out of ripe olives, according to Galen, it is temperate, and exceeds in no one quality. Of oils, some are simple, and some are compound. Simple oils are such as are made of fruits or seeds by expression, as oil of sweet and bitter almonds, linseed, and rape-seed oil.

Compound oils, are made of oil of olives, and other simples, as herbs, flowers, and roots. They are made thus:—Having bruised the herbs or flowers, put them into an earthen pot, and to two or three handfuls of them pour a pint of oil, cover the pot with a paper, set in the sun about a fortnight, or so, according as the sun is in heat, then having warmed it very well by the fire, press out the herb, &c. very hard in a press, and add as many more herbs to the same oil; bruise the herbs in like manner, and set them in the sun as before; the oftener you repeat this, the stronger the oil will be; at last when you think it strong enough, boil both oil and herbs together, till the juice is consumed, which you may know by its ceasing to bubble, and the herbs will be crisp; then strain it while it is hot, and keep it in a stone or glass vessel for your use.

The general use of these oils is for pains in the limbs, roughness of the skin, the itch, &c. as also for ointments and plasters. If you use it for wounds and ulcers, in two ounces of oil, dissolve half an ounce of turpentine, the heat of the fire will quickly do it; for Oil itself is offensive to wounds, but the turpentine qualifies it.

ELECTUARIES.

An Electuary is a preparation made up of powdered drugs made up with treacle, honey or syrup.

That you may make Electuaries when you need them, it is requisite that you always keep herbs, roots, flowers, seed, &c. ready dried in your house, to beat them into a powder when you need them. It is better to keep them whole than beaten; for beaten, they are more subject to lose their strength; as the air soon penetrates them. Having beaten them, sift them through a fine sieve, that no great pieces may be found in your Electuary. To one ounce of your powder add three ounces of clarified honey; If you would make more or less Electuary, vary your proportions accordingly. Mix them well together in a mortar, you cannot mix them too much.

The way to clarify honey, is to set it over the fire in a convenient vessel, till the scum rise, and when the scum is taken off, it is clarified. The usual dose of cordial Electuaries, is from half a drachm to two drachms; of purging Electuaries, from half an ounce to an ounce. Keep them in a jar. The time for taking them, is either in a morning fasting, and fasting an hour after them; or at night going to bed, three or four hours after supper.

CONSERVES.

The way of making conserves is twofold, one of herbs and flowers, and the other of fruits.

Conserves of herbs and flowers, are thus made; if you make your conserve of herbs, as of scurvy-grass, wormwood, rue, and the like, take only the leaves and tender tops; and having beaten them, weigh them, and to every pound add three pounds of sugar, you cannot beat them too much.

Conserves of fruits, as of barberries, sloes and the like, are thus made; first scald the fruit, then rub the pulp through a thick hair sieve called a pulping sieve; you may do it for a need with the back of a spoon; then take this pulp thus drawn, and add to it its weight of sugar, put it into a pewter vessel, and over a charcoal fire; stir it up and down till the sugar be melted, and your conserve is made. The way of keeping them is in earthen pots. The dose is usually the quantity of a nutmeg at a time morning and evening, or (unless they are purging,) when you please. Some conserves will keep many years, as conserve of roses; others but a year, as conserve of borage, bugloss, cowslips, and the like. Look at them once a day, and stir them, lest they ferment; conserves of borage, bugloss, and wormwood, are very liable to ferment.

OINTMENTS.

Ointments are made thus: Bruise those herbs, flowers, or roots, you will make an ointment of, and to two handfuls of your bruised herbs add a pound of hog's lard, beat them well together in a stone mortar, then put it into a stone pot, cover it with a paper; and set it either in the sun, or some other warm place, three, four, or five days, that it may melt; then take it out and boil it a little, and while hot strain it out, pressing it very hard in a press; to this composition add as many more herbs bruised as before, let them stand in like manner as long, then boil them as before. If the ointment is not strong enough you may do it the third and fourth time; for the fuller of juice the herbs are, the sooner will your ointment be strong: the last time you boil it, boil it so long till your herbs be crisp, and the juice consumed, then strain it, pressing it hard in a press, and to every pound of ointment add two ounces of turpentine, and as much wax, because grease is offensive to wounds, as well as oil.

POULTICES.

Poultices the Latins call CATAPLASMATA; now sometimes called Cataplasms. They are made of herbs and roots, fitted for the disease to which you are liable; they are to be chopped small, and boiled in water almost to a jelly; then adding a little barley-meal, or oatmeal, and a little oil, or rough sweet suet, spread upon a cloth and applied to the affected place.

Their use is to ease pain, to break sores, to cool inflammations, to dissolve hardness, to ease the spleen, to concoct humours and dissipate swellings. Use no poultices that are of a healing nature, before you have first cleansed the body, because they are subject to draw the humours to them from every part of the body.

TROCHES.

The Latins call them PLACENTULA, or little cakes, and the Greeks PROCHIKOIS, KULISKOI, and ARTISEOI; they are usually little round or oval flat cakes, like the Pomfret Cakes, or Lozenges.

Their first invention was, that powders being so kept, might resist the intermission of air, and so endure pure the longer. They can be better carried in the pocket of those who travel, &c.

They are made thus: Take two drachms of fine gum tragacanth; put it into a gallipot, and put half a quarter of a pint of any distilled water fitting for the purpose you would make your troches for, to cover it, let it remain ten hours, till it becomes a mucilage. With this you may make a powder into a paste, and that paste into a cake called troches. Dry them in the shade, and keep them in a pot for your use.

PILLS.

They are called PILULÆ, because they resemble little balls. This way of making medicines was invented only to deceive the palate, that so by swallowing them down whole, the bitterness of them might not be perceived, or at least might not be insufferable; and indeed most pills are bitter. But I think they were made in this form, that so they might be the longer digesting. The invention of pills is to purge the head; such infirmities as lie near the passage, are best removed by decoctions, because they pass to the grieved part soonest; so here, if the infirmity lies in the head, or any other remote part, the best way is to use pills, because they are longer in digestion, and therefore better able to call the offending humour to them.

The way to make pills is very easy, for with the help of a pestle and mortar, you may make any dry powder into pills, either with syrup, or jelly.

JULEPS.

A term now not much used in medicine; it formerly expressed what we now understand by mixtures. Thus Camphor Mixture was then called Camphor Julep.

Simple Juleps are thus made: Take a pint of such distilled water, as conduces to the cure of your disease, to which add two ounces of syrup; conducing to the same effect; mix them together, and drink of it at your pleasure. If you like tart things, add ten drops of oil of vitriol to your pint, and shake it together, and it will have a fine grateful taste.

DECOCTIONS.

Decoctions do not keep long. They are made of those leaves, roots, flowers, seeds, fruits, or barks, conducing to the cure of the disease for which you may make them, they are made in the same manner as Syrups. Decoctions made with wine last longer than such as are made with water; and if you take a decoction to cleanse the passage of the urine, or open obstructions, your best way is to make it with white wine instead of water, because it is penetrating.

Decoctions are of most use in such diseases as lie in the stomach, bowels, kidneys, passages of the urine, and bladder, because decoctions pass more quickly to those places than any other form of Medicines. The decoction may be sweetened with sugar or honey. If in a decoction you boil roots, herbs, flowers, and seed together, let the roots boil a good while first, because they retain their virtue longest; then the next in order by the same rule, viz. barks, herbs, seeds, flowers, spices, if you put any in, because their virtues come soonest out. Such things as by boiling cause sliminess to a decoction, as figs, quince-seed, linseed, &c. your best way is, after you have bruised them, to tie them up in a linen-rag, and boil them. Keep all decoctions in a glass close stopped, and the cooler place in which you keep them, the longer they will last before they turn sour.

The usual dose to be given at one time, is usually 2, 3, 4 or 5 ounces, according to the age and strength of the patient, the season of the year, the strength of the medicine, and the quality of the disease.

THE BOTANIC FAMILY PHYSICIAN.

☞ I have bestowed considerable labour upon this department, availing myself of the experience of the most celebrated and learned Botanical Doctors of Great Britain, the continent of Europe and America:—

ON STEAMING FOR THE CURE OF DISEASES.

Steaming is a very important branch of my system of practice, which would, in many cases without it, be insufficient to effect a cure. It is of great importance in many cases considered by the medical faculty as desperate; and they would be so under my mode of treatment, if it were not for the manner of applying heat to the body, for the purpose of re-animating the system, and aiding nature in restoring health. I had but little knowledge of medicine, when, through necessity, I discovered the use of steaming, to add heat or life to the decaying spark; and with it I was enabled, by administering such vegetable preparations as I then had a knowledge of, to effect a cure in cases where the regular practitioners had given them over.

In all cases where the heat of the body is so far exhausted as not to be rekindled by using the medicine, and being shielded from the surrounding air by a blanket, or being in bed, and chills or stupor attend the patient, then heat applied by steaming becomes indispensably necessary; and heat caused by steam in the manner I use it, is more natural in producing perspiration than any dry heat that can be applied to the body in any other manner, which will only serve to dry the air and prevent perspiration in many cases of disease, where a steam by water or vinegar would promote it, and add a natural warmth to the body, and thereby increase the life and motion which has lain silent in consequence of the cold.

Dr. Jennings has contrived a plan to apply heat to the body by dry vapour, caused by burning spirit, which he calls a vapor bath ; the idea of which was, I have no doubt, taken from hearing of my steaming to raise the heat of the body. It may answer in some cases and stages of the disease; but in a settled fever, and other cases where there is dry inflammation on the surface of the body, it will not answer any good purpose, and I think would be dangerous, without the use of my medicine to first raise a free perspiration ; for when the surface of the body is dry, the patient cannot bear it, as it will crowd the head and cause distress, the same as is produced by burning charcoal, or from hot stoves in a tight room, and will bring on a difficulty in breathing, which is not the case in steaming in my way. This machine can only be used in bed, where the vapour cannot be applied to the body equally at the same time, therefore it is no better than a hot dry stone, put on each side and to the feet of the patient, for he can turn himself and get heat from them as well as to have all the trouble of burning spirit and turning to the vapour of it, to get warm by this dry heat. When the patient stands over a steam raised by putting a hot stone in water, which gives a more equal heat all over the body than can be done in any other manner, it can be raised higher, and may be tempered at pleasure, by wetting the face and stomach with cold water, as occasion requires.

The method adopted by me, and which has always answered the desired object, is as follows :—Take several stones of different sizes, and put them in the fire till red hot, then take the smallest first, and put it into a pan or kettle of hot water, with the stone about half immersed—the patient must be undressed, and a blanket put around him so as to shield his whole body from the air, and then place him over the steam. Change the stones as often as they grow cool, so as to keep up a lively steam, and keep him over it ; if he is faint throw a little cold water on the face and stomach, which will let down the outward heat and restore the strength : after he has been over the steam long enough—which will generally be about fifteen or twenty minutes —he must be washed all over with cold water, and be put into bed, or may be dressed, as the circumstances of the case shall permit.—Before he is placed over the steam, give a dose of Nos. 2 and 3, or composition, to raise the inward heat. When the patient is too weak to stand over the steam, it may be done in bed, by heating three stones and putting them in water till done hissing, then wrap them in a number of thicknesses of cloth, wet with water, and put one on each side and one at the feet, occasionally wetting the face and stomach with cold water, when faint.

Many other plans may be contrived in steaming, which would make less trouble, and be more agreeable to the patient, especially where they are unable to stand over the steam. An open worked chair may be made, in which they might sit and be steamed very conveniently ; or a settee might be made in the same manner, on which they might be laid and covered with blankets, so as to shield them from the surrounding air. Such contrivances as these would be very convenient, in cases where the patient would have to be carried through a course of medicine and steamed a number of times, as is frequently necessary, particularly in complaints that have been long standing.

As I have frequently mentioned a regular course of medicine, I will here state what is meant by it, and the most proper way in which it is performed. Firstly give Nos. 2 and 3, or composition, adding a tea spoonful of No. 6, then steam, and when in bed repeat it, adding No. 1, which will cleanse the stomach and assist in keeping up a perspiration: when this has done operating, give an injection made with the same articles. Where there are symptoms of nervous affection, or spasms, put half a tea spoonful of the nerve powder into each dose given, and into the injection. In violent cases, where immediate relief is needed, Nos, 1, 2, 3, and 6, may be given together. Injections may be administered at all times, and in all cases of disease, to advantage; it can never do harm, and in many cases they are indispensably necessary, especially where there is cancer and inflammation in the bowels, and there is danger of mortification; in which case add a tea spoonful of No. 6. In cases of this kind, the injection should be given first, or at the time of giving the composition, or No. 3.

The use of steaming is good in preventing sickness as well as curing it. When a person has been exposed to the cold, and is threatened with disease, it may be prevented, and long sickness and expense saved by a very little trouble, by standing over a steam and following the directions before given, till the cold is thoroughly thrown off and a lively perspiration takes place; then go to bed, taking the stone from the kettle, and wrap it in wet cloths and put it to the feet. This may be done without the medicine, when it cannot be had; but is much better to take something to raise the inward heat at the same time. A tea made of may-weed, or summer savoury, or ginger and hot water sweetened, may be given, or any thing that is warming. This advice is for the poor, and those who have not a knowledge of the medicine; and will many times save them much trouble and long sickness.

Steaming is of the utmost importance in cases of suspended animation, such as a drowned person; in which case place the body over a moderate steam, shielded by a blanket from the weight of the external air, and rarifying the air immediately around them with the steam. Pour into the mouth some of the tincture of Nos. 1, 2, and 6; and if there is any internal heat remaining, there will be muscular motion about the eyes, and in the extremities. If this symptom appears, repeat the dose several times, and renew the hot stones, raising the heat by degrees; if the outward heat is raised too suddenly, so as to balance the inward, you will fail of the desired object, even after life appears. This is the only danger of any difficulty taking place—always bear in mind to keep the fountain above the stream, or the inward heat above the outward, and all will be safe. After life is restored, put them in bed and keep the perspiration free for twelve hours, by hot stones wrapped in cloths wet with water, occasionally giving the tincture as before mentioned the coldness and obstructions will be thrown off, and the patient restored to the enjoyment of his natural strength. Beware of bleeding, or blowing in the mouth with a bellows, as either will generally prove fatal.

In many cases of spotted fever, steaming is as necessary as in drowned persons; such as when they fall apparently dead; then the same treatment is necessary to lighten the surrounding air, till you can raise the inward heat so as to get the determining powers to the surface. Begin with a small stone, and as life gains, increase the steam as the patient can bear it; if the distress is great, give more hot medicine inside, and as soon as an equilibrium takes place the pain will cease. In all cases of this kind, the difficulty cannot be removed without applying heat to the body, and it is more natural by steam than by any other means that can be made use of. In cases of long standing, where the patient has been run down with mercury, and left in a cold and obstructed state, liable to rheumatism, and other similar complaints, they cannot be cured with medicine without heat applied by steam; as nothing will remove mercury but heat.

When a patient is carried through a course of my medicine, and steamed, who has been long under mercurial treatment, and while under the operation of the steam, when the heat is at the highest, the face will swell in consequence of the poisonous vapour being condensed by the air, the face being open to it. To relieve this, put him in bed, and take a hot stone wrapped in several thicknesses of cloth wet with water, pouring on a little vinegar, and making a lively steam; put it in bed and cover his head with the clothes and let him breathe the steam as hot as can be borne, until the sweat covers the swelled part. This will, in about fifteen or twenty minutes, throw out the poison, and the swelling will abate. This method, also, is of great service in agues, and teeth ache, caused by cold; and many other cases of obstructions from the same cause, especially young children stuffed on the lungs.

To steam small children, the best way is to let them sit in the lap of a person, covering both with a blanket, and sit over the steam, pouring a little vinegar on the stone; or it may be done in bed, with a hot stone wrapped in cloths wet with water, putting on a little vinegar, and covering them with the bed clothes laid loosely over them—but in this way you cannot exercise so good judgment in tempering the steam, as when you are steamed with them. If they appear languid and faint, the outward heat is high enough; put a little cold water on the face or breast, which will restore the strength; then rub them with a cloth wet with vinegar, spirit, or cold water, put on clean clothes and put them in bed, or let them sit up, as their strength will permit. This is safe in all cases of cold and obstructed perspiration. It ought always to be borne strongly in mind to give a child drink often, when under the operation of medicine, or while steaming; if this is not done they will suffer much, as they cannot ask for it.

In all cases of falls or bruises, steaming is almost infallible; and is much better than bleeding, as is the common practice, which only tends to destroy life, instead of promoting it. If the person is not able to stand over the steam, it must be done in bed, as has been described. Give the hottest medicine inside that you have, and keep the perspiration free, till the pain and soreness abates, and the strength will be soon restored.—If the advantages of this mode of treatment were generally known, bleeding in such cases, or any other to remove disease, would never be resorted to by the wise and prudent.

The use of steaming, is to apply heat to the body where it is deficient, and clear off the obstructions caused by cold, which the operation of the medicine will not raise heat enough to do:—for as the natural heat of the body becomes thereby lower than the natural state of health, it must by art be raised as much above it as it has been below; and this must be repeated until the digestive powers are restored sufficient to hold the heat by digesting the food; then the health of the patient will be restored by eating and drinking such things as the appetite shall require. In this way the medicine removes disease, and food, by being properly digested, supports nature, and continues that heat on which life depends.

Some who practice according to my system, boast of carrying their patients through in a shorter time, without the trouble of steaming; this is easily accounted for; steaming is the most laborious part of the practice for those who attend upon the sick, and the most useful to the patient; as one operation of steaming will be more effectual in removing disease, than four courses without it; and to omit it is throwing the labour upon the patient, with the expense of three or four operations more of the medicine than would be needed, did the person who attends do his duty faithfully.

I have adopted the plan of *numbering* the remedies, and describing them under their respective numbers. Nos. 1, 2, 3, are used to remove disease, and the other as restoratives.

Number One.

EMETIC HERB,—LOBELIA INFLATA.

IT IS USED TO CLEANSE THE STOMACH, OVERPOWER THE COLD, AND PROMOTE A FREE PERSPIRATION.

It is the most important article used in the Botanical system of medicine. It was first discovered as a medicine by Mr. S. Thomson of America. The faculty, with few exceptions, have opposed this remedy; but many of them have only expressed their ignorance. Some, like Dr. Graham, have stated its value. See page 161. Yet most of them have acknowledged its great use in Asthma.

In America the doctors were astonished at its beneficial effects, and they concluded that it must be poison. Such a conclusion is easily accounted for; they know nothing in all their medical science capable of producing a powerful effect upon the body except what is poisonous, and therefore they form their opinions after this erroneous theory. Mr. S. Thomson says, "Forming an erroneous opinion of this herb, they represented it as a deadly poison, and to destroy my practice, they falsely asserted that I killed my patients by giving it to them. Some of them made oath that it *was* poison. But the fact is very well known that *there is no death in it.* On the contrary, *there is no vegetable grown more harmless in its effects on the human system, and none* more powerful in removing disease and promoting health."

"While the faculty thought Lobelia to be poison they called it *my medicine.* But since they discovered its medicinable virtues to be so valuable, they are restless to rob me of the credit of making its value known. Dr. M. Cutler says, 'If the quantity be a little increased, it operates as an *emetic*, and then as a *cathartic*; its effects being much the same as those of the common emetics and cathartics. In this he is mistaken, for it is entirely different from every other emetic. I never knew it to act as a cathartic in all my practice for above twenty years, having administered it in every form in which it can be given, and for every disease that has come within my knowledge. Dr. Cutler cured himself of Asthma with it. I introduced the use of Lobelia, tinctured in spirit, for the asthma, and other complaints of the lungs, and cured many people. I cured a woman at Newington, of asthma, who had not lain in bed for six months. After taking the tincture she lay in bed the first night after; she recovered, has been in health twelve years, and has not been obliged to sit up one night since."

"Now the doctors have begun to say it is a good medicine in *skilful hands*. Dr. Thacher says that its fatal effects were owing to the quantity given, and charges me with having given a tea-spoonful of the powder; and when *he* gives directions for using it, he says, that from 10 to 20 grains, may be given with safety. Just look! If a tea-spoonful be given by an *empiric*, its effects are fatal; but if *it* be administered by a *learned doctor*, and called *grains*, it is *a very useful medicine!!*"

Mistakes have been made as to the *real* herb Lobelia. A poisonous root grows in the Southern States, called Lobelia and it has been used as a medicine; this may account for the true Lobelia having been called *poison*. This emetic herb may be found in the first stages of its growth, through the Summer from the size of a sixpence to that of a half-crown, round, and lying flat on the ground, (in America) pressed flat on the ground by the snow in winter, like a rose pressed flat. In summer it lifts up its leaves, and shoots forth a stalk a foot high, with branches, carrying up its leaves with its growth. In July it bears small pointed blue blossoms, followed by small pods, containing numerous small seeds. The pod is just like the human stomach, having an inlet and outlet higher than the middle; from the inlet it receives nourishment, and by the outlet discharges the seeds. It grows in highways and pastures, by waysides, and in stubble land. It is abundant in America, and grows in other countries, and in some gardens.

This herb may be prepared for use in three different ways,

viz—the *powdered leaves* and pods—a *tincture* made from the green herb with spirit—the seeds reduced to a fine powder and compounded with Nos. 2 and 6.

1. After the leaves and pods are separated from the stalks, pound or grind them in a mortar to a fine powder, sift through a fine sieve, and preserve it from the air. It may be given by itself, or compounded with other articles. *Dose*, a tea-spoonful of this powder, some quantity of sugar, in a tea-cup half full of warm water; or a tea-spoonful of No. 3, may be used instead of the water; to be taken two or three times, at intervals of 10 or 15 minutes. The liquid must never be more than blood-warm; hot water destroys its efficacy.

2. *The Tincture.* Take the green herb, (if the small plants are used take roots and all) pound them fine in a mortar; add a sufficient quantity of good spirit; when well pounded together, strain it through a fine cloth, and preserve the liquor in closely stopped bottles for use. It is an effectual counter poison, either taken inwardly, or externally applied. It is an effectual remedy for the asthma and all complaints of the lungs, nearly every docter now acknowledges it.—*Dose*, from half to a tea-spoonful. Its effect will be more certain if the same quantity of No. 2 be added, and where there are nervous symptoms, add half a tea-spoonful of nerve powder, (umbil) to the dose.

3. Reduce the seeds to a fine powder, and take half an ounce of it, or a large spoonful, with the same quantity of No. 2, made fine and put them into a gill of No. 6 and a tea-spoonful of umbil. Bottle for use. It is intended for violent attacks of disease, such as lock jaw, hydrophobia, fits, spasms, drowning, and in all cases of suspended animation, where the vital spark is nearly extinct. It will go through the system like electricity, giving heat and life to every part. Lock-jaw is relieved by pouring some of this liquid between the cheek and the teeth. As soon as it touches the glands at the roots of the tongue the spasms will relax, and the jaws be loosened, and the mouth be opened; then give a dose of it, repeating it as the spasms abate; afterwards give a tea of No. 3. "This course," says Mr. Thomson, I never knew fail of giving relief. It is effectual in bringing out measles, and small pox, and in the removal of warts, pimples, &c. I have cured three cases of canine

madness, by it; it is a specific for that disease. *Dose,*—a tea-spoonful.

Lobelia is most powerful to remove diseases, but perfectly innocent in its effects. It has been given to children of one day old and to persons 80 years old. There are two cases where this medicine will not operate, viz.—when the patient is dying, and where there is no disease. There can be no war where there is no enemy. When there is no cold in the body, there is nothing to contend against, and when there is no heat there is nothing to kindle; in both cases this medicine is silent and harmless. It is calculated to remove the cause, and no more. It clears all obstructions, until it produces an equilibrium throughout the system which is felt in the fingers and toes,—a prickling sensation like that caused by a blow on the elbow—an alarming symptom to those unacquainted with its operation; but it is always a certain indication of a turn of the disorder, and patients generally gain from that time.

The best way will be to give the smallest prescribed *dose* first, and repeat till it produces the desired operation. If the stomach is cold and foul, its operation will be expedited by giving No. 2. To patients in a decline, or to those who have chronic diseases, three to eight courses of the medicine are necessary to produce the favourable crisis; and the lower they have been, the more alarming will be the symptoms to those unacquainted with its effects. "I have seen some," says Dr. Thomson, "lie and sob like a child, for two hours, unable to speak, or raise their hands; and the next day quite well. If much opium has been taken, Lobelia will, in its operations, produce the same symptoms produced by opium, which, still lodging in the system, is roused into action by Lobelia, and the patient may be thrown into a senseless state, or be agitated so as to require holding. Sometimes they grow cold as though dying, and remain so from two to eight hours, and then awake like one from sleep after a good night's rest, as if nothing had ailed them. It is the last struggle of the disease, and they generally begin to recover from that time.——By taking a dose when first attacked by a disease, Lobelia will throw it off, and prevent long sickness. It requires, however, to be followed by some other medicine to hold the vital heat till nature is able to support itself by digesting the food as No. 2, and occasionally No. 3 to remove canker,* the great cause of disease, and then follow with No. 4, and 5, to correct the bile, restore the digestion, strengthen the system, and effect a cure."

Number Two.

CAYENNE—CAPSICUM.—SEE PAGE 61.

ITS USE IS TO RETAIN THE INTERNAL VITAL HEAT OF THE SYSTEM, AND CAUSE A FREE PERSPIRATION.

It is well known. It is desirable to have it pure, as it is frequently adulterated by red sand, red woods, and salt. It is best to buy it in pods, and grind it at home for use; though it may be obtained ground, and pure, from those who vend botanical medicines. It has been used principally for culinary purposes and latterly for medicinal purposes. It is one of the safest and best articles ever discovered to remove disease. The Edinburgh Dispensatory says, "There can be little doubt that it furnishes one of the purest and strongest stimulants that can be introduced into the stomach, while it has nothing of the narcotic effects of ardent spirits. It has been used with success in some diseases that had resisted all other remedies." Dr. Thacher gives the same opinion.

Mr. S. Thomson says, In the fall of 1807, I was in Newburyport, and saw a bottle of pepper-sauce. Being the first I had ever seen, I bought it, got some of the same kind of pepper that was dried, which I put into the bottle; this made it very hot. On my way home, I was taken unwell, and was quite cold. I took a swallow from the bottle, which caused violent pain for a few minutes, when it produced perspiration, and I soon grew easy. I afterwards tried it, and found that after it had expelled the cold it would not cause pain. From these experiments I became convinced that this kind of pepper was much stronger, and would be better for medical use than the

* The American faculty frequently use the word "*Canker*," which means a morbific state, or tendency to disease in any locality, internal or external.

common red pepper. Soon after this, I was again at Newburyport, and made inquiry and found some Cayenne; but it was prepared with salt for table use, which injured it for medical purposes. I became acquainted with a French gentleman who had a brother in Demerara, and made arrangements with him to send to his brother and request him to procure some, and have it prepared without salt. He did so, and sent out a box containing about eighty pounds in a pure state. I sent also by many others that were going to the places where it grows, to procure all they could; in consequence of which, large quantities were imported into Portsmouth, much more than there was immediate demand for.

I was only able to purchase but a small part of what was brought, and it was bought up by others, on speculation, and sent to Boston; the consequence was, that the price was so much reduced, that it would not bring the first cost, which put a stop to its being imported, and it has since been very scarce. When I first began to use this article, it caused much talk among the people in Portsmouth and the adjoining towns. The doctors tried to frighten them by saying that I made use of cayenne pepper as a medicine, and that it would burn up the stomach and lungs as bad as vitriol. The people generally, however, became convinced by using it, that what the doctors said about it was false, and it only proved their ignorance of its medicinal virtues, and their malignity towards me. It soon came into general use, and the knowledge of its being useful in curing disease, was spread throughout the country.

It has effectually cured the spotted fever. In all kinds of diseases, it has been given to patients of all ages, and under every circumstance almost. It is perfectly harmless, as those who have administered it for years can testify that they have never known it to produce bad effects. It is the most powerful stimulant, to raise and maintain that heat on which life depends. It is extremely pungent, setting the mouth on fire, for a few minutes, but even this is beneficial; for its effects on the glands, causes the saliva to flow freely, and leave the mouth clean and moist.

It must be ground to a fine powder. *Dose*, from a quarter to a tea-spoonful in hot water, sweetened; or it may be mixed with either of the other Numbers when taken. It will produce a free perspiration, to be maintained by repeating the dose, till the disease is removed. A spoonful of Cayenne, and one of salt, put into a gill of vinegar, makes a very good dinner sauce to assist the appetite, and strengthen digestion. A tea-spoonful of this preparation will remove faintings and flatulency. A tea-spoonful of Cayenne in a tumbler of Cider is better than ardent spirit. It is good to be combined with most medicines.

RED PEPPERS.

These are abundant in America. The pods are used in pickling. This pepper is of the same nature as Cayenne, but not so strong, and the best substitute for it.

GINGER.

See page 123. It may be used when a milder remedy than Cayenne is required. It is best to obtain the roots and grind or pound them to a fine powder. It makes an excellent poultice, mixed with pounded biscuit, or bread, or Slippery Elm Bark. To chew a little of the root constantly, and swallow the saliva, is good for a cough; and for those of a consumptive habit. It prevents the contagion attendant on sick rooms, &c.

BLACK PEPPER.

See page 208. This may also be used as a substitute for the preceding remedies, and administered in the same manner. These four maintain the heat of the body longer than any other prescribed remedy.

Number Three.

TO SCOUR THE STOMACH AND BOWELS, AND REMOVE CANKER.

I shall describe those remedies which are good to remove canker from the throat, stomach and bowels; caused by cold;

for when cold obtains the power over the inward heat, the stomach and bowels become coated with canker, which prevents its numerous little vessels from performing their duty. Some remedies proposed for this disease are too binding, and cause obstructions. The following is a good method to ascertain what is good for canker:—Chew some of the proposed article, and if it cause the saliva to flow freely, and leaves the mouth clean and moist, it is good; but if it dries up the juices, and leaves the mouth rough and dry, it is bad.

☞ The following articles may be purchased of the Medical Botanists, nearly in every town.

BAYBERRY, OR CANDLEBERRY.

It is a species of Myrtle, common in America. It produces berries which contain wax in abundance. The bark of the roots is used in medicine, in fine powder. It is an excellent medicine alone, or compounded with other articles, and a real specific for canker; probably the best. It is highly stimulating, and very pungent, pricking the glands, and causing the saliva, and other juices to flow freely. It is a first rate tooth-powder, cleansing the teeth and gums, and removing scurvy. As snuff it clears the head, and cures headache. It is good in relax, and all disorders of the bowels. When the stomach is very foul, it will often operate as an emetic.—*Dose*, a tea-spoonful in hot water sweetened.

WHITE POND LILY.

The roots are used. They are large. They should be well-washed, split into strips and dried; then pulverised, and preserved for use. It is a good medicine for canker, and all bowel complaints, given in tea alone, or mixed with other articles.

HEMLOCK.

The common Hemlock-tree grows in New England. The inner bark is used, an infusion of the bark in hot water is a good medicine for canker, and diseases arising from it. Mr. S. Thomson says, "I have constantly given it, and always found it a good medicine for complaints of the stomach and bowels. A tea made of this bark is very good, and may be used freely; it is good to give the emetic and No. 2 in, and may be used for drink in all cases of sickness, especially when going through a course of medicine and steaming. This, with bayberry bark and lily root, forms No. 3, or what has been commonly called coffee, though many other things may be added, or either of them may be used to advantage alone. The boughs, made into a tea, are very good for the gravel, or other obstructions of the urinary passages, and for rheumatism."

MARSH ROSEMARY.

This is good for canker and sore mouth. It has been used with Bayberry bark for No. 3 with good success. It should not be used without a large proportion of Bayberry bark.

SUMACH.

This is a new remedy. It has been found very effectual in dysentery. The bark is used; also the leaves, and the berries, when ripe; and when used as part of No. 3, should be pounded; and the three may be used separately, or altogether. A tea made of either of these articles is very good, safe in almost all complaints, and put into injections. It will cleanse or scour the stomach and bowels; is good for stranguary, relieves all obstructions in the kidneys, and strengthens them. The use of this article with Bayberry bark and Lily root, equal parts, for No. 3, or coffee, has been very useful.

WITCH HAZEL.

A tea made of the leaves may be taken freely with advantage. "It is the best thing for bleeding at the stomach," says Mr. Thomson," of any article I have ever found, either by tea made of the dry leaves, or chewing them when green. I have cured several of bleeding with it; and also in complaints of the bowels I have seen its efficacy. An injection of this tea, with a little of No. 2, is good for the piles, and many female complaints. In bearing down pains it will afford immediate relief, if properly administered.

RASPBERRY LEAVES.

See page 224. They may be used green, or dried. They have performed wonderful cures in relax, and the usual bowel complaints. An infusion alone, or as a component part of injections, never fails to give immediate relief. Its utility in travail is surprising. Give a strong infusion of the leaves, with a little No. 2, sweetened, and it will regulate every thing as nature requires. If the pains are untimely, it will make all quiet, if timely, and lingering, give more of No. 2, and Umbil in the infusion. When the child is born, give it some of the tea with sugar and milk in it; this prevents sore mouth; it is good to wash sore nipples with. A poultice made of the infusion and bread, or slippery elm bark, is very good for burns and scalds; if the skin is off, this poultice, or washing with the infusion will allay pain, and promote healing.

SQUAW WEED.

Indian name, *Cocash.* The roots and tops are used for medicine. Mr. Thomson says "It was given to me when I had the Canker-rash, and effected a cure. I have frequently used it for that complaint, and found it very good. Take the green roots and leaves, bruise them, pour on hot water, and give this tea sweetened. It may be kept by adding a little spirit, and is good for rheumatism, or for nervous affection. It is perfectly harmless, and may be used freely. It makes a very good bitter if tinctured with hot water and spirit; and when thus prepared, is good for dizziness, cold hands and feet."

Number Four.

Bitters to correct the Bile, and restore impaired Digestion.

BITTER HERB, OR BALMONY.

It is very good to correct the bile and create an appetite. The infusion of it may be used alone, or may be added to any of the other articles adapted to restore the digestive powers.

POPLAR BARK.

The bark of the stinking Poplar is the best, as it is the most bitter. An infusion of the inner bark is one of the best articles to regulate the bile, and restore the digestive powers. To make bitters, No. 4, it should be powdered very fine, and mixed with the other articles, or used alone. To make an infusion, take a handful of the bark pounded, put it into a quart mug, and fill it with boiling water. This infusion will relieve a relax, headache, faintness, and other complaints caused by indigestion. Those who have affections of the kidneys, or are consumptive, will find great benefit from its use.

BAYBERRY.

See page 33. The bark of the root or top, is a good bitter, and useful to correct the bile, and assist digestion. It is administered by infusion, which may be freely used in all cases of indigestion.

BITTER ROOT.

It is also called *Wandering Milk Weed.* The root is very bitter, and a sovereign corrector of the bile. It removes constipation, causing the bowels to move in a natural way. A strong infusion, with hot water, if drank freely, will operate as a cathartic, sometimes as an emetic. It is sure to throw off fever in its first stages, and should be used in all cases of constipation.

GOLD SEAL.

Called also *Kercuma.* It is a pleasant bitter. The powdered root is used. In weakness of stomach, where food distresses, a tea-spoonful of the powder given in hot water, sweetened, will give immediate relief. It is a powerful correction of the bile, alone, or with the bitter root, or may be compounded with either or all of the articles under this Number, to restore the digestive powers.

Number Five.

SYRUP FOR THE DYSENTERY, TO STRENGTHEN THE STOMACH AND BOWELS, AND RESTORE WEAK PATIENTS.

The articles are the bark of Poplar, Bayberry, Peachmeats, or meats of Cherry-stones, sugar, and brandy.

PEACH MEATS.

They are of great value to strengthen the stomach and bowels, and restore the digestion. Made into a cordial, with other articles, hereafter described, they effectually restore the tone of the stomach after long sickness, and restore weak patients particularly in dysentery. An infusion of the leaves will remove colic.

CHERRY STONES.

These may be used instead of Peach meats. An infusion with the cherries, pounded with the stones, sweetened, and a little brandy, promotes digestion, and a good appetite.

Number Six.

RHEUMATIC DROPS, TO REMOVE PAIN, PREVENT MORTIFICATION, AND PROMOTE NATURAL HEAT.

GUM MYRRH.

See page 190. Mr. S. Thomson had a lame ancle, and was told by an old man to apply the Tincture of Myrrh. It was squirted into the wound, which caused a temporary smarting. It was also taken inwardly, and it effected a cure. In cases of bad wounds and old sores, it affords great relief, and is a cure for worms. Its power is increased by using spirit, and a little Cayenne, for internal administration. If slightly boiled, it prevents the fumes from rising to the head, which otherwise would be injurious to the hysterical. It is a first-rate remedy for rheumatism.

SPIRIT OF TURPENTINE.

For external application. A portion of it should be added to the Rheumatic Drops, when used for the itch, or other bad humours. It should be used cautiously. See page 278.

GUM CAMPHOR.

For bad sprains, it may be added to the Rheumatic Drops, with great advantage.

The best Tincture of Camphor is the third Dilution, used by the *Homœopathists*. For a dose, they recommend one drop in water, or on loaf sugar, to be repeated every five or ten minutes, if need be. It is curative of Cholera in the first stage, colds, diarrhœas, epilepsy, faintings, poisoning by opium, ague. Allopathists order from 20 to 60 drops. An over-dose of Camphor may be relieved by strong Coffee. See page 60.

NERVE POWDER.—UMBIL.

American Valerian, or Ladies' Slipper, sometimes called Umbil, or Male and Female Nervine.

Mr. S. Thomson says, this powder is the best nervine known; I have made use of it, and have always found it to produce the most beneficial results, in all cases of nervous affection, and in hysterical symptoms; in fact, it would be difficult to get along with my practice in many cases without this important article. It is perfectly harmless, and may be used in all cases with safety: it is better than opium, which is generally given in cases of spasmodic affection, and which only deadens the feelings and relieves pain only by destroying sensibility, without doing any good. Valerian has been supposed by the doctors to be of a narcotic nature; but this is a mistake. They have drawn this conclusion, from its tendency to promote sleep; but this is owing to its quieting the nerves and leaving the patient at ease. When nature requires sleep to recover the natural tone of the system, half a tea-spoonful may be given in hot water, sweetened, and the dose repeated if necessary; or the same quantity may be mixed with a dose of either of the other numbers when given, and put into the injections; where there are nervous symptoms, it should never be dispensed with.

COMMON HERBS.

I call them common, because the preceding Articles were for a long time uncommon in America and especially in England; and because they are not so powerful as Lobelia, Cayenne, &c. Yet they are very efficacious in many complaints, of a warming nature, and capable of arresting disease. Some of them have already been described, and reference is made to each description.

SPEARMINT.

Described, page 180. It tends to stay vomiting. If an overdose of Lobelia should produce excessive vomiting, a strong infusion of Spearmint will stop it, and ease the stomach.

PEPPERMINT.

See page 179. It promotes perspiration, and overpowers a cold, if drank just before going to bed. The essence, or oil in warm water relieves pains in the stomach and bowels.

PENNYROYAL.

See page 207. It is of great value in medicine. An infusion may be used in all cases of sickness ; it warms and cleanses the stomach ; if drank freely, it produces perspiration, and removes obstructions. It will throw off colds and slight attacks of disease, and prevent sickness. In children, it removes wind and pain in the bowels. In going through a course of medicine, an infusion of it may be drank, and it will cause the medicine to have a pleasant operation.

SUMMER SAVOURY.

Page 245. An infusion is good for colds, and may be taken with benefit in sickness. The oil of the herb will cure tooth-ache.

HOREHOUND.

Page 139. The Horehound Candy is very useful for coughs, especially in old people and the asthmatical.

ELECAMPANE.

Its virtues are described, page 99.

MAY-WEED.

A hot infusion of this herb drank when going to bed, is good for a cold, and in slight attacks of fever, if used freely, and a hot brick put to the feet, will, in most cases, effect a cure.

WORMWOOD.

Described page 288. The green herb pounded and tinctured in spirit, is excellent for bruises and sprains.

TANSY

Described page 265. The green leaves pounded and applied will relieve sprains and bruises, and allay the swelling.

CAMOMILE.

Described page 59. An infusion is good for bowel complaints, and externally applied, will relieve sprains, bruises, and swellings, and remove callosities, corns, &c. and restore sunken kidneys.

BITTER-SWEET.

See page 193. It is a good external application. The bark of the root with cammomile and Wormwood, make an ointment of great value, very efficacious for a bruise, sprain, swelling, corns, and callosity.

MULLEN.

Page 186. The bruised leaves reduce swellings, and restore contracted sinews. Apply them warm. It is an important article in the strengthening plaster hereafter described.

BURDOCK.

Fully described page 54. The leaves are good applied to the feet in case of fever, to keep them moist and promote perspiration.

SKUNK-CABBAGE.

The root should be pounded or ground to a powder. This powder may be taken in tea, sweetened or made into a syrup, or a tea spoonful may be mixed with honey, and taken in the morning, or at night when going to bed. It is good for asthma, cough, difficulty of breathing, and all disorders of the lungs, and with other articles, makes one of the best preparations for those complaints I have ever found.

WAKE-ROBIN.

See page 87. This root is extremely pungent and stimulating and is often given for cholic and pain in the bowels, and to expel wind. I have mostly made use of it for coughs and disorders of the lungs, for which I have found it a very useful article, and it forms part of my composition for coughs. The root should be dried and reduced to powder, and may be mixed with honey or in syrup.

THOROUGHWORT.

This herb is well known in the country, and is made use of by the people in tea for many complaints. It is of a warming nature, and is good for coughs and other complaints of the lungs. It is used in my compound prepared for coughs.

FEATHERFEW

Fully described page 69.

CLIVERS.

A strong infusion is good for urinary obstructions. See page 73.

BLACK BIRCH BARK.

Page 41. An infusion of the bark cures complaints in the bowels, especially dysentery. Made into a Syrup with Peach-meats, or Cherry-stone-meats, it restores those who have been debilitated with the dysentery, &c, and strengthens the stomach and promotes digestion.

EVAN ROOT.

This is called by some people chocolate root, on account of its resembling that article in taste, and is made use of by some as a common drink instead of tea or coffee. It is good for canker, and may be used in No. 3, as a substitute for other articles. It grows common in this country and is too well known to need describing.

SLIPPERY ELM BARK.

The inner bark of this tree is of much value, and may be used to advantage in many ways. There are two kinds of the slippery elm ; one, the bark is rather hard and tough, and the other is very brittle ; the latter is the best for medical use. The bark should be peeled, the ross shaved off, then ground to a fine powder. If used internally put a tea-spoonful of this powder into a tea-cup with as much sugar, mix them well together, then add a little cold water to it and stir it till it forms a jelly thick enough to be eaten with a spoon. A tea-spoonful may be taken at a time, and is an excellent medicine to heal soreness in the throat, stomach and bowels caused by canker ; or more hot water may be put to it and made into a drink, and freely taken for the same purpose. I have made much use of this bark for poultices, and have in all cases found it a most excellent article for that purpose. Mixed with pounded cracker and ginger, it makes the best poultice I have ever found ; for burns, scalds, felons, old sores, &c., it is the best thing I have met with to allay the inflammation, ease the pain, and heal them in a short time.

BALSAM FIR.

This balsam is obtained from a tree well known in many parts of this country ; it is taken from small blisters which form in the bark. It is of a very healing nature, and is good to remove internal soreness. It forms an important article in my healing salve. When taken it may be dropped on loaf sugar.

GINSENG.

An American plant. It is a nervine, and useful in all cases of nervous affection alone, or mixed with other articles. From half to a tea-spoonful may be given for a dose, in hot water sweetened.

SNAKE-ROOT.

Page 251. It is of a hot nature; it is used in measles, and other eruptions, to keep the disorder out, which it does effectually by its warming qualities, which determine the disease to the surface. No. 2, and the Composition Powders have the same effect. An infusion of the root promotes perspiration, removes pain in the stomach and bowels, and expels wind. The roots powdered may be mixed with Ginseng or Umbil, for all nervous complaints.

MUSTARD.

Fully described page 187. It is frequently used for rheumatism, internally, and externally. Nos. 2 and 6 are superior for this purpose.

HORSE-RADISH.

Page 140, The leaves are sometimes applied to remove external pains; but they are apt to blister.

BALM OF GILEAD.

This tree is a species of the poplar and possesses some medicinal virtues. It resembles the black poplar, having similar tags; but the buds and leaves are larger. The buds bruised and tinctured in spirit, produce an effect something like the tincture of myrrh; and are good taken inwardly, as a restorative, and for bathing sores. The bark scraped from the twigs and steeped in hot water, is a good corrective of the bile, and will operate both as an emetic and cathartic; it is more harsh than the other kind of poplar, but may be used to advantage in disease.

BUTTERNUT.

American. It bears an oblong nut, nearly as large as an egg. The kernel contains much oil. The bark of the tree or roots, boiled down till it is thick, may be made into pills of an emetic and cathartic nature. A syrup may be made by boiling the bark in treacle and a little spirit; it is good for worm complaints in children. The buds and twigs have a milder effect. White Ash bark and Balm of Gilead, equal parts mixed, and made into a syrup or pills, form a strong purge, but it is safe. The green shell of the nut bruised forms a good blister; when applied it should be covered with a wet bandage, and kept moist; the blister, superior to that produced by flies, will rise in three hours. The bark of the Butternut is the principal ingredient in Dr. Hawke's Rheumatic and Cancer pills, and also in Chamberlain's Bilious Cordial, greatly celebrated.

BLUE AND WHITE NERVINE.

For a vomit, it ranks next to Lobelia. It is used alone, or combined with Thoroughwort. It prevents fever in its first stages, and has been successfully used in cases of consumption, which the doctors had declared hopeless. By infusion, or in powder.

PIPSISWAY OR RHEUMATIC WEED.

An infusion is good for cancers, and scrofulous humours, drinking it and bathing the affected parts. The roots of the *Wild Lettuce*, and those of the Pipsisway dried and powdered together, are good to cure all bad humours. Take a tea-spoonful of the powder in a glass of hot water, and bathe the affected parts with it. It is good to restore weak nerves.

GOLDEN ROD.

See page 125. The oil of this herb is a good medicine; and prepared in essence, it relieves headache; to be taken, or used as a fomentation.

MEADOW FERN.—AMERICAN.

The burs, pounded fine and simmered in cream, hog's lard, or fresh butter, are almost a sovereign remedy for itch or external poison, and all bad humour sores. When the burs cannot be had, take the bush and buds and make a strong decoction; drink of this and wash with the same. This liquor may be prepared in syrup, and by boiling it down may be made into ointment; the syrup should be taken and the ointment put on the affected parts. This ointment, or the wash, is good for salt rheum, or canker sores, and may be used freely.

YELLOW DOCK.

Page 94. The root is made into an ointment for the itch. The roots are to be finely bruised and mixed with cream; kept warm for twelve hours, and not to be scalded. Rub it on at night when going to bed. Three times using it will effect a cure. The foregoing described ointments, with No. 3, and Rheumatic Drops, prepared with Spirits of Turpentine, will cure any case of this complaint.

PRICKLY ASH.

American. The bark and berries are used. They are very pungent, a powerful stimulant, as also the tops and roots. It should be finely powdered, steeped in hot water, and put into wine or spirit. It makes a good bitter. It is very good for fever, ague, lethargy, cold hands and feet, and all cold complaints. *Dose*, half a glass two or three times a day.

BITTER THISTLE.

American. The leaves may be steeped in hot water, and drank, or they may be reduced to powder, and taken in treacle or warm water, or in wine or spirit. It is an excellent and safe corrective of the bile. The *Carduus Benedictus, Blessed Thistle*, may be used for the same purpose. See page 269.

ARCHANGEL.

See page 22. In America, there are two kinds growing near each other; they closely resemble, but are very different in taste. One is very bitter, and the other has no bitter taste, but is very rough and of a balsamic taste. They may be used together in a tea or syrup, and answer two important purposes; the rough removes the canker, and the bitter is a corrective of the bile. By adding No. 2, the compound contains the three great principles of the healing art, viz., *hot*, *rough*, and *bitter*.

DIRECTIONS FOR PREPARING AND USING THE VEGETABLE MEDICINE.

NUMBER ONE.—EMETIC HERB.

It is prepared and used in three different ways, viz. :—

1. The powdered leaves and pods. This is the common form of using it; and from half to a tea-spoonful may be taken in warm water sweetened; put into either of the other numbers when taken to cleanse the stomach, overpower the cold, and promote a free perspiration.

2. A tincture made from the green herb in spirit. This is used to counteract the effect of poison internally or externally used; and for asthma and other complaints of the lungs. For a dose, take a tea-spoonful adding about the same quantity of No. 2, in half a tea-cupful of warm water sweetened; and, in cases of nervous affection, add half a tea-spoonful of nerve powder. For the external effects of poison, take the above dose, and bathe the parts affected with the tincture, repeating it till cured.

3. The seeds reduced to a fine powder and mixed with Nos. 2 and 6. This is for the most violent attacks of spasms and other complaints, such as lock-jaw, hydrophobia, fits, drowned persons, and all cases of suspended animation, where the vital spark is nearly extinct. For a dose, give a tea-spoonful, and

repeat it till relief is obtained ; then follow with a tea of No. 3 for canker.

For children the dose must be regulated according to their age. If very young, steep a dose of the powder in half a tea-cupful of water, or tea of raspberry leaves, and give a tea-spoonful at a time of the tea, strained through a fine cloth and sweetened, repeating the dose every ten minutes, till it operates ; and give pennyroyal, or some other herb tea for drink.

NUMBER TWO.—CAYENNE.

This is a medicine of great value in the practice, and may be safely used in all cases of disease, to raise and retain the vital heat of the system, cause a free perspiration and keep the determining powers to the surface. The only preparation is to have it reduced to a fine powder. For a dose, take from half to a tea-spoonful in hot water, or a tea of No. 3, sweetened ; or the same quantity may be mixed with a dose of either of the other numbers when taken. The dose should be repeated every ten or fifteen minutes till the desired object is effected, and continued occasionally until health is restored. When this number is given, the patient should be kept warm, by sitting near the fire covered with a blanket, or in a warm bed.

NUMBER THREE.—FOR CANKER.

Take bayberry root bark, white pond lily root, and the inner bark of the hemlock, equal parts of each, pounded and well mixed together ; steep one ounce of the powder in a pint of boiling water and give for a dose, a common wine-glassfull sweetened.

If the above cannot be had, take as a substitute sumach, (bark, leaves or berries,) red raspberry or witch hazel leaves, marsh rosemary, or either of the other articles described under the head of No. 3 ; they are all good for canker, and may be used together or separate.

When the violence of the disease requires a course of medicine, steep one ounce of the above mentioned powder, No. 3, in a pint of boiling water, strain off a wine glass full while hot and add a tea-spoonful of No. 2, and the same quantity of sugar: when cool enough to take, add a tea-spoonful of No. 1 and half that quantity of nerve powder. Let this dose be given three times at intervals of fifteen minutes; and let the same compound be given by injection; and if the case requires it, again repeat it. If mortification is apprehended, a tea-spoonful of No. 6, may be added to each dose and to the injections.

After the patients have recovered sufficiently from the operation of the medicine, which is usually in two or three hours, place them over the steam as directed in page 21.

This operation is sufficient for one time, and must be repeated each day, or every other day, as the circumstances of the case may require, till the disorder is removed. Three times will generally be sufficient, and sometimes once or twice will answer the purpose; but in bad chronic cases it may be necessary to continue to carry them through a regular course two or three times a week, for a considerable length of time.

Great care must be taken to keep up an internal heat, so as to produce perspiration, after they have been through the operation, by giving occasionally No. 2, or the composition powder; for if this is not attended to, the patient may have a relapse, in which case it will be very difficult to raise it again, as they will fall as much below a natural heat, as they have been raised above it by artificial means.

During the operation, give milk porridge, or gruel well seasoned with a little Cayenne in it; and after it is over, they may eat any kind of nourishing food that the appetite may crave.

A tea-cupful of the tea of No. 3, should be taken night and morning to prevent a relapse of the disease, and during the day drink frequently of a tea made of poplar bark; and, if costive, use the bitter root.

As soon as the disorder is removed, use bitters, (No. 4.) to correct the bile and restore digestion; and half a wine glass-full of the syrup, (No 5,) taken two or three times a day, will strengthen the stomach, and assist in regulating the digestive powers.

The foregoing directions are calculated for the more violent attacks of disease, and such as have become settled; but those of a less violent nature must be treated according to circumstances. In the first stage of a disease, it may be most generally thrown off by a dose of the emetic herb, with No. 2, to raise a free perspiration, followed by a tea of No. 3, to remove the canker, and the bitters, or a tea of poplar bark, to regulate the digestion. For a sudden cold, take a dose of the composition powder on going to bed, and put a hot stone wrapped in wet cloths at the feet, which will, in most cases, remove the complaint; but if these applications do not answer the purpose, the patient should be carried through a regular course as soon as possible. Steaming is safe, and will always do good, and the injections must not be neglected, particularly where the bowels are disordered. In consumption and old lingering complaints, give the composition powder two or three days before going through a regular course.

NUMBER FOUR.—BITTERS.

Take the bitter herb, or balmony, bayberry and poplar bark, equal parts, pulverized, one ounce of the powder to a pint of hot water, and half a pint of spirit. For a dose take half a wine glassful. For hot bitters add a tea-spoonful of No. 2.

This preparation is calculated to correct the bile and create an appetite, by restoring the digestive powers; and may be freely used, both as a restorative and to prevent disease.

When the above articles cannot be had, either of those that have been before described under No. 4, which are all good for the same purpose, may be used as a substitute.

NUMBER FIVE.—SYRUP.

Take poplar bark and bark of the root of bayberry, one pound each, and boil them in two gallons of water, strain off and add seven pounds of good sugar; then scald and skim it, and add half a pound of peach meats, or the same quantity of cherry stone meats, pounded fine. When cool, add a gallon of good brandy, and keep it in bottles for use. Take half a glassful two or three times a day.

Any other quantity may be prepared by observing the same proportion of the different articles.

This syrup is very good to strengthen the stomach and bowels, and restore weak patients, and is particularly useful in the dysentery, which generally leaves the stomach and bowels sore. In a relax, or the first stages of dysentery, by using a tea of No. 3, freely, and giving this syrup, it will generally cure it, and will also prevent those exposed from taking the disease.

NUMBER SIX,—RHEUMATIC DROPS.

Take one gallon of good fourth brandy, or any kind of high wines, one pound of gum myrrh, pounded fine, one ounce of No. 2, and put them into a stone jug and boil it a few minutes in a kettle of water, leaving the jug unstopped. When settled bottle it for use. It may be prepared without boiling, by letting it stand in the jug for five or six days, shaking it well every day, when it will be fit for use.

These drops are to remove pain and prevent mortification; to be taken or applied externally, or to be put into the injections. One or two tea-spoonfuls of these drops may be given alone, or the same quantity may be put into a dose of either of the medicines before mentioned; and may be also used to bathe with, in all cases of external swellings or pains. It is an excellent remedy for rheumatism, by taking a dose, and bathing the part affected with it. In the headache, by taking a swallow, bathing the head, and snuffing a little up the nose, it will remove the pain. It is good for bruises, sprains, swelled joints, and old sores, as it will allay the inflammation, bring down the swelling, ease pain, and produce a tendency to heal; in fact, there is hardly a complaint in which this useful medicine cannot be used to advantage. It is the best preventive against mortification of anything I have ever found.

For bathing, in rheumatism, itch, or other humours, or in any swelling or external pain, add one quarter part of spirit of turpentine; and for sprains and bruises, a little gum camphor may be added.

NERVE POWDER.

This is the American valerian or umbil, and the preparation has been sufficiently described, (see page 328). This powder is a valuable and safe medicine, and may be used in all cases without danger; and where there are nervous symptoms, it must never be dispensed with. For a dose take half a tea-spoonful in hot water sweetened; or the same quantity should be put into a dose of either of the other medicines, and also into the injections in all nervous cases.

COMPOSITION, OR VEGETABLE POWDER.

Take two pounds of the bayberry root bark, one pound of the inner bark of hemlock, one pound of ginger, two ounces of cayenne, two ounces of cloves, all pounded fine, sifted through a fine sieve, and well mixed together. For a dose take a tea-spoonful of this powder, with an equal quantity of sugar, and put it to half a tea-cupful of boiling water; to be taken as soon as sufficiently cool, the patient being in bed or by the fire, covered with a blanket.

This composition is calculated for the first stages, and in less violent attacks of disease. It is a medicine of much value, and may be safely used in all complaints of male or female, and for children. It is good for relax, dysentery, pain in the stomach and bowels, and to remove all obstructions caused by cold, or loss of inward heat. By taking a dose on going to bed, and putting a hot stone to the feet, wrapped in wet cloths, it will cure a bad cold, and will generally throw off disease in its first stages, if repeated two or three times. If the symptoms are violent, with much pain, add to each dose a tea-spoonful of No. 6, and half a tea-spoonful of No. 1, and in nervous symptoms add half a tea-spoonful of nerve powder; at the same time give an injection of the same. If these should not answer the purpose, the patient must be carried through a regular course of the medicine, as has been before described.

COUGH POWDERS.

Take four tea-spoonfuls of skunk cabbage, two of horehound, one of wake-robin, one of No. 1, one of No. 2, one of bayberry bark, one of bitter root, and one of nerve powder, all made fine, and well mixed together. When taken, to be mixed with molasses. Take half a tea-spoonful of the powder on going to bed; keep warm and continue taking it until relief is obtained, particularly on going to bed.

Where the cough has been long standing, it will be the best, while taking this prescription, to go through a regular course of medicine, and repeat it if necessary.

CANCER PLASTER.

Take the heads of red clover and fill a brass kettle, and boil them in water for one hour; then take them out and fill the kettle again with fresh ones, and boil them as before in the same liquor; strain it off and press the heads to get out all the juice, then simmer it over a low fire, till it is about the consistency of tar, when it will be fit for use. Be careful not to let it burn. When used it should be spread on a piece of bladder, split and made soft. It is good to cure cancers, sore lips, and old sores.

SALVE.

Take one pound of beeswax, one do. of salt butter, one and a half do. of turpentine, twelve ounces of balsam fir; melt and simmer them together; then strain it off into a basin, and keep for use. It may be used to heal fresh wounds, burns, scalds, and all bad sores, after the inflammation is allayed, and wound cleansed.

STRENGTHENING PLASTER.

Take burdock leaves and mullen leaves, bruise them and put them in a kettle, with a sufficient quantity of water, and boil them well; then strain off the liquor, press or squeeze the leaves, and boil it down till about half as thick as molasses; then add three parts of rosin and of turpentine, and simmer them well together, until the water is evaporated; then pour it into cold water, and work it with the hands like shoemaker's wax; if too hard put in more turpentine, when it will be fit for use. It should be spread on soft leather and applied to the part affected; and is good to strengthen weakness in the back, and other parts of the body.

VOLATILE SALTS.

Take crude sal ammoniac one ounce, pearl ash two ounces, and pound each by itself, mix them well together, and keep them well stopped in a bottle for use. Damping it with spirit or essence will increase the strength. This applied to the nose is good for faintness and to remove pain in the head, and is much better than what is sold by apothecaries.

NERVE OINTMENT.

Take the bark of the root of bitter sweet, two parts of wormwood and camomile, each equal, one part, when green, or if dry moisten them with hot water; which put into any kind of soft animal oil, and simmer them over a slow fire for twelve hours; then strain it off and add one ounce of spirit of turpentine to each pound of ointment. To be used for a bruise, sprain, callous swelling or for corns.

POULTICE.

Make a strong tea of raspberry leaves or of No. 3; take a cracker pounded fine, and slippery elm bark pulverised, with ginger, and make a poultice of the same. This is good for old sores, whitlows, felons, and for bad burns, scalds, and parts frozen. Apply this poultice, and apply it as often as every twelve hours, and wash with soapsuds at every renewal; wetting it in the interim with cold water, or a tea of raspberry leaves, till it discharges; then apply the salve till a cure is affected.

INJECTIONS OR CLYSTERS.

This manner of administering medicine is of the greatest importance to the sick; it will frequently give relief when all other applications fail. It is supposed that the use of them is of great antiquity; but whether this be true or not, the using them to relieve the sick was certainly a very valuable discovery; and no doubt thousands of lives have been saved by it. The doctors have long been in the practice of directing injections to be given to their patients, but they seem to have no other object in administering them than to cause a movement in the bowels; therefore it was immaterial what they were made of.

According to the plan which I have adopted, there are certain important objects aimed at in the administration of medicine to remove disease, viz., to raise the internal heat, to promote perspiration, remove the canker, guard against mortifications, and restore the digestion. To accomplish these objects, the medicine necessary to remove the complaint must be applied to that part where the disease is seated; if in the stomach only, by taking the medicine it may be removed; but if in the bowels, the same compound must be administered by injection. Whatever is good to cure disease if taken into the stomach, is likewise good for the same purpose if given by injection, as the grand object is to warm the bowels and remove the canker. In all cases of dysentery, cholic, piles, and other complaints, where the bowels are badly affected, injections should never be dispensed with. They are perfectly safe in all cases, and better that they be used ten times when not needed, than once neglected when they are. In many violent cases, particularly where there is danger of mortification, patients may be relieved by administering medicine in this way, when there would be no chance in any other. I do, therefore most seriously advise that these considerations be always borne in mind; and that this important way of giving relief be never neglected where there is any chance for it to do good. In many complaints peculiar to females, they are of the greatest importance in giving relief, when properly attended to; for which purpose it is only necessary to repeat what has been before stated; let the remedy be applied with judgment and discretion, to that part where the disease is seated.

The common preparation for an injection or clyster, is to take a tea-cupful of strong tea made of No. 3, strain it off when hot, add half a tea-spoonful of No. 2, and a tea-spoonful of No. 6; when cool enough to give, add a tea-spoonful of No. 1, and the same quantity of nerve powder. Let it be given with a large syringe made for that purpose, or when this cannot be had, a bladder and pipe may be used. They must be repeated as occasion may require till relief is obtained.

Many other articles may be used to advantage in the injections; a tea of witch hazel and red raspberry leaves, either or both together, are very good in many cases. For canker a tea of either of the articles described under the head of No. 3, will answer a good purpose. When the canker is removed, the bowels will be left sore, in which case give injections of witch hazel or raspberry tea, with slippery elm bark. When injections are used to move the bowels only, No. 1, should be left out.—It is always safe to add the nerve powder, and if there are nervous symptoms, it must never be omitted.

STOCK OF MEDICINE FOR A FAMILY.

1 oz. of the emetic herb.
2 ozs. of cayenne.
½ lb. bayberry root bark, in powder.
1 lb. of poplar bark.
1 pint of the rheumatic drops.

This stock will be sufficient for a family for one year, with such articles as they can easily procure themselves when wanted and will enable them to cure any disease, which a family of common size may be afflicted with during that time. The expense will be small, and much better than to employ a doctor, and have his extravagant bill to pay.

GENERAL DIRECTIONS IN CURING OR PREVENTING DISEASE.

1. Be careful to always keep the determining powers to the surface, by keeping the inward heat above the outward, or the fountain above the stream, and all will be safe.

2. It must be recollected that heat is life, and cold death; that fever is a friend, and cold an enemy; it is therefore necessary to aid the friend and oppose the enemy, in order to restore health.

3. That the construction and organization of the human frame is, in all men, essentially the same, being formed of the four elements. Earth and water constitute the solids of the body, which is made active by fire and air. Heat, in a peculiar manner, gives life and motion to the whole; and when entirely overpowered, from whatever cause, by the other elements, death ensues.

4. A perfect state of health arises from a due balance or temperature of the elements; and when it is by any means destroyed, the body is more or less disordered. When this is the case, there is always a diminution of heat, or an increase of the power of cold, which is its opposite.

5. All disorders are caused by obstructive perspiration, which may be produced by a variety of means; that medicine, therefore, must be administered, that is best calculated to remove obstructions, and promote perspiration.

6. The food taken into the stomach, and being well digested nourishes the system and keeps up that heat on which life depends; but by constantly taking food into the stomach, which is sometimes not suitable for nourishment, it becomes foul, so that the food is not well digested; this causes the body to lose its heat, aad disease follows.

7. Canker is caused by cold, and there is always more or less of it in all cases of disease; continue to make use of such articles as are calculated to remove it, as long as there is any appearance of disorder.

8. When the disease is removed, make free use of those

things that are good to restore the digestive powers, not forgetting to keep up the inward heat by giving occasionally No. 2.

9. Keeping always in mind, that an ounce of preventive is better than a pound of cure; and give medicine on the first appearance of disorder, before it becomes seated; for it may then be easily thrown off, and much sickness and expense prevented.

10. In cases of fever, increase the internal heat by giving hot medicine, so as to overpower the cold, when the natural heat will return inwardly, and the cold will pervade the whole surface of the body, as the heat has done before; this is what is called the turn of the fever.

11. If No. 1 should sicken and not puke, there may be two causes for it, viz., the coldness or the acidity of the stomach.—For the first give No. 2 more freely, and for the latter, dissolve a piece of pearlash about the size of a large pea, in a wine glass of water, and let them take it, which will counteract the acidity. If this fail, make use of the steam, which will open the pores, extract the cold, and set the medicine into operation.

12. In giving medicine to children, give about one half, a little more or less, according to their age, of the quantity directed for a grown person. Be particular to offer them drink often, especially young children, who cannot ask for it.

13. Dysentery is caused by canker in the bowels, for which make free use of the tea of No. 3 with No. 2, and give the same by injection, in the first of disease, and afterwards give the syrup, (No. 5,) to strengthen the stomach and bowels, and restore the digestive powers.

14. The piles are canker below the reach of medicine given in the usual way, and must be cured by using a wash of No. 3, made strong, and by giving injections of the same, with No. 2. What are called bearing down pains in women, is from the same cause, and must be relieved by injections made of witch hazel, or red raspberry tea, steeped strong, with No. 2, strained. If this does not give relief, go through a regular course of medicine.

15. Women in a state of pregnancy ought to be carried through a regular course of medicine, especially when near the time of delivery. When in travail, give raspberry leaf tea, with a tea-spoonful of the composition powder, or No. 2, and keep them in a perspiration. After delivery keep up the internal heat, by giving the composition powder, or No. 2. This will prevent after-pains. If there should be symptoms of fever, carry them through a regular course of medicine, which will guard against all alarming complaints peculiar in such cases.

16. In all cases of a burn, scald, or being frozen, wrap the part in cloth wet with cold water, often wetting them with the same to prevent them becoming dry, and be careful to give hot medicine such as No. 2, or the composition powder, to keep up the inward heat. Pursue this plan for twelve hours, and then, if the skin is off, apply the poultice or salve. If there should be convulsions or fever, a regular course of the medicine must, without fail, be attended to.

17. When a scald is over the whole or greater part of the body, apply cotton cloth of several thicknesses to the whole body, wet with a tea of raspberry leaves, frequently wetting them with the same to prevent its becoming dry, and give them the hot medicine. When the scald is under the stocking, or any other tight garment, let it remain on, adding more cotton cloth, and wet the whole with cold water as often as the smart of the burn returns.

18. If the skin is off, or in case of an old burn, to guard against canker, apply a poultice of cracker and slippery elm bark made with a tea of raspberry leaves, washing it with soap suds, when the poultice is changed, and then with the same tea. When any part is frozen, the same method must be taken as with a burn.

19. For a fresh wound, cut, or bruise, wash immediately with cold water, and bind up with cloths wet with the same; keep a hot stone at the feet, and take medicine to raise a gentle perspiration; continue this till the inflammation is allayed, and the wound perfectly cleansed, then apply the poultice or salve till healed. The air must be kept from all wounds or sores, as it will cause pain, and prevent them from healing.

20. In spotted or deadly attacks, such as spotted or yellow fever, fits, drowned persons, croup, &c., the heat and activity of the patient is so much diminished, that the common administration will not give relief, the determining power to the surface being so small, through the loss of internal heat, that it will not give the medicine operation, as its effects are resisted and counterbalanced by the pressure of the external air. To counteract this pressure, keep the room, by aid of a good fire, about as warm as summer heat; and more fully to rarify and lighten the air, and aid the operation of the medicine, make a free use of the steam bath, and keep the patient shielded by a blanket, at the same time give Nos. 1 and 2. This course should be unremittingly persevered in till the patient is relieved. Keep always in mind to give the patient fresh air when steaming, and while going through a course of medicine, by making a quick fire of shavings, or very light wood, and opening a door or window at the same time; as this will immediately change the foul air in the room, by driving it out, and supplying its place with fresh air from the surrounding atmosphere. This mode is essential in all disorders, both in hot and cold weather. Steaming is not essential in hot weather, except when going through a course of medicine; after which a shower bath is good in the morning, as it lets down the outward heat, and gives power to the inward.

21. If the glands are dry, so that there is no moisture in the mouth, or if the patient is much pressed for breath, give a strong tea of No. 2, sweetened, and repeat it till the mouth becomes moist. No. 3 should be used while the mouth is dry, without adding a large portion of No. 2.

22. Be careful not to have the outward heat too high, by too many cloths or too much fire; for if this be the case, it will cause a balance of the outward and inward heat, and will prevent the medicine from operating, by stopping the circulation; and the patient will be very much distressed.—When this happens, throw cold water on the face and stomach, and give more hot medicine, which will let down the outward heat, and raise the inward.

23. If the patient is restless, wet the head and body with

cold water, and if there are convulsions or spasms, give the nerve powder with No. 2. Injections must also be used.

24. Never make use of physic in cases where there is canker inside, for it will draw the determining powers inward and increase the disease. I have seen so many bad effects from giving physic, that I have disapproved of the use of it altogether, but if any is given, after the operation, be careful to keep up the inward heat, so as to cause a free perspiration.

25. Avoid all minerals used as medicine, such as mercury, arsenic, antimony, calomel, preparations of copper or lead; and also nitre, and opium. They are all deadly poisons, and enemies to health.

26. Beware of bleeding and blisters, as they can never do any good, and may be productive of much harm, they are contrary to nature, and strengthen the power of the enemy to health. Seatons and issues should be avoided, as they only tend to waste away the strength of the patient, without doing any good; it is a much better way to remove the cause by a proper administration of medicine, which will be more certain and safe in its effects.

k

27. Be careful not to make use of saltpetre in any way whatever; it is the greatest cold of any thing that can be taken into the stomach, and was never intended for any other purpose than to destroy life. It is a very bad practice to put it on meat, for it destroys all the juices, which is the nourishing part and leaves the flesh hard and difficult to digest.

28. Never eat meat that is tainted or in any way injured, as it will engender disease; for one ounce in the stomach is worse than the effluvia from a whole carcase. Eat salt provisions in hot weather, and fresh in cold.

29. Be careful about drinking cold water in very hot weather, as it will tend to let down the inward heat so suddenly as to give full power to the cold. If this should happen, its fatal effects may be prevented by giving the hot medicine to raise the inward heat above the outward. Be careful also not to cool suddenly, after being very warm in consequence of uncommon exercise.

30. Remember that regularity in diet, is very important to preserve health ; and that if more food is taken into the stomach than is well digested, it clogs the system and causes disease. This is very important to those who have weak constitutions.

31. Ardent spirit is a slow poison ; it is taken into the stomach to stimulate, but the effect is soon over, and much use of it destroys the tone of the stomach, injures the digestive powers, and causes disease. It is therefore much better, when the feelings require any thing of the kind to make use of stimulating medicine, such as No. 2 and 6, for these will answer a far better purpose.

By a strict observance of the foregoing directions, you may save much pain and expense, and enjoy good health, and long life which is the earnest wish of the writer.

DESCRIPTION OF SEVERAL DISEASES, WITH DIRECTIONS FOR THEIR CURE.

BY M. ROBINSON, M. D.

FELONS.

A felon always comes on a joint, and is often caused by some strain or bruise, which makes a leak in the joint or muscle, and the sooner it has vent the better. If it comes on the inside of the hand, and is brought to a head by poulticing, it will often break through the back of the hand before it can get through the thick skin on the inside. The best way to give it vent is to burn a piece of spunk* the size of half a pea, on the place affected. If you think the flesh is dead down to the matter, you may stick the point of a needle into the dead skin and raise it up, and cut out a piece under the needle sufficient to let out the matter ; then apply poultice or salve ; if painful, wrap it in cloths of several thicknesses, wet with cold water, and repeat this as it becomes hot or painful. Take the composition or warm medicine, and keep up the inward heat.

If the sore has been several days coming, and appears nearly

*Rotten wood, or touchwood.

ripe, applying a piece of unslacked lime to it, and wet the cloth with cold water, till the lime is slacked; and repeat this till the skin looks of a purple colour; then open it as before directed. This method is safer and quicker in causing a cure, than laying it open with a knife, as is the practice of some doctors. Cutting the live flesh, forms a leak, and often spoils the joint; but by searing by either of the above modes, it secures and prevents the leak, and makes a speedy cure.

FREEZES AND BURNS.

These two disorders are one and the same thing, and require the same treatment. Take a cloth wet with cold water, and wrap several thicknesses round the part, to be wet as often as the pain increases. Give warm medicine inside. If the scald is dangerous, carry them through a regular course of medicine, as though they had a fever, or any other acute disorder; keep the cloth or poultice on to secure it from the air, from 12 to 14 hours, till the soreness or pain is entirely gone.—If the skin is off, a poultice of wheat bread, wet with any of the articles composing No. 3, keeping it wet with the tea till the sore discharges, then wash with soap suds; when dressed wash with the tea of No. 3 and continue the poultice or salve until a cure is effected.

A freeeze is a direct cold, and a burn is an attractive cold; for as much as the heat opens the pores more than usual, the cold follows and closes them as much more than they were before the operation of the heat—this stops the perspiration from going through the surface, and the water collects under the grain of the skin, which is called blistering: the water applied on the outside opens the pores and lets the water out by perspiration, and the grain adheres to the skin—the pain ceases and the cure is completed.

CURE OF A SCALD.

The patient was 14 years of age, and was taking from the fire a kettle of boiling cider, which he tipped, and poured it boiling hot into a large bed of live embers, which covered his feet with this hot mass; he was obliged to hold on till the kettle was set on the floor, and then jumped into a pail of cold water, and stood there till his father procured some cloths, in which he immediately wrapped his feet; his father attended to pouring on water to keep the cloths filled. This keeps the air from the surface, and eases the pain; for as the water wastes and lets the air to the burn, the pain will increase. By pursuing this course for about two hours, the boy fell asleep. Water was poured on the cloths but two or three times during the rest of the night, and in the morning preparation was made to dress the wound, when to the surprise of all present, no blister had risen, nor a particle of skin broken. He put on his stockings and shoes as usual, and went about his work perfectly well.

CASE OF A BOY WHO WAS BADLY SCALDED.

A lady took from the fire a tea-kettle filled with boiling water, when her little son, about six years old, turned the contents on both his feet, and falling, one hand went into the tea-kettle; both feet and one hand were very badly scalded. I happened to be present, and immediately tore up cloth sufficient to do up each part, wetting them with cold water. He was put to bed and I gave him some warm medicine, put a warm stone at his feet, and wet the cloths as often as he complained of pain. In about two hours he fell asleep, after which two or three times wetting the cloths, kept him easy through the night. In the morning, on taking off the cloths, there was no appearance of blisters, nor any skin broken, and he put on his stockings and shoes, and appeared as well as he was before the accident. It was the opinion of the family, the night before, that the boy would not be able to go to school for a fortnight; but on finding him well the next morning, they were hardly able to believe their senses, or that the child had been scalded.

FURTHER REMARKS ON BURNS.

Burns are the most easily cured, if rightly managed, of any wounds I ever attended; and are most difficult and dangerous when not understood, and wrongly treated. How often have we seen these sores continue all the winter, and could not be healed? as also, burns by blisters made with Spanish flies, which amount to the same thing.—By not being treated in a proper manner in season, the canker gets in and eats out the flesh, after which, what is called proud flesh, fills up the sore. The doctor applies his sugar of lead, vitriol, red precipitate, to eat out the dead flesh; this effects the cords and draws them out of shape, and often makes a sore that they cannot cure, which terminates in a mortifying canker sore. Therefore immediately attend to the canker, which always awaits such cases, and where the skin is off, in cases of burns or blisters, apply a poultice of cracker, or elm bark wet with a tea of No. 3, until the canker is gone. Sometimes add ginger, keeping the poultice wet with cold water; when the sore discharges, apply salve until a cure is effected.

Observe the evil effects of blistering. I knew a case where a doctor drew a blister on a child's breast up to the neck, for stuffing at the lungs. It lingered with this scald near its vitals about a week; I was then called to visit the child and found it to be dying. The mother asked me what I thought was the matter with it. I took off the dressing and showed her the mortified flesh over the blister, and told her that was the disorder; she seemed much surprised, and I then asked her if the child had been scalded, and had mortified in the same manner, whether she would have had any doubt of its being the cause of her child's death! She said she would not. I gave her my opinion that it was exactly a similar case, and that the child's death was caused as much by the blister, as it would have been by a scald. The child died before morning. I had declined doing any thing for it, as I was satisfied I could do no good; if I had made the attempt, it would have been said that I killed it.

I have seen many cases where I was perfectly satisfied that the patient died in consequence of blisters, not only on the stomach, but on the head. In many cases where a blister was drawn on the head, as it began to draw, their senses were gone, and they died raving or stupified. More than half the cases where the head was shaved and blistered that have come within my knowledge, have proved fatal. I can see no reason why a scald on the head or the body, done designedly, should have a tendency to effect a cure, when persons are sick, and the same thing happening to them by accident, when well, should destroy their health or cause their death. If a person should have his head or stomach so badly scalded, as to take off the skin, we should consider him in a most dangerous condition; but nothing is said about it when it is designedly done. I shall leave it to the reader to reconcile, if he can, this inconsistency, —I have known most dangerous stranguries caused by blisters; and those who applied them did not know the cause, and many have applied to me for relief.

MORTIFICATION OF THE LIMBS.

I was called on to go on board a vessel to see a young man, who had a block fall from the mast head on his foot weighing 13½lbs., which bruised all his toes to pieces, except the little one. The accident happened on Friday, and I did not see him till the Tuesday following, during which time he neither ate nor slept. His nerves were much affected, and he had spasms and convulsions through the whole system. I took off the dressing from the foot, and found it black, and the smell very offensive. The captain of the vessel appeared to be very anxious about him, and asked me if I could help his foot—I told him I must try to save his life, for his whole body was as much disordered as his foot. He requested me to do what I thought best. I put a poultice of meal on his foot, and wet the cloths with cold water to allay the heat; then gave him medicine the same as though he had been attacked with nervous fever. The captain attended him through the night, and I went to see him the next morning, and found him much better. The captain said he was astonished at the operation of the medicine, for his vomiting and sweating had carried off all the pain in his body and foot, and had also reconciled the nerves.

I unbound his foot and found that the black and yellow streaks up the leg had disappeared, and on the foot all the flesh that was alive seemed to receive fresh support from the body;

and the living and dead flesh appeared as though two colours were painted by the side of each other. I then made a ley of pearl ash and warm water, and soaked his foot in it, which caused a slimy glaze over his foot; this took away all the offensive smell. I then washed it with vinegar to kill the alkali, and keep it from irritating the skin. The acid cleared off all the slimy matter, so that it wiped clean. I then cut off the great toe at the middle joint, and the two next at the upper joint, and set the next which was broken. I cut out the dead flesh, to stop in part the putrefaction. I then put on another poultice, and ordered it to be kept wet with cold water, and a warm stone wrapped in a wet cloth, to be put to his feet to keep a steam, giving him warm medicine inside to keep up the inward heat; and by wetting the foot with cold water, it kept the determining power to the surface, thus raising the fountain and lowering the stream. By this treatment it is as impossible for mortification to go from the limbs to the body, as it would be for the log that floats over the dam to go back into the pond, when the fountain is kept full. The next day I dressed his foot and found that the dead flesh had digested very much; I again soaked it in the ley, and next washed in vinegar as before, which was of great service in allaying the bad smell. I then caused him to be carried through a regular course of medicine, which completely restored him to bodily health; his appetite was good, and all pain and soreness abated, so that he took food regularly, and lost no sleep afterwards, till he got entirely well which was in about four weeks. The captain was a very good nurse, and was faithful in attendance on the young man till he got well; and expressed the highest gratitude for my attention and success; and as a proof of his confidence he very handsomely remunerated me.

OLD CANKER SORES ON THE LEGS.

When I was a young man, I was much troubled through the winter, for many years, with sores on my legs. At the commencement of cold weather, if I broke the grain on my shin, it would become a bad sore, and continue through the winter; the canker would get into it and eat into the bone, and sometimes spread under the grain like a burn, and feel the same, being extremely sore, with stings and twinges like a cancer. These sores were so troublesome, that it lead me to invent a cure. Finding the cause to be canker, I took some of the articles composing No. 3, steeped strong, and washed the parts affected with it; if there was a bad smell, I first washed the sore with strong soap suds, taking off all the loose skin, which was blistered with cankery humour, and then washed with a tea of No. 3, to destroy the canker and harden the sore; sometimes wetting it with drops. My present mode of treatment is as follows: If the inflammation runs high, and the sore spreads fast, I put into it a pinch of fine No. 2, then put on a poultice of white bread and ginger, wet with the above tea, wrapping it up with several thickenesses of cloth, and wetting it with cold water as often as it becomes so dry as to be painful, being careful to exclude the air for twenty-four hours. In this time it generally discharges ripe matter, and the inflammation and canker abate. When next dressed, the sore should be first washed with soap suds as before, then with the tea. If the soreness is gone, you may apply the healing salve, with the wet cloth. On going to bed, be careful to exclude the cold air, by occasionally putting a hot stone wrapped in wet cloths, to the feet, so as to keep up the steam. If the sore is painful, wet it with cold water. Give the medicine to keep up the inward heat, such as composition of hot bitters, and when these do not answer the purpose, go through a course of medicine, and repeat as occasion may require. This method, if persevered in, I seldom knew to fail of success.

I was called to attend a case of this kind not long since, where the inflammation and pain were very great, and fast spreading under the grain of the skin. There had been applied an elm and ginger poultice, made with a tea of No. 3. I took off the dressing and applied a pinch of No. 2, to the sore, after which I laid on the same poultice, putting on a cloth which I kept wet with cold water till the next morning, when on dressing it, I found the inflammation abated, the sore discharged ripe matter, and by two dressings more of the same, the cure was completed.

CASE FROM THE BITE OF A RAT SUPPOSED TO BE MAD.

Not long since I was sent for to attend a man who had been bitten on one of his elbows by a rat, supposed to be mad. The wound healed in a few days, then turned purple round it, as though the blood had settled and turned black, until he was blind. He was sick at the stomach, and had a high fever. I carried him through a course of medicine, but with little advantage. The swelling and dark colour progressed most rapidly, till his face became *very black.* These appearances led me to suspect that the madness of the rat was caused by eating ratsbane, and this poison was communicated to the man by the bite, as he appeared the same as a person I had once seen who had been killed by taking that poison. I then washed his face with a strong tea of Nos. 1 and 2, and gave the same inwardly with No, 3, carried him through another course of medicine, keeping a cloth on his face wet with the tea, as before, to keep out the air, when under the operation of the medicine, to sweat his face and throw the poison out. I kept him in a sweat for several days, occasionally with his face secured from the air, which method had the desired effect, by bringing the poison out. By continually keeping up the perspiration, the swelling abated, but whenever this was not attended to, so as to keep the determining powers to the surface the spasms would increase to such a degree that his life was frequently despaired of. He was carefully attended in this manner about one month before I could determine in my own mind whether the disease or nature would gain the victory; after which he begun gradually to regain his health, and in about six months he appeared to be clear of poison. The man was sixty years of age; and the accident happened in the fall of the year, which rendered it more difficult to conquer this cold and deadly poison, than it would have been in warm weather.

BAD WOUND IN THE EYE CURED.

A man cutting turf, and accidentally had a pitchfork stuck into one of his eyes, by a person who was pitching the turf near him. It passed by the eye ball and stuck fast in the skull, so that it was with considerable exertion that he could draw it out. The eye swelled and closed up immediately, and the people were much frightened, and sent for me; but I could not go. I gave direction to the man who came for me, to return and carry him through a course of medicine as soon as possible, keeping several thicknesses of cloth wet with cold water, on his eye, and not to open it for twelve hours; and to keep him in a perspiration the whole time. This was faithfully attended to, and on opening the wound after the above time, the swelling was all gone, the eye was open, and a large quantity of blood was in the wet cloth, which had been drawn from the eye. They continued to wet the cloth, and gave him warm medicine inside, keeping him in a gentle perspiration for the next twenty-four hours, which cleared the eye of all the blood, restored the sight, and amended his health, so that he was well in about a week, to the astonishment of all who saw him.

CANCER SORES.

The cause of this sore is very little understood. In all sores of an eating nature there is more or less canker, according to their violence. A cancer is the highest degree of canker, being the most powerful effect of cold, and consequently the greatest degree of inflammation, therefore the remedies ought to be those of a warming nature, as the greatest preventive against canker. Whenever a violent inflammation is discovered, it is supposed that heat causes the difficulty; but the fact is, it is only an evidence of war between heat and cold, for there is no inflammation where there is perfect health, because heat then bears complete rule; and no disease can take place until the cold makes an attack on the body, which causes an unnatural heat to oppose an unnatural cold. Whenever the cold takes possession the inflammation shows itself, by stopping the circulation; the effect is, swelling, inflamed callous, arising from some leak, caused by the natural course being stopped. If it suppurates and discharges it is called ulcer, bile, and the like, and the canker goes off with the putrefaction. If the leak is so low as to get callous as fast as it discharges, it becomes a hard, dead lump of flesh, and not having circulation enough to support it, begins to rot; here the canker shows its heating nature, being seated in the dead flesh, and eating on the live flesh, which is intermixed with it, causes pain and distress, in proportion as the body is filled with coldness and canker; if this is sufficient to keep the power above the natural circulation, the patient will continue in this distressed situation, being eaten alive, until worn out with the pain, death comes as a friend to relieve him. This is the natural termination of this dreadful malady, which is far better than to combine with it the common form of practice in using arsenic, which only helps to eat up and distress the patient.

In order to give a more correct idea of the dangerous effect of making use of arsenic in cancers, I shall make a short extract from Thacher's Dispensatory, on the subject. "Arsenic has long been known to be the basis of the celebrated cancer powder. It has been sprinkled in substance on the ulcer, but this mode of using it is excessively painful and extremely dangerous, fatal effects having been produced from its absorption." This fact I have known in several instances, where Davidson's agents, and others, have undertaken to draw out cancers, when the patients would absorb enough of this poison, which seating on the lungs, caused them to die of consumption in the course of one year. My wish in exposing such nostrums, is to benefit those who may be ignorant of the imposition; for it may be relied on as truth, that there is more or less poison in all those burning plasters used to cure cancers. I would advise all to beware of them. It would be much better to risk the cancer than the cancer quack.

The principal object aimed at is to take out the bunch, and in doing that by the above method, a worse evil is inoculated, which is more fatal than the cancer. The tumour is a mixture of live and dead flesh, and is often under a live skin; if it be necessary to make an incision through the live skin, in order to dissolve the dead flesh, the best way is to burn a piece of spunk* on the place, and repeat it till the flesh is dead enough to suppurate. The smart will be but two or three minutes, and not so painful as the arsenic for the same time, which lasts for

*Rotten wood, or touchwood.

twelve hours. Where the tumour is small, the cancer balsam will be found sufficient, by repeating the plaster for two or three weeks to take out the dead flesh and remove the canker; after this is done, apply a ginger and elm poultice wet with a tea of No. 3. If the system appears to be generally affected with the cancer humor, carry them through a common course of medicine, and repeat the same while attending the sore.

I had a cancer on my foot about the size of an Indian corn, which had troubled me twice, by acute darting pains and twinges. I cured it by applying a plaster of the cancer balsam, repeating it twice at each time. When there is dead flesh under the skin, it is best to burn the spunk first, and then apply the poultice or balsam; it is also recommended to give medicine to eradicate the canker from the system, both before and after the operation on the sore.

Three cancers on the breast have come under my care, that I could not cure. One of them was as large as a half-peck measure, and grew fast to the breast bone. I carried the woman through a course of medicine several times. and applied a poultice of butternut shucks to dissolve the dead flesh, and continued this course for some months, until the bunch had more than half dissolved, and had grown off the bone, so that it was quite loose, and I was in hopes to have effected a cure; but she was taken with a fever in my absence, and died. The other two I could relieve, and keep them free from pain, making them comfortable as long as they lived; but nature was too far exhausted to complete a cure. I have had under my care other cases of cancers on the breast and other parts of the body, which I had no difficulty in curing in the manner before stated.

I shall conclude the subject by a few general remarks, viz.: Guard thoroughly against canker and coldness—attend to the canker by a course of medicine, and repeat it—use the ginger poultice if the inflammation is great, putting some No. 2 on the raw sore, then apply the poultice, keeping it wet with cold water—not forgetting the composition and No. 2 inside at the same time. Let all poisonous drugs, burning plasters, and caustics alone—attend faithfully to the directions here given—honour your own judgment—keep your money—and bid defiance to doctors.

PILES,—HOW CURED.

I was called to attend an elderly man who had been confined to the house, and much of the time to his bed, for seven weeks, with the piles. Seven doctors attended him before I was sent for, and he continued to grow worse. The doctors had operated on one side, and said they must on the other; it was their opinion, as well as his, that he was in a decline. The side that they had operated upon was much worse to cure than the other. I carried him through a regular course of medicine twice in three days, when he was able to go out of doors. The injection composed of No. 3 steeped, and a small quantity of No. 2, was used; warm tallow was applied several times in a day, sometimes washing externally with the same tea. He had been dieted very low; I restored his digestive powers, and he recovered his appetite; his sores healed, his general health mended to such a degree that he was no more confined with that complaint. A little tallow used when going to bed prevents piles and chafes in young and old. Remember this. For chafes FULLERS EARTH and water is a never-failing remedy.

SORE HEADS IN CHILDREN,—SCALD HEADS.

This sore often comes after having the itch; it is contagious, being caused by canker and putrefaction. The most effectual way to cure this disease is to carry them through a course of medicine several times, as the case may require, previous to which, the head must be oiled and covered with cabbage leaves, or draw a bladder over the head to keep out the cold air. The head should be covered so as to make it sweat as much as possible, in order to dissolve the hard scabs. After laying all night the smell will be offensive; wash the head in soap suds, when clean, wash it also with a tea of No. 3, after which, wash with a tea of No. 1. Sometimes anoint it with the rheumatic drops and nerve ointment—let it come to the air by degrees. Be careful to guard the stomach, by giving composition, warm bitters, &c. The ointment, drops, and No. 1, in powder or juice, may be occasionally used together or separate. Continue to wash with soap suds, and then No. 3, occasionally, until a cure is effected.

SORE BREASTS.

Some women suffer much from this complaint, which is caused by cold, occasioning obstructions in the glands of the breast When they are swelled, bathe with the rheumatic drops, or pepper vinegar ; if this does not remove the swelling, and it should be necessary to bring it to a head, apply a poultice of lily root made thick with ginger, or slippery elm bark ; at the same time give the composition powder, or No. 2, to keep up the inward heat. If the woman is sick, carry her through a regular course of medicine, which will remove the complaint and restore health in a short time. I have cured a great many who were very bad, by pursuing the above plan, and never met with the slightest difficulty. I attended a woman who had both breasts badly swelled. She was sitting by the window with it up, and could hardly get her breath ; she could not bear to have any fire in the room, complaining that it made her faint. I told her that if I could not make her bear heat, I could do her no good. I gave her some No. 2, to raise the inward heat, and caused a good fire to be made in the room. The inward heat, gained as fast as the outward, and in one hour she could bear as warm a fire as I could. I carried her through three regular courses of medicine in five days, and at the same time applied the lily poultice, which brought them to a head without pain ; and she was soon well.

TO STOP BLEEDING.

Internal bleeding is from the stomach and lungs, and is caused by canker, or soreness of the stomach ; it often takes place very suddenly, and creates much alarm. The patient sometimes trembles with fright, and often has fits of the ague, which is caused by the cold increasing in proportion to the loss of blood. In the first place shield them from the air with a blanket by the fire, and give the hottest medicine you have : if nothing better can be had, give hot water or any kind of tea ; and get a perspiration as soon as possible ; then apply the steam bath ; giving ginger tea, or No. 2, if you have it, if not, black pepper. As soon as there is an equilibrium in the circulation, there will be no more pressure of the blood to the stomach or lungs, than to the extremities, and the bleeding will cease. It has been my practice in cases of this kind, to give some of the rheumatic drops, shield them from the air with a blanket placed by the fire, then give a dose of composition powders, and No. 2, and if this does not answer the purpose, give a dose of No. 1, which, with the steam, I never knew to fail of stopping the blood ; and by giving medicine to remove the canker and to restore the digestive powers, I have always been able to effect a cure. The same application will answer for other weakening and alarming complaints in women.

External bleeding, caused by wounds in the limbs, may be stopped by placing the wound higher than the body. One of my sons cut his leg very badly ; I placed him on the floor and took his foot in my lap ; as soon as the wound was higher than the body the bleeding ceased. I then poured on cold water till the wound was white, then put in a few drops of No. 6. took two or three stitches to bring the wound together, dressed it with salve, and it soon got well with very little soreness. Another case of a little girl who cut off the main artery of the middle finger, and it bled very fast. I put my thumb above the wound and stopped the blood, then poured on cold water with my other hand, and washed the wound well, then placed her hand above her head, which prevented it from bleeding, till I could get ready to dress the wound. It bled no more, and soon got well.

RUPTURE.

This difficulty is caused by a hurt or strain, which makes a breach in the tough film or membrane that supports the bowels in their place, and the intestines come down in the cavity between this membrane and the skin ; being sometimes very painful, and difficult to get back ; and have to be kept from coming down by a truss. When the bowels come down and remain any length of time, they become swelled, and are very painful, causing great distress and danger, and sometimes have proved fatal, as they cannot be got up again till the swelling is removed, This may be effected by a course of medicine without danger.

A gentleman was troubled with rupture, his bowels came down, swelled and were very painful, a doctor was sent for from Por smouth, who applied a bag of snow, which drove the pain to the stomach, and caused puking. The swelling increased, and became very hard. The case now becoming desperate, and the family being alarmed, I was sent for, and on hearing the circumstances, sent some medicine, and gave directions to sweat him as soon as possible. My directions were faithfully attended to, and as soon as he became warm, the nerves slacked, the swelling abated, and all the appearance of mortification disappeared, the bowels went back, and in twelve hours he was restored from a dangerous situation, to almost his usual state of health. In this case may be seen the difference between the artificial doctor and nature's physician; which is the same as between fire and snow.

AGUE IN THE FACE.

This is caused by cold in the glands of the mouth, which keeps back the saliva till it causes swelling and soreness; the canker becomes prevalent at the same time, which causes severe pain in the face and throat. The sooner a cure is attempted the better; to effect this take a dose of the tea of No. 3, with a teaspoonful of No. 6 in it, for the canker; then tie a small quantity of No. 2 in a fine piece of cloth, wet with No. 6, and put it in between the teeth and cheek, on the same side where the pain is; sit by the fire covered with a blanket, and breathe the warm air from the fire; this will prick the glands and cause the saliva to flow very freely, which will take out the soreness, and relieve the pain. The face may be bathed at the same time with No. 6. If the case is of long standing, so that the system is affected, and if this does not remove the complaint, give a dose of No. 1. If it is caused by decayed teeth, fill the hollow with cotton wool, wet with the oil of summer savoury, or spirits of turpentine, which will deaden the nerve, and stop its aching. This is good in all cases of teeth-ache, and will generally effect a cure without extracting.

TO RELAX THE MUSCLES IN SETTING A BONE.

This may be done by bathing the part with warm water, and is much better than the method that is generally practised, of extending the muscles by the strength of several persons, which weakens the part so much, that the bones are liable to get out of place again ; besides the operation causes severe pain to the patient and much trouble to the operator, which is all obviated by my method. In cases where a joint is put out, or a bone broken, give a dose of No. 2, or the composition powder, with half a tea-spoonful of nerve powder, which will promote a perspiration, prevent fainting, and quiet the nerves ; then wrap the part in cloths wet with water as hot as it can be borne, and pour on warm water for a short time, when the muscles will become relaxed, so that the bones may be put in their place with little trouble.

I was once called to a woman who had put her elbow out of joint by a fall from her horse. It was badly out, being twisted about one quarter of the way round. I ordered some water to be made hot immediately, stripped her arm, and as soon as the water was hot, put a towel in a large tin pan, and poured on the water till well wet ; as soon as cool enough, wrapped it round her arm, and poured on the water from the pitcher, as hot as she could bear it, for about 15 minutes. I then took off the towel and directed one person to take hold of the arm above the elbow, and another below to steady it ; and then placed my fingers against the end of the bone on the upper side, and my thumb against that on the upper side, and by a gentle pressure each way, set the joint without pain or force on the muscles, to the astonishment of all present, who calculated that it would require the strength of several men. I then wrapped it with the same towel, which had become cold ; this brought the muscles to their proper tone, and kept the joint firm in its place ; I put her arm in a sling and she walked home that night about a mile, and the next day was well enough to knit all day.

In case a shoulder is out of joint, I relax the muscles in the same manner, and put the arm over my shoulder and lift it up, which has always put the joint in its place, without any danger, and very little pain to the patient ; and then by applying cold water, the muscles will become braced, so that there will be no danger of its getting out again. I know of a case where a man had his hip turned out, and several doctors had exhausted their skill in vain to set it ; when one of my agents being present undertook it by my plan of treatment, and after he had relaxed the muscles sufficiently, and put his knee against the hip joint, turned the leg out and crowded the joint into its place, without any difficulty.

MEASLES.

This disease is very common, especially among children, and is often attended with bad consequences, when not properly treated. It is a high state of canker and putrefaction; and if the determining power is kept to the surface, it will make its appearance outside, and go off itself; but if cold overpowers the inward heat, so as to turn the determining power inward, the disease will not make its appearance, and the patient will become much distressed, frequently producing fatal consequences, if some powerful stimulant is not administered to bring the disorder out. To give physic in cases of the kind is dangerous, as it strengthens the power of cold, and keeps the canker and putrefaction inside, which sometimes seats upon the lungs and causes consumption; or turns to the stomach and bowels, when they die suddenly, as has been the case with hundreds, for a few years past. I have attended a great many cases of the measles in the course of my practice, and never lost one, and never have known of any that have died of this disorder, who were attended by any of my agents.—When the symptoms make their appearance, give a dose of the composition powder, or of No. 2; then give the tea of No. 3, to guard against canker, and add some No. 2, to overpower the cold; and when the second dose is given, add No. 1, to clear the stomach and promote perspiration; as soon as this takes place, the disorder will show itself outside. By continuing to keep the determining power to the surface, nature will take its regular course, and the disease will go off without injuring the constitution. If the bowels appear to be disordered, give an injection; and be careful to keep the patient warm.

I once had a case of a young woman who had the measles; she lingered with the symptoms four or five days, then became very sick, turned of a dark purple colour, and had a high fever when I was called to attend her. I gave her a strong dose of

No. 3, steeped, and put in it a tea-spoonful of the third preparation of No. 1, which caused such a violent struggle that I had to hold her in bed ; but it was soon over, for in about ten minutes she vomited, and a perspiration took place, which was followed by the measles coming out, so that she was completely covered with the eruption. She was soon well and about her work.

SMALL POX.

This disease is the highest state of canker and putrefaction which the human body is capable of receiving, and is the most contagious, being taken in with the breath, or communicated by inoculation, in which case it is not so violent and dangerous as when taken in the natural way. The distressing and often fatal consequences that have happened in cases of small pox are more owing to the manner in which it has been treated, than to the disease. The fashionable mode of treatment in this disease, has been to give physic, and reduce the strength, by starving the patients and keeping them cold. This is contrary to common sense, as it weakens the friend and strengthens the enemy ; and the same cause would produce similar effects in any other disorder. All that is necessary is to assist nature to drive out the canker and putrefaction, which is the cause of the disease, by keeping the determining powers to the surface, in which case there will be no danger. The same manner of treatment should be used in this complaint as has been directed for the measles. The canker rash, and all kinds of disease that a person is not liable to have but once, such as chicken pox, &c., are from the same cause, and must be treated in a similar manner

COUGH.

The general opinion is, that cough is an enemy to health, and ought to be treated as such ; but this idea I hold to be altogether an error, for it is the effect, and not the cause of disease. When the lungs are diseased, there will be a collection of matter which must be thrown off, and the cough is like the pump of a ship, which discharges the water and prevents her from sinking, so also the cough throws off what collects on the lungs, which if suffered to remain there would soon putrify and cause death. It is a common saying, that I have a bad cough, and can get nothing to stop it, and the doctor often says if I could stop your cough, I should have hopes of a cure, but this is as unreasonable as it would be to stop the pumps of a ship, which would cause her to sink the sooner. Ask a sailor what he would do, and he would say keep the pump going till you can stop the leak, and when that is stopped the pump will become useless, as there will be nothing to throw off. Such medicine should be given as will promote the cough till the cause can be removed, which is cold and canker on the lungs; after this is done, there will be no more cough. If a cough is caused by a sudden cold, it may be removed by taking the composition powder on going to bed, with a hot stone wrapped in wet cloths to produce a perspiration, and at the same time taking the cough powder, which will make the patient raise easy, and also help to remove the cause. When the cough has become seated, and the lungs are diseased, they must be carried through a regular course of the medicine, repeating the same as occasion may require, till a cure is effected, at the same time giving the cough powder, especially on going to bed.

Whooping-cough must be treated in the same manner—continue to give the powders till cured.

JAUNDICE.

Much has been said about the bile, or gall, being an enemy in case of sickness; but this is a mistake, for it is a friend, and should be treated as such. It is the main-spring to life, and the regulator of health, as without it, the food could not be digested. When people have what is called the jaundice, it is the prevailing opinion that they have too much bile, and it is said they are bilious; this is a mistaken notion, for there is no such thing as there being too much gall—it would be more correct to say there was not enough. The difficulty is caused by the stomach being cold and foul, so that the food is not properly digested, and the bile not being appropriated to its natural use, is diffused through the pores of the skin, which becomes of a yellow colour. The symptoms are, want of appetite, costiveness, faintness, and the patient will feel dull and sleepy; these are evidences of bad digestion and loss of inward heat. The only way to effect a cure is to promote perspiration, cleanse the stomach, and restore the digestive powers, which will cause the bile to be used for the purpose nature designed it.

Nature has contrived that each part of the body should perform its proper duty in maintaining health, and if there were no obstruction there would never be disease. The gall-bladder grows on the liver, and is placed between that and the stomach, so that when the latter is filled with food, the bile is discharged into the stomach to digest it. The bile never creates disorder, for it is perfectly innocent, being nature's friend; and those appearances called bilious, show the effect of disease, and not the cause. The gall is a very bitter substance, and it is the practice of the doctors to order bitter medicine to cure the jaundice, and this seems to be the universal opinion, which is correct, but it certainly contradicts the notion that there is too much bile, for if there is too much, why give medicine to make more? I have attended many cases of this kind, and never had any difficulty in effecting a cure. My method is to give No. 2, or the composition powder, to raise the inward heat, and No. 1, to cleanse the stomach and promote perspiration, then give the bitters, (or No. 4,) to regulate the bile and restore the digestive powers. If the complaint has been of long standing and the system is much disordered, they must be carried through a regular course of the medicine, and repeat as occasion may require, at the same time give the bitters two or three times a day, till the appetite is good and the digestion restored. Any of the articles described under the head of No. 4, are good, and may be freely used for all bilious complaints.

WORMS.

A great deal is said about worms causing sickness, and there is scarcely a disease that children are afflicted with but what is attributed to worms. The doctors talk about worm complaints, worm fevers, worm cholics, &c., and give medicines to destroy the worms, and, by so doing, they frequently destroy their patients. There was never a greater absurdity than their practice, and the universal opinion about worms causing disease.

The fact is, they are created and exist in the stomach and bowels for a useful purpose, and are friendly to health, instead of being an enemy; they are bred and supported by the cold phlegm that collects in the stomach and bowels. This is their element, and the more there is of it, the more there will be of the worms. They who are in health are never troubled with worms, because they are then quiet, and exist in their natural element. Every one has more or less of them and the reason why children are more troubled with what is called worm complaints is because they are more subject to be disordered in their stomach and bowels, than grown persons. When children are sick and their breath smells bad, it is said they have worms, and everything is laid to them, but this is owing to disease caused by canker, for there is nothing in the nature of worms that can affect the breath. In cases of this kind, the only thing necessary is to cleanse the stomach, by getting rid of the cold phlegm, and restoring the digestive powers, when there will be no difficulty with the worms.

The common practice of the doctors is to give calomel and other poisons to kill the worms. This must appear to any one who examines the subject to be very wrong as well as dangerous, for the worms cannot be killed by it, without poisoning the whole contents of the stomach. I once knew a case of a child, who, after eating a breakfast of bread and milk, was taken sick; a doctor was sent for, who said it was caused by worms, and gave calomel to destroy them, which caused fits. The child vomited and threw up its breakfast. A dog that happened to be in the room, ate what the child threw up; he was soon taken sick and died—the child got well. The fortunate accident of the child throwing off its stomach what it had taken, probably saved its life, for if there was poison enough to kill a dog, it must have killed the child. The absurdity of such practice is like the story related by Dr. Franklin, of a man who was troubled by a weazel in his barn, and, to get rid of the weazel, he set fire to his barn and burnt it up! I had the following relation from the doctor who attended the case:—

Three children had what he called worm fever, and he undertook to kill the worms. One of them died, and he requested liberty to open it to see what would destroy worms, in order to know how to cure the others, but the parents would not consent. The second died, and the parents consented to have it opened; but, after searching the stomach and bowels, to their surprise no worms could be found. The third soon after died. The fact was, their death was caused by canker on the stomach and bowels, and the medicine increased the difficulty by drawing the determining powers inward, which aided the cold to promote the canker. Where children die by such treatment, the blame is all laid to the worms, and the doctor escapes censure. I have had a great deal of experience in what are called worm complaints, and, after having become acquainted with the real cause have had no difficulty in curing all that I have undertaken. I began with my own children. One of them was troubled with what was supposed to be worms; I employed a doctor, who gave pink root, and then physic to carry it off together with the worms. It would shortly after have another turn, which would be worse. He went on in this way, and the worms kept increasing, till I became satisfied he was working on the effect and neglecting the cause, when I dismissed him and undertook the cure myself. I first gave the warmest medicine I then knew of, to clear off the cold phlegm, and gave bitter medicine, such as poplar bark, wormwood, tansy, and physic made of twigs of butternut, to cleanse the stomach and correct the bile. By pursuing this plan, the child soon got well, and was no more troubled with worms. A child in the neighbourhood where I lived, about six years old, was taken sick in the morning, and the doctor was sent for, who gave medicine for worms; soon after it had fits, and continued in convulsions during the day, and at night died. I was satisfied that its death was hastened, if not caused by what was given. When the stomach is diseased, or when poison is taken into it, the worms try to flee from the danger, which causes distress, and they sometimes get into knots, and stop the passage into the stomach.

My practice has been, in cases of worm complaints, to give the composition powders or No. 2, to warm the stomach; a tea of No. 3, to remove the canker, and the bitters of either of the articles described under No. 4, to correct the bile. If they are bad carry them through a course of the medicine, and give the bitters. When there are nervous symptoms, give the nerve powder. Injections should also frequently be given. The butternut syrup is very good. If there should be danger of mortification, make use of No. 6, both in the medicine given, and in the injections.

The tape worm is from the same cause as other worms, and may be cured in the same manner. They are, when single, about half an inch long, and one-third as wide; they join together and appear like tape, and often come away in long pieces of several yards. I was once troubled with them, and used to be faint and had no appetite; I cured myself by taking butternut physic, which brought away several yards at a time; and by taking the bitter medicine to correct the bile, was never troubled with them again.

I have often heard about people having a greedy worm; but this is a mistaken notion, for there never was any such thing. The difficulty is, the stomach is cold and disordered, so that food is not properly digested, but passes off without nourishing the system, and this creates an unnatural appetite. Remove the cause by warming the stomach and correcting the digestive powers, and there will be no further difficulty. I was called on to see a young woman, who it was supposed had a greedy worm. It was thought to be very large, and would frequently get into her throat and choke her almost stopping her breath. Her mother told me that the day before, one of the neighbours was in and told a story about a person having a monster in their stomach, which was taken in by drinking at a brook; this terrible account so frightened her daughter that the worm rose into her throat and choked her so that she had fits. I took the girl home with me and gave her a dose of hot bitters, with some of the nerve powder that night; the next morning I carried her through a course of the medicine as well as I knew at the time, which cleared the stomach and bowels, and strengthened the nervous system. I told her there was no worm that troubled her, and she had faith in what I said. I gave her medicine to correct the bile and restore the digestion and she soon got well, being no more troubled about the worm. The difficulty was caused by a disordered stomach and want of digestion, which produced spasms in the stomach and throat.

CONSUMPTION.

This complaint is generally caused by some acute disorder not being removed, and the patient being run down by the fashionable practice, until nature makes a compromise with disease, and the house becomes divided against itself. There is a constant warfare kept up between the inward heat and cold, the flesh wastes away in consequence of not digesting the food, the canker becomes seated on the stomach and bowels, and then takes hold of the lungs. When they get into this situation, it is called a seated consumption, and is pronounced by the doctors to be incurable. I have had a great many cases of this kind, and have, in all of them, where there was life enough left to build upon, been able to effect a cure by my system of practice. The most important thing is to raise the inward heat and get a perspiration, clear the system of canker, restore the digestive powers, so that food will nourish the body and keep up that heat on which life depends. This must be done by a regular course of medicine, as has been directed in all violent attacks of disease, and persevered in till the cause is removed.

This complaint is called by the doctors a hectic fever because they are subject to cold chills and hot flashes on the surface; but this is an error, for there is no fever about it; and this is the greatest difficulty—if there were, it would have a crisis, and nature would be able to drive out the cold and effect a cure. The only difficulty is to raise a fever, which must be done by such medicine as will raise and hold an inward heat till nature has the complete command. When such patients are very weak and low, they will have what is called cold sweats. The cause of this is not understood; the water that collects on the skin does not come through the pores, but is attracted from the air in the room, which is warmer than the body, and condenses on the surface; the same may be seen on the outside of a mug or tumbler in a hot day, when filled with cold water, which is from the same cause. It is of more importance to attend to the preventing this complaint, than to cure it. If people would make use of those means which I have recommended, and cure themselves of diseases in its first stages and avoid all poisonous drugs, there would never be a case of consumption, or any other chronic disorder.

FITS.

These are produced by the same cause that other complaints are; that is, cold and obstructions, and may be cured by a regular course of medicine, which overpowers the cold, promotes perspiration, and restores the digestive powers. Poison, or any thing else which gives the cold power over the inward heat, will cause fits, because the natural tone of the muscular power is destroyed, which produce violent spasms in the whole system. So much has already been said on this subject that it is unnecessary to say more, to give a correct idea of the manner of cure.

ST. ANTHONY'S FIRE, OR ERYSIPELAS, NETTLE SPRING, OR SURFEIT.

These are all caused by overheating the system, and cooling too suddenly, which leaves the pores obstructed, and then by taking more cold, will bring on a warfare between cold and heat, when they break out, and itch, and smart, as if stung by an insect. When the heat gets a little the ascendancy, so as to produce perpsiration, it will disappear till they get another cold. The only way to effect a cure is to give the hot medicine, and steam, till they are brought to the same state of heat as that which first caused the disease, and then cool by degrees. This I have proved in several instances, and never had any difficulty in entirely removing the cause in this way. Make use of a tea of No. 3, for canker, and the bitters to correct the bile, and a little nerve powder to quiet the nerves, and they will soon be restored to perfect health.

STRANGURY OR GRAVEL.

This disorder is often caused by hard labour and exposure to the cold in the early part of life, and when they grow old, their heat diminishes, the bile becomes thick, and a sediment collects on the bladder, which obstructs the passages; the glands through which the urine passes are clogged and become diseased, so that there is difficulty in voiding the water, which causes great pain. It is seldom that there is a cure in such cases, but relief may be obtained by a course of the medicine, and making free use of the poplar bark tea. A tea of the hemlock boughs is very good ; and also I have known great relief from using the wild lettuce and pipsisway, the tops and roots bruised and steeped in hot water. Many articles that are good to promote the urine may be used to advantage.

DROPSY.

There are two kinds of this complaint ; one is caused by losing the inward heat so as to stop the natural perspiration, which causes the water that is usually thrown off in this way to collect in the body and limbs. This may be cured by raising the internal heat and causing a profuse perspiration, when the water will pass off in the natural way ; then make use of such medicine as will remove canker and restore the digestive powers when the food being digested, will keep up the natural heat of the body, and also the perspiration. The other kind is caused by cold and obstruction ; but instead of the water collecting and remaining in the body and limbs, a leak forms in the glands and lets it into the trunk of the body, where there is no vent to let it off. This cannot be cured without tapping, and is very seldom completely cured. I have never known but two who were in this situation to be perfectly restored. One was a girl whom I attended. I tapped her and took away seventeen pounds of water, and then swathed her up close, and gave medicine to keep a perspiration ; she did not fill again and was completely cured. The other was a man—he had been tapped twice. I carried him through a course of medicine several times and gave the juniper ashes with molasses and gin, which carried off large quantities of water, and entirely removed the disorder. I have cured a number who had the first mentioned complaint, by the common course of medicine ; one woman was cured by taking the wild lettuce, bruised and steeped in hot water. Dropsy is referred to in several parts of this book, and particularly under the *Herbal* department. Refer to the Index.

BILIOUS COLIC.

The name of this complaint is erroneous, for bilious means the bile, and no one ever heard of a bile cholic, or pain caused by gall, as it is a friend to health, and never causes disease or death. This pain is caused by a disordered stomach, and want of digestion ; the stomach is filled with canker, which gets into the narrow passage from the stomach, when the action of the bowels cease ; after the pain subsides, those parts where it was are very sore. To cure it raise the inward heat by giving the hot medicine ; remove the canker with No. 3, and giving the bitters to correct the bile, and repeat it till a cure is effected. If the case is bad, carry them through a course of medicine, and often give injections.

PLEURISY.

This distressing complaint is caused by cold or want of inward heat. I never had any difficulty in curing it by my common practice. The only remedy made use of by the doctors is to bleed ; this only increases the disease by reducing the strength of the patient, without removing the cause. I was once called to a soldier who had a violent pain in his side ; the doctor that attended him had bled him five times, without removing the pain, which made him so weak that it was with difficulty he could be held up in the bed. I relieved him in one hour by a common course of medicine, and bathing his side with the rheumatic drops. It took three weeks to get up his strength which might have been done in three days if he had not been bled. I was called to another case of the kind, of a soldier at the same place. He had been bled, and a large blister put on his side to remove the pain, which caused a strangury and he was in great distress. I declined doing any thing for him without the consent of the commanding officer, who was not present. The soldier begged of me to tell him what would do for the latter complaint, as he could not live so. I told him to take off the blister, which was immediately done, and it gave him instant relief. By carrying them through a course of medicine, as has been directed for other violent attacks, will cure all cases of this complaint without danger; and is much better than bleeding or blisters, which increases the difficulty.

RELAX.

This complaint is caused by indigestion, or loss of the powers of the gall; which becomes thick in consequence of cold, or loss of inward heat, when the stomach will be sour. The best remedy is to give No. 2, which will thin the gall; cleanse the stomach with No. 1, and give the bitters to correct the digestion. A dose of composition powders with a tea-spoonful of No. 6 in it, will in most cases effect a cure. The bayberry and poplar bark are good, and also many other articles that have been described as good to restore the digestive powers.

DYSENTERY.

This is a distressing complaint, and very common, especially among children; although much has been said on the subject, yet its importance will justify some further directions. It is caused by cold, which gets the ascendancy over the inward heat so as to draw all the determining powers inward; the stomach is disordered, the digestive powers are lost, and the bowels become coated with canker; the food is not digested so as to afford any nourishment or heat to the system, and all the juices flow inward and pass off by the common passage. The canker makes the bowels very sore, and when any thing passes them it causes excruciating pain. The best plan of treatment is to carry the patient through a regular course of medicine, and repeat it, if occasion requires, every day till relief is obtained. During the operation give chicken broth, and after the disease is checked, give occasionally a little brandy and loaf sugar burned together, and a strong tea of poplar bark. Give the syrup, (No. 5,) two or three times a day, until entirely recovered; the bitters (No. 4,) may be given night and morning to restore the digestion. Care must be taken to keep up the inward heat, in the interim, by giving occasionally No. 2, in a tea of No. 3, sweetened. Steaming is very important in this complaint, and injections must often be administered.

RHEUMATISM.

This complaint is caused by cold obstructing the natural circulation, which causes pain and swelling. It often affects the joints so that they grow out of shape. A cure is easily effected if timely and properly attended to, which must be done by such medicine as will cause perspiration and remove obstructions. In common cases taking the rheumatic drops, and bathing the parts affected with the same, will remove the complaint. When the case is bad, carry them through a course of the medicine, and bathe with the drops, repeating it as occasion may require till cured. At the same time give a tea of poplar bark or hemlock boughs; and many other articles which have been described as good for this complaint, may also be made use of to advantage.

The gout is from the same cause, and the stomach being greatly disordered and very sour, produces a burning sensation. I have cured several cases by the common course of medicine, and giving the bitters to restore the digestive powers.

SORE LIPS.

They are common in very hot or cold weather, when there is nearly a balance of power of outward and inward cold, which produces canker. To cure it, take a strong dose of tea No. 3, with a tea-spoonful of No. 2 in it, when going to bed, and wash them with the same, then wipe them dry to take off the matter collected; then wet them with tea, and put on as much ginger as will stick; repeat the same two or three times, till the coat is sufficient to keep out the air; when this comes off repeat the same process again, until the soreness is gone; then wash again with tea and wipe them dry, and apply warm tallow till a cure is completed.

SORE EYES.

This is generally caused by being exposed to sudden changes of heat and cold, which produce canker, and where this is, there will be inflammation. There are many things good for this complaint, but the best that I have found, is white pond lily root, marsh rosemary, witch hazel, and red raspberry leaves; make a strong tea with all or either, and add one third as much of No. 6, with a little of No. 2; bathe the eyes several times in a day; every morning put your face in cold water, open and shut the eyes till well washed, repeat this till a cure is effected. At the same time take the tea to clear the system of canker.

HEAD-ACHE.

This pain proceeds from a foul stomach, the bile loses its power, the food clogs, by not being digested, and the effect is felt in the head, which is the fountain of sense. Sometimes there is sickness at the stomach. In such a case it is called the sick head-ache; and when they vomit the head is relieved. This proves that the cause is in the stomach. It must be cured by cleansing the stomach, and restoring the digestive powers. A dose of composition powders, sitting by the fire, wrapped in a blanket, will generally give relief; but if it should not, take a dose of No. 1, in a tea of No, 3, and take the bitters to correct the bile; No. 2 should also be taken to warm the stomach, and if it be sour take the pearlash water. It is very fashionable with the doctors to tell about dropsy in the head, but in this I have no belief; for there is no disease in the head but what proceeds from the stomach, except from external injury. If they understood the real cause, and would give the proper medicine to remove it, there would be no difficulty in the head; but when a child is sick they give calomel and other poisons, which increases the disease, and if they die it is laid to the dropsy in the head, and this is satisfactory, because the doctor says so.

CORNS.

These come on the joints of the toes and are very troublesome. They may be cured by soaking the foot in warm water till the corn is soft, shave it thin, take a strip of bladder or skin of suet, eight or ten inches long, and half an inch wide, rub it till soft: then supple it well in rattlesnake's oil, or the nerve ointment, wrap it round the toe and keep it on till worn out; if this does not cure, repeat the same till the corn is removed. I have seldom known this to fail of effecting a cure.

VENEREAL.

The disease that is called by this name, is more common in seaports than the country, because there is more promiscuous and illicit intercourse of the sexes than in other places. It is a high state of canker and putrefaction, which takes hold of the glands of those parts that are first affected with it, and, if not checked, the whole system will become diseased by the venereal taint. It is more common among sea-faring men, because of their being long absent at sea, and on coming on shore, they give free scope to their passions, without being very scrupulous about the manner of the indulgence. It originates probably with those common women who have connexion with many different men, and going beyond the impulse of nature, this impure connexion causes uncleanness, which produces the disease; and when seated, is contagious.

The reason why this disease causes so much fright and alarm is owing to two cases: the first is the disgrace that is attached to dishonesty in getting it, and the other is the manner in which it has generally been treated, in giving mercury to cure it—the remedy becomes worse than the disease. That this disorder cannot be cured by any other means is altogether an error, for I have cured a number of cases by very simple means. The first symptom felt is a scalding sensation of pain when voiding the urine; and within twenty-four hours after this is experienced, it may be cured by applying cold water and making use of the rheumatic drops; if there be much soreness, make use of a tea of No. 3, with the drops in it, which must be taken as well as applied to the parts. If the disease has been of long standing, and the whole system has become affected, they must be carried through a course of medicine. Where there has been mercury made use of, and there is all the attendant consequences of such treatment, it is much more difficult to effect a cure, and is also done by a full course of medicine, and repeating it a number of times; raising the heat by steam each time, as high as they can bear, to throw out the mercury and remove the canker, at the same time applying the poultice, then give the bitters to correct the bile.

I had the case of a woman who was brought to me on a bed fifteen miles. She was in a very putrid state, and as bad as she could be, with all the consequences that are caused by being filled with mercury. Different doctors had attended her for eleven months, and she had been constantly getting worse. She had been kept ignorant of her state till a few days before brought to me, on account of her husband. I carried her through five courses of medicine in two weeks, and applied a poultice of white bread and ginger, made with a tea of No. 3. This completely broke up the disorder, and by giving medicine to correct the bile and restore digestion, she was cured, and returned home in three weeks after coming to me. By taking things to restore her strength, she has enjoyed good health ever since. Another woman was cured in the same manner, who had been in this way for six years, and unable to do any business. I attended her three weeks, when she was restored to health, and returned home. In less than a year after she had two children at a birth, and has enjoyed good health to this day.

This disease may be produced by other means than what have been described. It may be taken in with the breath by being much exposed in attending on those who are in a very putrid stage of the complaint : or may be communicated to parts where the skin is broken, and in many other ways ; when they will have many of the symptoms the same as when taken in the common way. Children will sometimes be affected with the venereal taint, whose parents have had the disease. A disease similar in appearance, with much the same symptoms, may be brought on by overdoing and being exposed to the cold. I once had a case of a young married man, who by straining himself from loading mill-logs and being exposed to wet and cold, caused a weakness in the back and loins, and he had what is called a gleet, and an inflammation, with all the symptoms common in the venereal. His wife became affected in the same manner, and they continued in this situation three months, when I was called to attend them, and by making use of such things as I then had a knowledge of to strengthen the loins and remove the canker, I was able to cure both in a short time. The man had all the symptoms that appear in the venereal, except hard bunches in the groin, called buboes. These I am satisfied are caused by mercury; for I never knew any to have them except they had taken mercury. Syringing with mercury and sugar of lead, dries the glands and contracts the passage, and stops the discharge, when the putrid matter instead of going off, collects in the groin and forms hard tumors, which remain a long time and have to be brought to a head to let off the putrid matter. Bunches of a similar kind often come on different parts of the body, caused by mercury.

A COURSE OF MEDICINE.

In all cases regulate the quantity of the doses, and the times of administration according to the coustitution and strength of the patient. In case of an attack of fever, if the mouth be dry, give cayenne in warm water sweetened, with nerve powder and a little bitter root, until the mouth and throat become moist, and the patient continues to spit freely. In the mean time have some strong canker tea prepared from the best articles you have, (bayberry alone, is the best in this case,) and give the patient freely of this, together with the cayenne, nerve powder, and a little bitter root, frequently wetting the face, hands and feet, with cold water, until the fever turns, or, in other words, until you raise the internal, and let down the external heat (raise the fountain and lower the stream) sufficient to produce a natural action, when perspiration will make its appearance on the forehead and breast, by which time the correct practitioner will have stones and water hot, and other things in readiness for applying the steam.

If the patient should have vomited so as to have thrown up the medicine given, the doses should be repeated until the stomach retains a sufficient quantity to enable the patient to bear the steam, when he should be divested of all his clothing, except the shirt, and placed over the steam as has been before directed, and the steaming continued as long, and raised as high as it can be borne, always bearing in mind, that the higher the heat can be raised in the system, the more free and thorough will be the operation of the medicine. The patient then must be put to bed, with a stone that has been partially cooled in steaming, at the feet, and the emetic immediately given. If the heat has been sufficiently raised, and the stomach now contains plenty of cayenne, the emetic may be given in the canker tea alone; but if from any cause the steaming shall not have been thoroughly performed, or if the cayenne shall have been thrown from the stomach, there should be cayenne added with the emetic. Continue giving the emetic until the stomach is thoroughly cleansed; three doses will be generally sufficient. If the process has been conducted to the best advantage, the patient will, soon after the commencement of the vomiting begin to run down, that is, he will grow pale and weak, and continue to sink, as it were, until he has not strength to move, or even speak; his breathing may vary from short and soft, to long and loud, and from the most free and easy to the most laborious jerking, in short, every symptom and appearance that can well be imagined, calculated to alarm and terrify those who are unacquainted with the true cause and effect; yet the experienced practitioner beholds those scenes with pleasure, because he knows this to be a certain presage of the recovery of the patient, and his heart swells with gratitude to the persecuted and much injured Dr. Thomson, who alone is entitled to the credit of discovering and furnishing the means of gaining so easy a victory.

Sometimes, instead of the symptoms above described, the patient will appear to be much distressed, will tumble in every direction, and talk in the most incoherent manner, even raving to insanity—these extraordinary symptoms, however, seldom appear, unless in desperate and deadly attacks, or in cases of long standing, where the system has become very much obstructed, and the vital heat and action nearly overcome. The most desperate case of the kind which we ever witnessed was of about fifty hours' continuance; language is totally inadequate to describe this scene. The patient, a little girl, recovered from that time, and is now in the enjoyment of health.

We have known some instances where practitioners, who were unacquainted with the full operation of the medicine, have become alarmed, when, as a matter of course, consternation would seize the mind of the relatives and friends of the patient, and a medical doctor would be sent for, and by the time he arrived, the medicine given would have completed its operation, and the patient being on the turn, would soon revive, and finding himself perfectly relieved, is easily persuaded to believe that the *steam* Doctor had administered the fatal dose, but that the *god of Health*, the *medical* Doctor, had arrived *just in time to save his life.* The practice has suffered much in this way.

We have probably dwelt much longer upon this part of our subject than may be deemed necessary by some, yet the imporance which we attach to a knowledge of the wonderful operation and effect of the emetic herb, must be our apology, if, indeed any is required. Dr. Thomson, has said enough to quiet the fears of any one, were it not that the force of early prejudice renders it necessary that we should have "line upon line, and precept upon precept."

We will now turn to our patient, whom we will suppose to have recovered strength sufficient to converse, when a dose of bitters should be administered, and some gruel, or other light food given; then if he wish, he should be permitted to sleep until he naturally awakes. The heat (and consequently strength,) will continue to gain, and by giving a few doses more of the bitter, with cayenne, (not forgetting the food) the perspiration will soon begin to flow, and the patient will soon be impatient to change his wet, and *now* uncomfortable situation for the steam bath. If the doctor has performed his part thus far, he will now have every thing in readiness for the *second steaming*, and will set his patient over the steam as before, and again raise the heat as high as possible, when the shirt should be taken off, the blanket held loose around the patient, and two or three quarts of cold water poured quickly over him, so as to spread as much as possible on every part of the body and limbs, then immediately wipe dry, and as a clean shirt is put on, let the blankets be dropped, and the patient get immediately into bed, or if he prefer it, be dressed, but by no means to sit in, or otherwise be exposed to a current of air.—Care should now be taken to administer the bitters and cayenne freely ; the former to correct the bile and strengthen the digestion, in order that food, the natural fuel, may keep up the heat, until a sufficient quantity of food should be taken and digested, to render the cayenne no longer necessary for that purpose. If the disorder returns, repeat the course as above directed.

REMARKS.—The above is for a case of fever, and may answer as a general text for a course of medicine in all cases, yet the ingenious practitioner will, in many instances, at once see the propriety of numerous variations from, and additions to, the *minutia* as here laid down, yet, the leading objects to be arrived at, are in all cases the same.

In cases of long standing, particularly in consumption, where the digestive powers have been deranged for a considerable length of time, and the system consequently filled with morbid matter, it is indispensably necessary to have some good broth, beef tea, or other like food, giving it as soon as the emetic commences operating, in order that the glands may be supplied with nourishment, as fast as the morbid matter with which they are charged shall be removed by the medicine.

By this means the strength of the patient may be materially increased with every course of medicine.

Care should be taken in selecting stone, to get those of a coarse, open grain. Limestone, or those containing coal or sulphur, must *never* be used, as they give out no steam, but, cause the patient to sicken and faint.

N. B.—Give as much cold water as the patient wishes, at all times.

POETICAL DIRECTIONS.

First steep the coffee, number Three,
With number Two, then use it free ;
To clear the cold, and raise the heat,
Now place a hot stone at the feet.

The inward warmth now oft repeat,
And change the stone when lost its heat;
The fountain 'bove the stream keep clear,
And perspiration will appear.

Then take the emetic number One,
Until its duty is well done;
The stomach cleansed, and head made free,
From filth and pain both equally.

Then lie a while in sweet repose;
Then wash all o'er and change your clothes;
Again to bed both clean and white,
And sleep in comfort all the night.

Now take your bitters by the way,
Two, three, or more times in a day;
Your appetite, if it be good,
May be appeased by wholesome food.

Physic I would by no means choose,
To have you first or last to use,
For if you take it much in course,
It will disorder reinforce.

Should the disorder reinforce,
Then follow up the former course;
The second time I think will do;
The third to fail, I seldom knew.

Th' Emetic, number One's designed
A gen'ral med'cine for mankind,
Of every country, clime or place,
Wide as the circle of our race.

In every case, and state and stage,
Whatever malady may rage;
For male or female, young or old,
Nor can its value half be told.

To use this med'cine do not cease,
Till you are free from your disease;
For Nature's friend this sure will be,
When you are taken sick at sea.

If any one should be much bruis'd,
Where bleeding frequently is used,
A lively sweat upon that day,
Will start the blood a better way.

Let names of all disorders be
Like to the limbs join'd on a tree;
Work on the root, and that subdue,
Then all the limbs will bow to you.

So as the body is the tree,
The limbs are cholic, pleurisy,
Worms and gravel, gout and stone,
Remove the cause, and they are gone.

My system's founded on this truth
Man's Air and Water, Fire and Earth,
And death is cold, and life is heat,
These tempered well, your health's complete.

LIFE AND MOTION.

ALTERED FROM DR. THOMSON.

Clearly to understand the laws of life and motion, the radical principles of animalization, is of infinite moment. Without some adequate conception of these, the nature of disease cannot be correctly understood, so as to prescribe a rational, safe, and certain remedy for the removal of disease in the human system.

Through many long and tedious seasons, these subjects had revolved, in my mind, before I could form a correct opinion. I witnessed many distresses in the family of man; my heart was pierced with many sorrows, until my mind was established in those simple truths that have laid the foundation of my practice, that has been so successful in subsequent years.

Persecution raged against me—all the presses in the country were closed against me—priests, doctors, lawyers and legislators, were combined against me—*ex post facto* laws were put in operation—prosecution commenced—false witnesses arose—bigotry, prejudice and superstition, waved their magic wand, but all in vain—truth has prevailed. The darkness of the ancient philosophers is passing away, and those simple truths, which are the genuine *philosophy of life*, and the fruits of the labours of my life begin to prosper beyond my former expectations.

Among those physicians called regular, I have found many who appeared to be as ignorant of the laws of life and motion, and how the functional powers of life are kept in operation, as though they themselves had never possessed an animal body.

My text is recorded in the mouth of everything that breathes. "BREATHING" is my text. Some have treated on respiration, but if they have not understood their subject, they might as well have been silent. *Breathing* is a demonstration of the existence of animal life. The principle of life has been taught to be SUPER-natural; leave out the SUPER, and say the cause of life and motion is NATURAL, perfectly and entirely natural, and we will concede to the truth of the assertion. The cause of breathing, or of animal life and motion, where there is no animal life, we shall carefully examine. Steam machinery is propelled by steam, which is a species or kind of breathing; these possess not the capacity for animalization.

In animal or human bodies, the constituent or component parts are essentially the same in man or beast. Animal bodies are composed of earth and water; these constitute the substances, dimensions, shape, and the size of bodies, &c. and give or constitute solidity, in what are denominated SOLIDS. These elements being constituted of various, still more simple elementary principles, which may be subdivided again and again, does not militate more against our position, than the infinite divisibility of numbers by decimal arithmetic destroys the unity of numbers.

FIRE and AIR are properly the fluids that pervade and fill and actuate the living animal; their operation is life—the elementary principle of life which keep the animal machine in motion. Where heat is extinct the animal is dead. HEAT and AIR combined, are so modified in the living, moving animal, as to constitute the living state, and justify the assertion that cold and inaction is a state of death, or rather death itself; and a specific degree of heat and motion so combined and modified, is the essential principle of life in the living animal, yea, rather life itself.

Waving all the minutia of chemical divisions and subdivisions, in simplyfying elementary combinations that constitute BODIES *dead or living*, the four great original elements of AIR, EARTH, FIRE, and WATER, contain and comprise all the more simple elements of which they may be respectively composed. A specific association, due proportion, mixture or combination of these four great elements, in an organic animal body, constitutes the living state, and prolongs life; an improper disproportion, combination, and modification destroys life.

To illustrate the nature and cause of respiration, or breathing of the living animal, we will refer to the operation of fire and water. Put a skillet of cold water over the fire; in a few minutes examine it by immersing your hand therein, you will perceive the first warmth of the water is on the top or upper surface; the coldest water is at the bottom of the skillet, nearest to the fire; the reason is, as soon as it becomes warm, it becomes rarified and lighter, and rises; just in proportion as it grows warm it becomes active, until it is all in a fluttering, fluctuating state of ebulition, and wastes by steam, sweat or breath, perspiring or respiring, until it will evaporate. This shows that heat rarifies and lightens water.

The subject may be further illustrated by reference to the effect of heat on the atmospheric air. You build your house in the open atmosphere—the house is filled with air within—the air within is a counterbalance, or resistence to the weight or power of the surrounding air without; the balance within and without is equal in coldness and inaction, resembling a state of death. To produce action, motion, or breath, kindle a fire in the house, the doors and windows being closed in the usual manner, in a few minutes every door and window begins to hum and sound the march of air. The air within becomes rarified and lighter than the air without; the air without presses in at every crevice to restore or form an equilibrium with the air within; the hotter and stronger the fire, the stronger will be the current of breath, or force of breathing air—as the heat diminishes the noise and breathing current of air will decline in force of operation, and the noise and motion will cease when the heat becomes extinct, and the equilibrium is restored.

The effects of heat rarifying and lightening the water and air, and occasioning a breathing motion, resemble and illustrate in some good degree, the breathing, sweating, and functional motions of the animal machine. The constituent, or component parts of men's bodies, give organic shape and size, and form, and functional structure or organization to the machine. The peculiar mixture, composition, proportion, and modification of these elements, constitute its aptitude or adaptation to the animalizing influence of fire, lightening air, and exciting breathing motion, and all the concatenations of motion, connected with this original or primary action, all evincing that heat is an essential principle of life; and cold, or an extinction of heat, is death.

A still-born child was resuscitated by placing the placentia or after birth on live embers, still connected with the child by the umbilical cord or navel string, and as the after birth began to heat, and had gained warmth sufficient to begin to fill and dilate the navel cord with warmth and moisture, it was stripped towards the body of the child, and through this medium a sufficient degree of warmth was conveyed to the body, the lungs expanded, and life was restored. This may serve in some measure to illustrate and confirm our ideas of life and motion.

In every thing that breathes, the breathing is from the same general cause. The principle of life and motion is radically the same in all animated bodies. Without heat there is no breathing; but when heat is continually generated or evolved in a confined room, excepting at one avenue, as in the lungs, there must be breathing, or what is the same, an inhaling of cold air, and an exhaling of a gaseous vapour from them.

Every animated body has its proportion of caloric or heating principle, suited to its size, adapted to its nature, proportioned to that degree of living power requisite to keep up the operation of all the animal functions, essential to the perpetuating of the peculiar specific form and mode of being in such animal.

The heat of animal fire, or that degree and condition of it that constitutes the living state of animalized existence, is maintained and continued by a suitable supply of appropriate fuel, or materials naturally adapted to that end or use; these are, *food and medicines.* These harmonize with each other in their salutary effect, or natural influence on animal bodies. Food and medicine originate from the same munificent hand, grow in the same field, and are adapted to the same end or design, viz., to supply fuel to the fire of life, to sustain and nourish the animal machine, by warming, dilating, filling the vascular system, maintaining the action, and supplying the wasting powers of the living state. Medicine removes disease, not only by removing obstructions, but by restoring and repairing the waste and decay of nature.

On these supplies our life depends, viz., the continuance of that state of warmth and action which constitute the living state. When food is masticated and taken into the stomach, the process of digestion commences. By the warmth and action of the organs of digestion, and the gastric juices, the food is decomposed or consumed, like fuel consuming in a fire. The breath and perspirable vapour are the smoke arising from this fire. The fœcal matter of dejections are as the ashes or earthly substance remaining after the consumption of fuel.

To understand the cause and nature of life and death, or of warmth and motion, of cold and inaction, it is necessary to advert to general principles, and the analogies of nature.—There is one general cause of the natural sensations of hunger, and one general method to relieve that want, or satisfy and relieve that sensation. Suitable food relieves hunger when taken into the stomach.

In perfect accordance with this, there is but one immediate cause of disease—however varied the remote cause may be, the immediate cause of the sensation of disease is uniformly and invariably the same, differing only in degree, and incidental diversity of symptoms, occasioned by local injuries, organic lesion, or functional derangement, dependent on these or whatever might predispose to a diseased state. As there is one general cause of the sensation of hunger, to be relieved by one general method, viz. by food; and this food may consist of sundry articles adapted to the same general end, so there is one general, or immediate cause of the sensation of disease, to be relieved or removed upon one general principle, though a variety of articles may be used. But as a few simple articles of diet are better suited to mantain a healthy state of body than an epicurean variety, so disease is more readily and certainly removed by a few simple remedies, that are best adapted to the human constitution.

That medicine which will most readily and safely open obstructions, promote perspiration, and restore a salutary operation of the digestive powers, by exciting and maintaining a due degree of heat and action through the system, is best suited to every state or form of disease, and must be universally applicable to a diseased state of the human system. Thus, the power or faculty of breathing is a capacity or condition to be acted on with effect, rather than any inherent power or faculty of acting. HEAT *rarifying and lightening air*, excites respiration—rarifying and lightening water, excites perspiration. Rarifying and lightening air and water, the vapour of breathing and sweat are produced and thrown off.

By heating water in the stomach, we lighten the air in, and expand the lungs—the weight of the cool, condensed and weightier external air, presses out the light and rarified air; these circumstances of the living state of the animal body, occasion the alternate contractions and dilations of the lungs, that constitute the action of breathing, indispensable to the living state.

By heating water in the stomach, and air in the lungs, we put the steam engine into operation. The operation of the animal machine strongly resembles the mechanical operations of the steam engine. Some of the fundamental principles of action are the same. In inspiration, cool fresh air is inhaled; in respiration, the rarified lightened air and vapour are exhaled, or thrown off, out of, or from the *steam pipe.* This action, by which steam is expended, the whole machinery of the living animal is kept in operation—the great fountain pump of the heart is kept in play, and pumps the blood through the lungs and arteries to the extremities, deep in the flesh and near the bones, which is returned in the veins. The warmth and action commencing at the fountain, are propagated through the system to the remotest extremities. So long as the fire keeps up that state, and degree of warmth essential to the living state of the animal body, or, to speak figuratively, so long as the fire is kept good in the boiler, to keep the engine at work, so long the pump will go.

Our regular meals supply regular fuel to keep up animal heat, as the regular tending a fire with wood or coal, will keep it burning. Drink supplies the boiler with water, which creates the steam; condensed water is discharged through its natural channel. On these principles of the philosophy of life we may expect a regular well formed machine to continue its operation until worn out, or broken by indiscretion and bad management of the engineer.

If the machine be entrusted to the management of an ignorant, incompetent engineer, who has no correct conceptions of the principles of life and motion, and is negligent in the discharge of his duty, your *steam boat* if I may so speak, will begin to fail in its speed, for lack of fuel to keep up the fire and water to supply the steam, or the engineer may conclude the *cholera* affects the machine, and will cast ice into the boiler to cool it down, or tap the boiler as a preventive, or remedy, and draw off the hot water—his boat begins to sink rapidly down the stream. This is often done by the lancet. If you would keep your steam boat's *steam breath* motions going on, keep up a supply of water in the boiler, and a supply of fuel to keep it sufficiently warm; raise the steam, and the actions of life will proceed regularly.

Concerning the doctrine of *vital principle* diffused through the whole organic structure of the animal machine, inducing an elementary mode of union or specific union of the component elements, differing in nature from all chemical union and affinities, and from all the laws of physical union with which we are acquainted,—this subject has employed the minds and pens of many talented writers, who have cast but little valuable light on the intricate theme.

When we are asked what constitutes a living fibre, we might as well ask what constitutes any other property of living matter. What constitutes that in which the life of a leaf or stem of a living tree consists ? "What can we reason, but from what we know ?" Every living thing has something peculiar to the nature or life with which it is endowed in the living state, whether vegetable or animal—but a living animal has heat and motion ; without this animal heat and motion, the animal becomes dead—without a due proportion of heat inward and outward, or outward and inward, there is no animal motion, no animal life. We know not of any vital principle, except a capacity to be brought into that peculiar mode, state and degree of warmth and action, constituting animalization, or the sensitive living state of animal bodies.

Warmth and action do not constitute animal life, in unorganised matter—they do not constitute animal life without an organised animal structure, to which heat gives the impulse applied to and connected with the animal structure, caloric or the principal of heat rarifying and lightening air, excites action, which circumstance of being, constitutes animalization, or the living state.

Warmth and action do not constitute animal life, only as applied to, connected with, and exercised in an organized animal body, possessing a capacity inherent in its nature to be put in operation, in which state or condition of being, sensation, perception, and consciousness of identity, or individual existence, are gradually developed ; but these circumstances of life are not like itself—there may be animal life, viz. breath and motion, in an animal body where these functional powers are totally deranged or utterly extinct. Fire and steam are necessary to propel a steam boat, but notwithstanding the capacity or adaptation of the mechanical structure to be propelled, the boat will not go until the fire is kindled and the steam raised to put it in motion.

The animal body is the machine so constructed, so modified, endowed with such a capacity for life, call it vital principle, or what you please, that heat rarifiying and lightening air, stimulating and expanding the lungs, puts the machinery in motion, and pumps the tide of life through all its crimson channels. This combination of circumstances constitutes the living state of the living animal: for where these circumstances do not exist, there is no animal life—the animal form is dead.

Suppose a man in all the vigour of life falls into the water and sinks; in a few minutes he is taken out apparently dead, the warmth and motions of life, if not extinct, are at a low ebb—as soon as you can kindle up the decayed spark, and restore inward heat by medicine, friction, or any appropriate means, if the capacity for the action of life is not utterly extinct, an energy is given to the system, the air in his lungs becoming warm, rarifies and expands, and heaves them into action—the machinery begins to move—the wheels of life no longer wallow in back water—the proper state and proportion of heat inward and outward is recovered—nature rises to its wonted strength and vigour.

All that is requisite in such a case is, to supply fuel to raise the latent spark of the fire of life. The same holds good in a collapsed state of disease, whether it appears in a cholera form, or whatever shape it may wear. The vascular system loses its wonted tone—the whole system is sinking—the power of life is unable to distend and expand the lungs—the heart and arteries no longer propel their contents by mantaining the requisite action. The spark of life is becoming extinct—the water that should breathe, exhale and perspire away, becomes congestively condensed, and extinguishes the spark of living fire. The coolness and weight of the internal air is too much for the small degree of heat remaining in the lungs, heart, &c.; the power of life, or rather the power of capacity to live, to keep the powers of animal life in their warm, and moving, or living state, becomes measurably extinct. For lack of heat, the air in the lungs is not rarified and lightened, so as to give the necessary action, &c.

In this case shield the sufferers from surrounding cold air, by wrapping in a blanket, and placing warm in bed, and gradually raising a steam around him; administer gradually, frequently and perseveringly, the warming medicines, and give injections, which all acquainted with my system will readily understand—proceed until you can gain a sufficient degree of inward heat to expand freely, to rouse the sinking, fainting, I might say, drowning patient, to a proper degree of warmth and action ; when they have had a proper course, they will sweat freely ; and when they crave food, give them enough to keep up the steam ; the pump of life will begin to work freely, and the patient to rejoice in the warmth and action arising from the resuscitated powers of departing life.

Much has been said about drawing in the breath ; but the fact is, you cannot keep the breathing air out so long as there is a due degree, or natural proportion of heat in the lungs ; neither can you prevent the motion of the pump-like action of your heart in its systole and diastole. But when the heart decays, or state of living warmth declines, the lungs begin to labour like a wheel wading slowly in back water. The pump has not power to roll the blood along the arterial canals—the pulse falters—the extremities grow cold—the blood that maintained the warmth, by its active circulation, recedes from the extremities—there is not heat enough at the fountain or boiler to keep up the steam, and continue the living action—blood settles in the veins, not being supplied and propelled by pulsation in the arteries—the fire becomes extinct—the pump no longer plays at the fountain ; the man dies * * * for want of breath, for want of capacity to breathe, or because the inward heat is reduced below the living point. The proper and natural proportion and modification of the inward and outward heat, as they exist in the living animal, become deranged, destroyed, and life is extinct. The disease is as contagious as though the man had been * * * hanged or drowned ! !

The regular faculty are requested to inquire whether the depleting antiphlogistic practice, that has been popular, and notoriously mortal in its results, has not been the cause of producing much disease, and many of the most fatal results that have attended on what has been called scarlet fever, yellow fever, cold plague, and *now* cholera. Thus "the breath of life" is inhaled or breathed into man ; and by heat rarifying air, breathing commences, and man thus becomes, and is thus sustained, a living animal.

In conclusion, the cause of vegetable and animal life is the same, viz., one common principle produces similar effects; nutritive life in animals and vegetables bear a striking resemblance to each other—vegetables, like animals, are constituted or formed of the four great cardinal elements—all vegetable life is under the control, influence and operation of similar principles, as that of an animal. Without earth, water, fire and air, nothing like vegetation could exist. The winter season is a state of death to vegetation; just in proportion to the loss of heat is the degree of the suspension of life, we mean a loss of heat in that peculiar modification or elementary combination thereof, that constitutes the living state of a vegetable; this is a degree of death, or a degree of the suspension of vegetable life. In many instances the suspension is total.

In cold countries, after the winter has passed away, and the spring returns, suspended vegetation, and suspended animation, are again restored; the torpid reptile again inhales the breath of life. Heat in this case is not only an agent of restoration to life and vigour, but is so adapted to the condition of the being on which its influence is exerted, as to constitute a living principle. So, on the other hand, cold is not only an approximation to death, but that degree of cold which is inconsistent with, and contrary to the living state, is death itself.

Heat does not act alone and independent of its fraternal elements, but in harmony and accordance with the whole family. But without their elder brother, there is no life in the material universe. The elements would rest in everlasting silence and inactivity, if destitute of this generative principle of life and motion.

Abstract the element of fire from all the other elements; stillness and silence would be universal—the life of all that breathes and moves would be swallowed up in the stillness of eternal death. Earth and sea would be and remain a solid, unmoving and immovable mass—the fluid air would be consolidated, would be a blank!

AIR.

Air, an invisible elastic fluid, of which there are several kinds, varying from one another as much in their properties as the grosser fluids, oil, water, and mercury, differ from one another. The term *air*, when used without any addition, is now restricted to mean common air, or the air of the atmosphere; other elastic fluids being called *gases*, when cold does not condense them; and *vapours* when it does. Thus we have hydrogen *gas*, or inflammable air, permanent at all temperatures; and the *vapour* of water, or steam, which is condensed by cold. We shall now mention some particulars respecting atmospherical or common air. The researches of modern chemistry have determined, that the atmosphere is not a uniform fluid, but a mixture of two principal elastic fluids, with a few others in very minute proportions, and holding in solution a varying quantity of watery vapour. The composition of one hundred parts of atmospherical air, freed from all adventitious mixture, is seventy-nine parts of gas called azote, or nitrogen; and twenty-one parts of another gas called oxygen gas. Atmospherical air is indispensably necessary for the breathing of animals; and, though inflammable bodies will burn in some other gases, yet as these gases are rare, except when artificially produced, air may also be considered as the great supporter of combustion. When, by various methods familiar to chemists, the oxygenous portion of the atmosphere is separated from the azotic, it is found that an animal dies, and a burning body is extinguished; we hence conclude that it is only the oxygenous part of the atmosphere that is fit for the purposes of respiration and combustion. Air is, by these processes, continually becoming more and more unfit for the use of breathing; hence the danger of continuing long in a small room without changing the air, or admitting a fresh portion of oxygen.

Change of AIR *in apartments necessary.*—Independently of its chemical properties, air that has been long unchanged, and in which one or more human bodies have been confined, is possessed of qualities highly dangerous and even destructive, as we see in many instances in jails, ships, and other confined apartments. Hence the necessity of free ventilation in houses of every description; of daily admitting a thorough current of air into sleeping rooms, and indeed, into every room of a house. From the neglect of this ventilation, arise the dangerous and malignant fevers in the confined and ill-ventilated dwellings in the closes, alleys, and courts of large towns. Since attention has been called to this circumstance, how seldom do we hear of the ship or the jail fevers! Though the fever, which was formerly so fatal in ships and jails, is still lamentably prevalent somewhere or other, and though we still hear of towns or tracts of territory being visited with its depopulating scourge, it is not in ships and jails that it is suspected to take its rise, but in the abodes of slothful and squalid poverty, where no judicious and directing mind enforces the necessity of ventilation and cleanliness. Even in the apartment where a patient is in bed, the fear of his catchiug cold should not prevent us from occasionally changing the air of it, by opening the doors and windows for a few minutes at a time, taking care not to expose the sick person to the current of air, but closing the curtains and using such other precautions as common sense will readily suggest.

Air, considered with reference to the cause, the cure, or the mitigation of diseases.—Many circumstances connected with air, which chemistry is unable to trace or explain, are much to be attended to in a medical point of view. The bad air from marshy grounds produces ague; and fevers are generated by the malignant effluvia from animal bodies; and the air seems to carry the infection of other diseases, as small-pox, measles, hooping cough, scarlet-fever, &c. The air of certain places is supposed, justly, to have an influence in giving a tendency to certain diseases, or to bring them on directly. The croup is frequent in cold, damp situations, exposed to the east wind, or near the sea. The sea air is unfavourable in certain states of consumption, or in affections of the breast, which would probably end in that disease. The mild, equable air of the country, is unloaded with the endless variety of matters mixing with the air of large towns, is favourable to recovery from many ailments, as indigestion, dropsy, jaundice, breast complaints, asthmas, and the wasting diseases of children, as also to that feeble state of constitution which has not received any appropriate name. It is remarkable that some persons in asthma are not better in air, which we should think the purest.—*Change of air*, even to a worse, has been of service in hooping-cough; but it is useless to attempt this, at an early period of the disease, as it is hardly possible by any means to prevent it from running on a considerable time. In general, it is hardly worth while to try a change of air till it has continued distinctly at least a month or six weeks. A good deal of the influence of the air on the skin and lungs must depend on its degree of moisture or dryness. When there is much watery vapour in the air, it is less able to receive more, and the perspirable matter from the skin not being carried off, we shall appear to perspire more, though in reality the perspiration is less. In like manner, the watery vapour which is continually thrown off by the lungs is not carried away fast enough by a heavy, moist atmosphere; and in certain diseases of the lungs, in colds, consumptions, asthmas, &c., some patients, according to the quantity of watery vapour, or mucus, exhaled from the lungs, will be benefited either by a dry air, or the contrary. It is wrong, therefore, to lay down any general rule about a particular spot or climate, as its good or bad effects will vary according to the state of the disease in each particular patient.

CLOTHING.

The choice and regulation of clothing is of great importance both to health and comfort. It will readily be supposed that the physician does not meddle as to its form and decoration, but that his instructions are chiefly confined to what is worn next the skin; and that he will forbid all such articles of dress as are likely to prove injurious by pressing on tender parts, and altering their structure, or impeding functions. In this variable and uncertain climate of ours, *woollen* garments are by far the best kind of clothing. They enable the body to resist the effects of the frequent changes of the weather; being what the chemists call bad conductors of heat, they both prevent the natural warmth of the body from escaping, and the external heat from reaching it, and thus preserve it in a steady temperature. When sweating occurs spontaneously, or is induced by artificial means, flannel does not take up the moisture in a fluid form, but rather as a vapour, and thus the coldness of the fluid is not perceived. Flannel is sometimes debilitating by the perspiration it excites too constantly; or, it is irritating by its roughness on some tender skins. It requires, in the first case, either to be worn of a very thin texture, or to be exchanged for cotton; and, in the second case, it must be discontinued, and linen must be used. Flannel, which is worn next the skin, should be frequently changed; it should be washed in water not very warm, which prevents its becoming too thick—*Cotton* has all the good properties of flannel, though in an inferior degree.

Chamois is used next the skin by many people, as uniting the advantages of both the former materials. *Linen* forms inner clothing of great comfort to the strong and healthy, being highly conducive to cleanliness; and if it be frequently changed, it renews the air between the linen and the body.

Silk should not be worn next the skin, as it has no affinity for water, and the sweat not being absorbed is apt to fret the body, and to cause a shivering when it cools. It should be worn above flannel or linen. *Fur* is necessary in very cold climates, but it is apt to harbour insects; and it is one of the most powerful retainers of contagion.

In our climate much caution is required in changing of dress. The winter clothes should be worn till summer is unquestionably arrived. A few days of sunshine in April or May should not tempt us to lay aside our warm clothing. It is of the greatest importance to health, to keep the extremeties dry and warm; and in those who are subject to gout, to any complaint of the head or chest, or bowels, particular attention should be paid to the feet. The shoes should be carefully kept from admitting moisture; the stockings should be warm, and frequently changed. The feet should be washed often, and not in very hot water. If we proceed to the more exterior part of our clothing, we shall find that the principal thing to be attended to is to prevent undue pressure on any part by ligatures, bandages, garters, or stays. The blood-vessels are liable to be compressed, or the abdomen and chest, with the important organs contained in them, to be hindered in the free exercises of their functions. In the regulation of the female dress, much is sacrificed to fashion and appearance. But the physician ought to be heard when he warns the delicate young lady of the danger of cold, consumption, and sore throat, from the insufficient covering of the neck, the breast, and the arms; and when he points out the danger of stays and tight lacing, to induce disorders of the liver and other viscera of the abdomen, or to cause headaches and spitting of blood, by hindering the due performance of the circulation.

EXERCISE.

The necessity of exercise to the health and comfort of the animal body is demonstrated by the instinctive desire for it which appears both in man and in the lower animals; as also by the pernicious and lamentable consequences of sedentary habits, and a life of indolence. Even from the moment of birth some exercise is necessary, and this is supplied to the infant by the washing and dressing to which it is subjected; and its vigorous crying, when we are sure it is not from the feeling of pain, is to be regarded as a salutary mode of dilating its chest, and of putting many muscles into action. In the progress of its days, the dandling of the nurse, and then its own exertions, succeeded by the active play of the schoolboy, conduce, by the motion given to the limbs, to the digestion of the food, the circulation of the fluids, and to the growth and health of the body; while the bad effects of the want of exercise are seen in the ill health of the imprudent student, the plodding merchant, and the indolent and luxurious man of wealth. As exercise is of the most essential use in preserving the health, so it is a very important agent in the cure of disease. The disorders of digestion receive most decided benefit from exercise. The feeble constitution which scrofula attacks, is invigorated by exercise, and enabled to resist that very prevailing malady. Even hereditary gout may be mitigated or kept off, if the subject of it has fortitude to resist the blandishments of luxury and indolence.

The modes of exercise are various, and, in the case of disease, a choice is necessary. That exercise is the best which employs the greatest number of muscles, and as the most useful objects are, by the kindness of Providence, the most easily attained, so walking, which is the best of all exercises, is in the power of all. Walking, in a degree proportioned to the strength of those who employ it, is useful in the cure of various diseases, as of those of the stomach, in gout, and some others; but there are other complaints in which it is unsafe, as in inflammatory affections, and in those where there is a tendency of blood to the lungs. It is, therefore, a hazardous plan to drive away a cold by walking it off, instances have been known where violent inflammation of the lungs has been brought on by such an attempt. All the more violent exercises, as fencing, dancing, running, wrestling, and the like, are to be avoided in diseases of excitement; and in those of debility, exercise is to be prescribed at first with great caution, and to be taken very gradually; and thus by prudence and perseverance, very feeble persons have become able to take exercise of the most active kind. When a patient, for whom exercise is good, is unable to take it by his own exertions, we must direct some mode of exercise, as riding on horseback, or in a carriage, sailing, or springing on an elastic board. Riding on horseback has been much celebrated in consumptive diseases; and, provided it be taken in fine weather, and before the disease has made much progress, it will assist the other means of attempting to arrest its progress; but we must not expect from it the great and signal benefit which Sydenham ascribed to it. Sailing, also, has been much famed as a remedy in consumption, and though it has failed in numberless instances, it is worth a trial. The sea air appears to be beneficial, and the sickness and vomiting which accompany a voyage, have the effect of improving, in many cases, the action of the stomach and bowels, in removing tumours, and stopping discharges of blood. Riding is to be avoided in diseases of the kidneys, as it is apt to occasion much pain, and a discharge of blood. Riding in a carriage is an exercise of body and mind, well adapted for a variety of chronic ailments, stomach complaints, and low spirits. The exercise is good, and the change of scene prevents the patient from brooding over his real or fancied maladies. Exercise should generally be taken in the best and purest air, and a moderate degree of cold, provided it be not attended with moisture, adds to the strengthening effects of exercise, In some cases of disease neither exercise nor gestation is in the patient's power, and we must substitute for them rubbing with the flesh brush, or with the hand. Such treatment is sometimes necessary in rheumatism, sprains, tumours, white swellings, and dropsical limbs.

SLEEP.

That state in which the powers of sense and voluntary motion are suspended, in order to recruit the powers of the system, exhausted by the continued actions which they exert. All animals generally sleep in the night, when the silence and darkness remove the ordinary impressions on the senses; and the continuance of sleep varies much according to the age, constitution, habit, and other circumstances of the individual. New-born children sleep a great deal, and thus their nutrition in the very early periods of life is favoured, while the parent in her weakened state is not fatigued. It is impossible to specify a period for the duration of sleep, which shall be adapted to all constitutions; but in an adult healthy person, from six to eight hours may be reckoned sufficient. Too much sleep blunts the faculties, and disposes to listlessness and inactivity of mind and body; it also gives rise to flabby, corpulent, and unwieldy habits. A disturbed and unsound sleep arises from a variety of causes; from the presence of feverish and other diseases, from disordered bowels, from too great fulness of stomach with meat or drink. Sleep is also prevented by uneasiness of mind, by a certain degree of cold; by light, noise, and other impressions on the senses; and in some persons by the use of green tea, or of coffee. To bring on sleep is often an essential object in several diseases. The medicines which have this power are called narcotic, and are of primary importance in the practice of physic. Of these, the most generally useful are opium and its various preparations, henbane, and hemlock.

EXTERNAL APPLICATIONS.

Heat.—A certain degree of external heat is necessary to promote the vital manifestations of all warm blooded animals. It is frequently employed as a remedial agent externally, The *Hot Air Bath*, at a temperature of from 100° to 130° Fahr. is a powerful stimulant, and principally valuable when the blood has receded from the superficial parts of the body, and the internal organs congested; as in some cases of fever, in spasmodic cholera, in drowning, in chronic rheumatism, and stiffness of the joints.

Bottles filled with hot water, are applied to the feet, to excite the circulation and augment the animal heat in diseases attended with cold extremetics, for which purpose nothing is better than common wine bottles, filled with boiling water and wrapped round several times with flannel to prevent them from burning the patient. Hot bricks may be used in a similar manner. The same are applied to the stomach to relieve spasmodic pain. Hot sand, inclosed in a bag, may be employed for similar purposes.

Cold Bath.—The cold bath, though popularly esteemed one of the most innocent remedies yet discovered, is not however to be adopted indiscriminately. On the contrary, it is liable to do considerable mischief in all cases of diseased *viscera*, and ought not to be used during costiveness. As a general bracer of the system to persons of a relaxed fibre, especially females, it generally proves highly beneficial, and in most cases, when not carried to excess, is a great means of promoting a good state of health. When beneficial, a glow of heat succeeds the bathing; if chilness and headache are the result, it should immediately be abandoned, as being evidently pernicious. Cold water is a powerful tonic, but, like all other valuable things, may be abused. Sea water, in general, is preferable to fresh, though when not attainable, the latter is a valuable substitute not to be despised.

Hot Bath.—By which is understood any degree of heat between 93 and 96 degrees. It has a peculiar tendency to bring on a state of repose, to remove local irritation, promotes personal cleanliness, and is excellent to children affected with convulsions and diseases of the skin. It restores suppressed perspiration, relieves gouty, rheumatic, and hectic patients, and is useful in complaints of the kidneys and liver. It is also especially useful in swellings of the legs, and in obstructions peculiar to females.

The **Shower Bath** is very similar in its effects. In insanity it is used with the greatest benefit, to allay mental excitement. When the patient appears overcome it should be discontinued, and renewed when the violent symptoms recur. After four or five applications of this kind, the patient becomes entirely subdued, when he should be taken out of the bath, rapidly dried, warmly covered up, and put into bed. Calmness and sleep generally follow, with many days of tranquillity and ease. The daily use of the shower bath is very beneficial.

Tepid Bath—A bath at about 90 degrees. It is often useful in fevers and in diseases of the skin, is quite sufficient to produce a salutary reaction, with a degree of perspirability on the surface of the skin. It is useful in gout, rheumatism, headaches, colds, &c.

The Vapour Bath is employed in the same way as hot air, but it is more soothing and sudorific. It softens and relaxes the skin, producing copious perspiration. It may likewise be employed during the cold stage of intermittent fever, cholera, dropsy in old debilitated persons, liver complaints, rheumatism, gout, slight colds from checked perspiration, and chronic skin diseases accompanied with a dry state of the cutaneous surface. It is of great value in producing a relaxed state of the skin, and profuse perspiration.

The Inhalation of the Vapour of Hot Water proves highly serviceable as a soothing remedy in irritation or inflammation of the membrane lining the throat, or bronchial tubes and tonsils.

Warm Fomentations and Poultices are employed to relieve inflammation, pain, tension, and spasms.

Warm Water has been highly extolled as an application to burns and scalds, especially those on young children. The water must be applied with flannels, repeatedly changed, but at the same time preventing as much as possible the exposure of the burnt surface to the air. In every case it soothes and mitigates the pain, and lessens the inflammation and constitutional disturbance that usually follows injuries of this kind.

Cold Affusion is often recommended for use, when it is desirable to make a powerful and sudden impression on the system. In inflammatory affections of the brain (even of young children), in violent delirium, in poisoning by opium or prussic acid, or in torpor from the fumes of burning charcoal, it may be used most advantageously. In hysteria, epilepsy, or lockjaw, it is often serviceable in diminishing the duration of the fit, and in relieving the deadly sleep that follows. The mode in which cold affusion is effected, is as follows:—Water is poured on the head (inclined over a pan or tub), from a pitcher held a height of two or three feet. If the person be in bed, the head should be placed over the side of it. In children, it is sufficient to squeeze a large sponge, filled with cold water, at some height from the head. The time that it should be continued varies from one to two or three minutes, afterwards the body should be carefully wiped dry, wrapped up warm, and placed in bed.

Tepid Affusion is frequently employed, and by some regarded as a safer, though less powerful means than cold. Sponging the body with tepid water in scarlet fever is very beneficial; in continued fever, it diminishes the frequency of the pulse and of respiration, and causes a tendency to sleep.

Cold is frequently used as a remedial agent. Cold air, in fevers, is both grateful and efficacious. In the admission of fresh and cold air to patients affected by febrile disorders, consists one of the most important features of the improved methods of treating fevers.

The Cold Bath is employed with the view of obtaining the plunge or shock, and the reaction or glow after it. In general the immersion being only temporary, reaction quickly takes place, and a sensation of warmth is soon felt: the circulation of the skin is speedily re-established, a glow ensues, perspiration comes on, and the body is invigorated.

In weakly persons, however, this reaction may not follow, or only imperfectly, and on such the cold bath will be found to act injuriously. As a general rule, it should only be used when there is a sufficient degree of tone and vigour in the system to cause a *reaction.* Even with the strong, long immersion renders the pulse small, and ultimately imperceptible, the respiration difficult and irregular, a feeling of langour succeeds, the joints become rigid and inflexible, pain in the head, drowsiness, and cramps are experienced, the temperature of the body falls rapidly, and faintness, followed by death, may ensue. The treatment of such a state, must be the same as in

Drowning.—Keep the head raised, dry the body and rub with hot cloths, let one person press on the chest with his flat hands and another also with his flat hands, shove the belly up to the chest, then suddenly take away their hands, and in this way, by performing the action of respiration, endeavour to restore breathing. A hot bath is also of great value Have several assistants to rub the body with their hands. Clear the mucus from the mouth, hold the nose, and then suck out the foul air with a tube, and blow in fresh air, as represented in the cut. Place hot bricks and bottles of hot water in the armpits, between the thighs, and at the feet, keeping up the friction the whole time; irritate the nostrils with a feather, or hartshorn, and administer a clyster of warm turpentine. If possible, apply electricity. When swallowing can be performed, give weak warm wine, or spirit and water, and soon afterwards a mustard emetic. After restoration, purge or give such medicines as seem to be required. Persons have been recovered who have been under water twenty-five minutes. Twelve hours' exertion may result in restoring a person to society. Bleeding is often required during the progress of recovery, particularly when the respiration is laborious, the brain oppressed, and when delirium or wandering, the frequent attendant on restored animation, is present.

Cold Lotions.—Water and spirit lotions are employed to generate cold by evaporation, and thereby to relieve local irritation and inflammation. They should be applied by a single layer of thin linen, and not made to confine the part. Cold lotions are applied to the head in brain fever in severe bruises, fractures, dislocations, and erysipelous inflammation.

Ice is sometimes employed to stop long continued bleedings from the nose and other parts. In cases of madness, inflammation of the brain, and in fever, where there is great excitement of the brain, with a hot dry skin, it is often used with the greatest benefit. Ice is also taken internally in the latter stages of typhus fever.

FOOD.

There is a period in the life of man in which the organs of digestion are weak, and yet, at the same time, there is a necessity for much nourishment. This period is infancy; for as at this time the body increases fast, much nourishment is required to help and forward the growth; milk being naturally provided and therefore probably adapted to it, we may suppose it to be a food of easy digestion and considerable nourishment. Examining then the properties of milk, will give us some insight into the nature of food in general.

Milk is not a simple substance; it is a mixture of three; namely, coagulable matter, expressed oil, and sugar. Coagulable matter is that which will unite, and become solid, leaving the rest thinner and more fluid, viz. the curd; and expressed oil is such as can be procured from any substance by pressing, as oil of almonds, olives, and the like: by expressed oil in milk, we understand the cream.

The most simple food, then, does not appear to be the easiest of digestion; if it were, we should have expected that milk would have consisted of one substance only.

That coagulable matter is capable of affording considerable nourishment, may be gathered from our experiencing that animal mucilage nourishes the most; mucilage being that substance which has sufficiant moisture to keep it together: as, for, example,—sound, good meat.

This coagulable matter in milk is fluid indeed when taken, but there is a juice peculiar to the stomach, very different from an acid, that renders it solid. We find the stomach of a calf, though clear of every thing that is acid, to have this property. An infusion of a few grains of the inner coat will coagulate or curdle several quarts of milk.

Dr. Cullen says, this coagulating or curdling of milk in the human stomach, is more owing to a weak acid in the stomach, of healthy persons, the relicts of vegetable food; but in different stomachs it has a different effect, giving a sense of weight and heaviness. Dr. Mosley says this sense of weight may be removed by mixing milk with sugar; but I have tried it and found no such effect, probably because I did not add enough sugar, which to me is unpleasant. When young, I ate much milk and found no weight; now I am old, I find this weight; therefore refrain from milk.

Milk new drawn is best and most wholesome for weakly persons and infants. Milk is of a costive nature and boiling it renders it more so, and as boiled milk is less acescent in the stomach, it is better for the robust and vigorous, particularly as it is in this state more cooling. As sugar prevents the spontaneous separation of the several parts of milk in the stomach, it is proper to give sugar along with it to convalescents.

Cheese.—With respect to cheese, for we shall not have a better opportunity to mention it, it has in general, a costive quality; but it differs, in proportion to the quantity of oil in the coagulable part. The more rich and oily parts there are in cheese, the more nutritive it is and soluble; that is, the readier it will digest; the leaner the cheese, the more difficult it digests. Cheese is liable to become rank and putrid; we must then consider it as having all the effects of animal food when advanced to putrefaction; at this time it ceases to be nutritive, and can only be considered as an assistant to digestion. Cheese, indeed, as food, is only fit for the laborious and robust.

Butter.—A quantity of pure cream eaten is undoubtedly unwholesome; being, from its dispositions to get acid and rancid, very difficult of digestion; but, in the form of butter, it may be used with advantage. It is a strong nutriment, fit to accompany our vegetable diet, especially such vegetables as are naturally dry of themselves; in this case, it gives them the properties of rich, oily substances.—But, to return,

It appears then that milk, and, of course, all other food, must become solid in the stomach, and, after that, undergo a fresh change, that is, be redissolved, for digestion; for which purpose, it must remain some time there, before it be passed off.

Now, that the expressed oil, which is the cream, helps digestion, is evident from milk's not digesting so well when it has been skimmed, the curd being harder; for the cream and the sugar, being mixed with the curd, separate the different parts of it more from one another, so that the natural fluid of the stomach will penetrate the easier, and fermentation go on better.* And as to sugar, it being from its nature more apt to ferment, will of course facilitate digestion.

That expressed oil affords much nourishment, we find from

* If new milk be too rich or heavy for a child's stomach, let it be diluted or mixed with water; it should never be skimmed.

men and animals being able to live a long time upon nuts, almonds, &c., such containing a quantity of this oil. But, expressed oil alone produces sense of weight in the stomach, owing to a relaxation it brings on, preventing the stomach's contracting and expelling its load; and, if taken in quantities, it will bring on sickness.

That sugar also affords great nourishment, is evident from animals thriving on the shoots of young plants, which contain a great deal of sugar; and from some negroes living wholly on the sugar-cane. But sugar alone is viscid, and by adhering to the sides of the stomach, will stimulate it, disorder the system, and, if diluted with any watery fluid, would be so thin as not to be retained in the stomach long enough for digestion; but mixed with the coagulable part of the milk, it is sufficiently retained. Either of these substances alone then, viz. coagulable matter, expressed oil or sugar, would be *hard* of digestion; but blended, as in milk, they are *easy* of digestion.

Immediately after child-birth, when the milk begins to flow in the mother's breasts, it contains a larger quantity of sugar and water, for there is always a small quantity of water in proportion to the coagulable matter. Some months after childbirth the coagulable matter increases, and the sugar proportionably diminishes. For as the infant-stomach is weak, the solid part of the milk is at first less, so that a looser mass is formed, much easier to be dissolved. As the child grows stronger, its stomach can bear more of this coagulate matter, and digests it, if it be firmer. This points out that a young child, one of a month old, will not thrive, in general, on breast milk eight or nine months old.

We also learn from this, that weak stomachs require food of easy digestion; strong stomachs, food of harder digestion. Thus, chicken, &c., will nourish people most recovering from sickness; and bacon, &c. will best recruit a labourer.

For breakfast, milk is the most proper food, provided it agree with the stomach and bowels. If it give a sense of weight and disagrees, as sugar soon ferments and facilitates digestion, Dr. Mosley, as I have said, recommends to those who feel weight and fulness after milk, to use a good quantity of sugar with it, which will correct this inconvenience.

Milk is equally fit at every period of life, being, in general, easy of digestion, and occasioning less heat to the system than any other animal or vegetable food, producing less feculent matter, and not offending the stomach, unless it form into too firm a coagulation, which occasions the fulness and weight I have mentioned. In such cases, if it be not corrected by sugar, it should be avoided.

Boiled milk has been found, by experience, more costive than raw. When milk is boiled, a considerable quantity of air is detached, evident from the froth on the surface; and air is the chief instrument of fermentatiou in bodies; of course, after boiling, it is not so apt to turn sour in the stomach. We find that boiling it will keep it sweet some days; for these reasons it is proper for the robust and vigorous, but not so proper for weak stomachs.

The bad effects of milk, I conceive, says Dr. Cullen, to be in the cream; the quarter part of which is not pure oil, the rest coagulable and saline parts. In the form of butter, the oil is much more pure and more nutritious, taken with vegetables, particularly such as are least farinaceous.

Milk when new drawn from the cow does not so easily separate into parts as when it has been some time exposed to the air, and, of course, it is more nutritious. A mixture of sugar will prevent this spontaneous separation, therefore gives it the advantage of new drawn milk. Convalescents therefore should mix it with sugar, as I have before observed.

Whey carries with it a great part of all the ingredients of milk, though it may not seem so, and is more nourishment than the milk itself. Farmers fatten pigs solely upon whey.

VEGETABLE FOOD.

Taste and smell generally direct our choice in vegetables, and it may be said, with very few exceptions, that those esculents which are most agreeable to the taste and smell are most salutary, and *vice versa*. But as the taste and smell in certain constitutions are often depraved and vitiated, we had best say, that those which sit easiest on the stomach are most wholesome.

Vegetables tend to reduce plethoric and full habits; abate heat, and are, of course, very proper for corpulent people, and those troubled with feverish heats and distensions of the blood vessels.

That vegetables correct putrescency, is evident from their curing what is called the sea-scurvy, brought on by living on flesh meat, which, without a mixture of vegetable food, is apt to continue long enough in the stomach to putrefy.

Vegetables are particularly proper in hot climates, being less stimulant; and though less nutritive, and have been accounted flatulent, they are more cooling than animal food: but as flatulency is seldom experienced by persons in a healthy state, it may reasonably be imputed rather to the weakness of the stomach and bowels than to the vegetables themselves.

The vegetable substances capable of nourishing are as follow:

1. Farinaceous matter or flour. This is generally contained in grain; but sometimes we find it in the stems of plants, and sometimes in their roots, much of it in potatoes.

2. Vegetable mucilage; as for example, gum-arabic, &c. That this is capable of nourishing, is evident from whole caravans living on it, for a long time, when they can procure no other food.

3. Sugar.

4. Expressed oils. And

5. Native vegetable acid; or the juice of sour fruits, which tends to take off the putrescency of animal food; that is, to prevent meat from corrupting or putrefying, whilst it continues in the stomach.

For animal food, without a mixture of vegetable, is apt to continue too long on the stomach, before it ferments. In this case, it will sometimes begin to putrefy before it is passed off, which putrefaction getting into the blood, will often bring on a putrefaction of all the fluids of the body. This is a complete sea-scurvy, which, if not timely remedied, always terminates dreadfully. Salting provisions makes them harder of digestion; and though it prevents meat from corrupting soon out of the body; yet, as the salt seldom, if ever, penetrates sufficiently into the substance of the meat, so as totally to secure it against putrefaction, when in the body; if it be not immediately made to ferment, by the addition of vegetable food, or some vegetable acid thrown in with it, it will be apt to putrefy before it digests, and contaminate the whole system. Hence we see, how liable mariners are, on a voyage where there is a scarcity of vegetables, to be afflicted with the scurvy, and how soon they get rid of that disorder, when they once get on shore again, to the free use of herbs and roots.

Now, those five vegetable substances, we have mentioned, go naturally through fermentation, and are converted into blood.

With respect to the fibres, the solid part of vegetables, we find them frequently pass through the body, without being altered. As for example, peas and the skins of gooseberries, currants, &c. Now, as the texture of the strongest tendons of animal food is constantly destroyed in their passage through the body, while such parts of vegetable food shall be evacuated as they are taken in, it is a question whether these last are digested; if any of them are, it must be such only as are young and tender.

In the East, they eat rice; in England, wheat; in Germany, rye; in some parts, oats and barley; and in Africa, Indian wheat. This is the grain commonly used for food, and it appears to be well adapted to digestion.

Rice has of late years been introduced into this country as a cheap food. Whole nations in the east subsist wholly on rice and other vegetables, yet live long and are healthy. The universal opinion that rice is an astringent is founded in error. It is generally prescribed, and judiciously, as a diet in lax habits and debility of the digestive organs, because it produces less disturbance to the stomach and bowels in digestion than any other food; yet it is highly nutritious, and more easily digested than bread, seldom occasions acidity or flatulency, and perhaps is the most wholesome grain used by man.

Farinaceous matter is, in its nature, solid, capable of being dissolved in water, and forming a jelly. If, before we dissolve it in water, we expose it to heat, it coagulates or becomes solid, thus if we bake it, we convert it into bread; after which, it will not so readily dissolve. But bread dissolved by long boiling, is less viscid than a solution of flour would be; and consequently more wholesome. Were flour used, with water, raw, it would be so viscid as to clog and cloy the stomach; we therefore prepare it, to take off this viscidity.

Flour is not apt to undergo that fermentation in the stomach so as sufficiently to correct the putrescency of animal food; we therefore ferment it first; that is, we make it into bread. Another reason for converting it into bread, is that, in fermentation extrication of air takes place, which leaves a number of holes, making the bread spongy; by which means, when eaten, it soaks up the fluid of the stomach and facilitates digestion.

In order to coagulate the flour, that is, make it into bread, and give it a whiteness, which is the nature of all coagulants to do, bakers sometimes mix it with a quantity of alum, which if not so great as to give the bread a taste, can do no harm to adults; but a small quantity will do much mischief to infants. Panada, therefore, for children, should by no means be made of bread in which any alum has been mixed. It is for this reason physicians prescribe biscuit-powder.

Sometimes bakers use whites of eggs, and sometimes spirits of wine, to coagulate the flour, as in French bread; the first is innocent, and the last evaporates during the baking; and can produce no ill effect. For if bread be not perfectly coagulated, and well baked, it will sometimes ferment a second time in the stomach, particularly if it continue long, as in weak stomachs, and turn sour: but baking it a second time will totally prevent this. Thus, rusks and toasted bread are often prescribed for disordered stomachs, as being least liable to do mischief; for the least extrication of air in weak stomachs is injurious.

But farinaceous seeds and roots are not sufficient to correct the putrescency of meat; we therefore make use of vegetables, that were not originally designed for food, namely, pot-herbs. Of these,

The one sort are cabbages, cauliflowers, brocoli, and all the varieties of this class of plants. They naturally contain a stimulating oil, and a bitter astringent juice, so as not to be fit for use; but we find this only in wild cabbages, &c. By cultivation, this oil and bitter juice are destroyed, and such as grow in our gardens consist of little more than mucilage and sugar; and, of course, are fit for food.

The method taken to destroy these noxious juices, is, to grow the plants in the dark, or, with as little air as possible; this is done by planting them in a rich soil, and thus making them so luxuriant, that the leaves shall embrace one another; by which means the body of the plant grows in the dark, and with little or no air. Hence the inner leaves becomes white, and are free from those hurtful juices. The outer leaves may be eaten, but the inner ones are most wholesome. So young plants are more wholesome than old ones, as whatever of these juices they contain, they are not near so rank.

Another kind of plants we use, is parsley, fennel, thyme, mint, sage, &c., and some others of the same kind. These contain a stimulating oil that would be injurious to the constitution, if eaten in any quantity; and, on that account, are only used as condiments with a seasoning to other foods. Celery is of the same kind; but, by earthing it up, and thus making it grow in the dark, and with little or no air, we destroy its noxious oil. Wild celery, if eaten, will blister the mouth.

The several species of onions, garlic, shalots, &c. are of another class; we cannot destroy the oil in these, but by boiling.

Lettuce, endive, dandelion, &c. contains much opium, and when wild are very bitter and dispose to sleep, consequently are unfit for food; but by cultivating them in rich soils, and covering them from light and air, by tying them up, we render them wholesome.

Spinage, beets and other plants of that kind when wild, contain also a bitter oil, so as not to be eatable; but, by cultivation in rich soils they lose this oil.

In the same manner asparagus contains oil so stimulating, that if eaten wild, it would blister the tongue; but, by cultivating it in rich ground, and making use only of the young shoots, we avoid this inconvenience.

None of these plants alone afford much nourishment; we use them to correct the putrescency of animal food, and particularly in the summer, as not stimulating.

They are apt to ferment, and turn sour in a weak stomach,

and in fermenting, will let loose the air contained in them, become flatulent and occasion wind: when persons find this, they should refrain from eating them, till the stomach grows stronger; for, by continuing to take down such things as disagree with them, they not only disorder themselves for the present, but will, in time, so injure their digestive organs, as to be hereafter attended with dreadful consequences.

Peas, beans, kidney-beans, &c. are more flatulent or windy still; especially, when eaten unripe, they are very windy: such persons therefore with whom they disagree, should by no means eat them.

With respect to esculent roots; these contain mucilage, sugar, and farinaceous matter, that is, flour. The last two afford much nourishment, but the mucilage does little else than forward fermentation. The more mucilaginous and watery these roots are, the more apt they are to ferment and correct the putrescency of animal food, and consequently the fitter to be eaten in warm weather. But the more sugar and flour they contain, the more they nourish.

Turnips, radishes, onions, &c. are equally as liable to ferment and correct putrescency, as the herbs springing from these roots; and as they contain a greater quantity of sugar than their respective herbs they are more nutritive.

Carrots, parsnips, artichokes, Jerusalem artichokes, beetroots, &c. contain much sugar and farinaceous matter, but very little mucilage. These are wholesome, nutritive, and easy of digestion.

The sugar adds much to the nutritive quality of the farinaceous matter in all these substances.

Potatoes, yams, earth-nuts, &c. contain flour almost alone, with very little sugar, but more water than we find in farinaceous seeds. However the farinaceous matter is the same in both, and is coagulable by heat. We boil them and roast them, to destroy their viscidity.

Potatoes are more easily digested than bread, and very rarely disagree with the most delicate stomach; but they afford less nourishment than either rice or bread; which proceeds chiefly from the large quantity of water contained in their substance;

yet many of the Irish, a strong, healthly people, live wholly on potatoes and milk.

Potatoes, artichokes, asparagus, often agree with weak stomachs, when cabbage, carrots, onions, &c. will not.

It is not yet determined whether mushrooms are animals or vegetables. They have all the properties of animal food, and must be considered as such.

FRUITS.

A proper use of fruits greatly contributes to the preservation of health. Ripe fruit extinguishes thirst, moderates heat, and opens the body.

Acids, particularly the native, vegetable ones, moderately used in diet, are grateful to the stomach, assist the appetite, promote digestion, cool the body and correct a tendency to putrefaction; but the too free use of them will disorder both the stomach and the bowels.

Fruits contain sugar, native vegetable acid, and mucilage; and their skins contain more or less an astringent juice; but so little of it, as not to render them unwholesome. Nay, it is rather of service, as it stimulates the stomach, causes it to contract strongly, and thus prevents the fruit becoming acid and flatulent. The sugar, acid and mucilage are capable of fermenting and being converted into blood. As sugar affords more nourishment than any other substance, such fruits as are sweetest are the most wholesome, viz. figs, grapes, &c.

Sugar is even more nutritive than flour, but it is seldom thoroughly digested; being so very soluble, it passes off from the stomach before any change can take place in it, but entangled in the cells of fruit, it is retained longer in the stomach, so as to yield some nourishment. So again, it is not apt to ferment in the stomach alone, but mixed with the mucilage of fruits, fermentation readily takes place. Besides, the acid of fruits helps to correct the putrescency of animal food.

The more diluted sugar is, the more apt it is to ferment. Hence, watery or mucilaginous fruits, with little sugar, as gooseberries, currants, cherries, &c., afford but little nourishment, but then they tend more to correct the putrescency.

Such as contain more sugar and less water and mucilage, are not so apt to ferment, consequently are not so proper to correct putrescency; but then they are more nutritive than such as contain more mucilage and water, and less sugar. They afford so much nourishment, that in many countries they are used as food: thus figs, dates, &c., in Portugal, are eaten as common food.

By evaporating the water from fruits, that is by drying them, we lessen their disposition to ferment, consequently, we make them less flatulent and more nutritive, if eaten moderately.

The fermentation of some fruits in the stomach, has, by letting loose the air, sometimes so distended it, as to prove fatal; but we may correct this by adding sugar to them, or spices. However, such as find they disagree with them, if they value their health, should refrain from eating them.

Fruits containing a great quantity of native vegetable acid, afford so little nourishment, (as lemons, oranges, &c.) that we seldom use them, but as a power acting on the stomach, to correct the bad properties of other food; as will be shown hereafter.

Sour fruits, eaten in autumn, have been accused of bringing on violent continued purgings, but without any reason. Indeed, some sour fruits will act as purgatives, and the purging shall continue; but this must be owing to the state of the body, predisposed to purge; for we find, that when fruit purges a body, not predisposed to purge, no purging continues when the fruit is evacuated. In hot summers, when there is great plenty of fruit, dysenteries or continued purgings are apt to be general; but this is owing to the heat of the weather; for persons will be afflicted with dysentery, who eat no fruit. In short, in such disorders they counteract; and those who eat no fruit, are more apt to purge, than such as do. Nay, if large quantities of fruit should purge, it will not prove dangerous; it will act no further than as a dose of physic.

Lord chancellor Bacon, one of the best writers on the preservation of health, condemns the use of cucumbers and melons.

He says they are cold and bad, and that a French physician, who had great practice from such persons as ate much of them, built a country-seat, and wrote over it in gold letters, in French, the English of which is, "Cold cucumbers built this hall, and crude-musk-melons furnished it."

ANIMAL FOOD.

Let us first consider the difference between animal and vegetable food. Now, as we said before, fermentation which takes place in food, within the stomach, is different from that which takes place out of it. If the stomach then be weak, so as not to bring on the fermentation which is natural to it, the fermentation that would take place out of the stomach, will take place in it, and bring on certain diseases. Thus the mischiefs of animal food putrefying, are greater and more dangerous than such as arise from undigested vegetable food; as this turns sour only.

Another difference is this. Vegetable food, during digestion, stimulates less. When the stomach is distended with food, the whole system, during digestion, is more or less stimulated; but more so with animal food than with vegetable. Now the more our system is stimulated, the quicker is the circulation, and the more feverish we become.

As animal food fills the vessels fuller, and with denser blood, than vegetable, it naturally increases our muscular strength: but then it loads the brain, (every part being fuller of blood in proportion) and occasions heaviness and stupor; whereas, vegetable food, from not loading the system with blood, rather diminishes muscular strength, but enables the mind to act with greater force. Vegetable food, therefore, is fitter to give clearness of ideas; and animal food is best adapted to labour. A physical demonstration might be given of this; but, to a general reader it would be idle. However, habit has a great effect in this case. Men, accustomed to labour, and to eat vegetable food, (as are the porters of Constantinople,) may be capable of great muscular exertion; but this does not prove the power of vegetable food over animal, So a horse fed on grass, and kept in exercise, will be better able to work, than one fed on hay and corn for twelve months together, without exercise: but neither is this any proof.

That food which contains the greatest proportion of liquid creates the greatest evacuation by stool; but it must be recollected at the same time, that though liquids have the above good quality, and promote secretion, yet, the sooner food is evacuated the less nutritive it becomes of course, those who use least drink are most nourished.

The more vegetable food a person eats, the less drink he requires; and that drink should be pure water; the substance with which water is impregnated is of little consequence: but those who eat much animal food may require fermented liquors; but it must be remembered, that, though fermented liquors contain an acid proper to correct putrescency, they also contain an alcohol, which, though it stimulates, is hurtful to the stomach.

The chief nourishment drawn from food, as I have observed, is the oil it contains; and there is more oil in animal food than in vegetable. A proof of this is evident, there being more corpulent persons in England, where animal food is eaten in larger quantites, than in any other nation of twice the population in the world.

In time of digestion, perspiration is stopped, and more so when we have eaten much vegetable food; but in general, vegetable food is more perspirable than animal. Nature, in the structure of the body, has designed man to live on both kinds of food, and reason should teach him which to choose and when.

Dr. Cullen has accurately considered this subject, and says, that the more a man labours with his body, the more animal food he should eat, and the more he labours with his mind, the more vegetable. Too much animal food eaten produces dulness, laziness, and yawning.

Dr. Cullen's doctrine on animal food is as follows:—Though it gives strength, it is hazardous to the system, as it produces plethora and all its consequences; and by its stimulating powers, sooner wears out the system; and if we take exercise sufficient to render this diet salutary, such an accumulation is made of putrescent fluids, as in after life to lay a foundation of the most inveterate chronic distempers. It is therefore a question whether we should desire this high degree of bodily strength, with all its inconveniences and dangers. Certainly, those who lead a sedentary life, should avoid an excess of animal food. In hysteric and hypochondriac constitutions animal food is absolutely necessary; but it should be used with as much vegetable food as is found requisite: and when a cure is performed, this diet may be changed. If this luxurious age could be persuaded, continues the Doctor, this disease might be removed, with much less danger, by exercise, fresh air, and avoiding warm chambers, venery, and late hours.

Such persons should eat a great deal of bread, the safest of all vegetable food. Vegetable food is not only necessary to secure health, but long life. In infancy and in youth we should be confined to it mostly, in manhood and decay of life, use animal food, and near the end vegetable again.

Variety of food, adds Dr. Cullen, seems to me necessary, and liquid and solid food should temper each other; the only danger of variety is eating too much.

Animal food, though seemingly of greater cohesion, is readier dissolved in the stomach than vegetables; not quicker, but more effectually or entirely: but though some vegetables never dissolve, yet their juices are more quickly extracted than those of animal food, and pass sooner off; for solubility does not depend so much on firmness of texture as on viscidity of the juices. Thus the younger the animal, the less soluble it is; veal than beef; lamb than mutton, &c. Young food being more viscid than old.

Heaviness, as it is called, in the stomach, is seldom felt from vegetables, except eaten with tough pastry, or the more viscid substances.

Vegetable food continues longer in the stomach than animal, and gives little stimulus; and the system is affected in proportion to the extent of this stimulus, which is incomparably greater from the animal viscid, oily food, than from the vegetable, firmer, and more aqueous.

Dr. Cullen says, where neither putrefaction nor acidity has gone a great length in the stomach, animal food keeps the body more regular and less costive than vegetable food; and thus, those who are costive from vegetable food, having recourse to animal, are, in this respect better.

The Hindoos, we are told, who live wholly on vegetable food, cannot work so long as Europeans; they may, as the porters of Constantinople, have muscular strength, but they soon tire.

The chief of the fluids in the body is oil. Now, as animal food is easier converted and longer retained in the system, and as it contains a greater proportion of oil, it will afford more nourishment than vegetable, and repair best the waste of the solid fibres.

Next, as to perceptibility, of which I shall give some explanation hereafter, Sanctorious, to whom we are indebted for this knowledge, says, mutton is the most perspirable of all foods, and that vegetables rather check perspiration.—This is owing to less stimulus in vegetables, so that persons who live on vegetables have not their perspiration so suddenly excited. In time of digestion, as before observed, perspiration is stopped from whatever food we eat—much more from cooling vegetables.

Next, as to the quantity of these mixed foods, animal and vegetable, of which most is best to be eaten. It is an aphorism of Sanctorius, that weight gives strength. Men, in some measure, are able to work in proportion to their food. The English labour more than the Dutch, and wherever men are exposed to hard labour, their food should be animal: but animal food, though it gives strength, loads; hence it is only proper for bodily labour, and entirely improper for mental exercise; for whoever would keep his mind acute and penetrating, should eat rather more vegetable food than animal. The body is even oppressed by animal food; a full meal always produces heaviness, dulness, and inactivity.

Animal food, though it gives strength, tends to produce plethora and all its consequences; it urges the circulation, stimulates the whole system, and excites fever; but promotes perspiration. By the repetition of these stimuli the machine is sooner worn out and life shortened.

Vegetable diet has this advantage over animal, that it whets the appetite, and we can hardly suffer from a full meal of it. Upon the whole, it must be concluded, that a larger proportion of vegetable food is useful and more wholesome to the generality of mankind.

There is no error in this country more dangerous or more common, says Dr. Cullen, than the neglect of bread; it may well be called, "the staff of life." It is the safest vegetable and the best corrector of animal food; and in a hypochondriac state, a large proportion of it will obviate its bad consequences. The French, by their great use of bread, avoid this state, and therefore it should be particularly eaten by the English, who are so voracious of animal food.

Buchan advises families, where they have convenience, to make their own bread, and mix it with a little rye, for baker's bread is often found unwholesome.

Spices, as cinnamon, cloves, nutmegs, mace, pimento, &c., which are the produce of warmer climates, and mustard, anise, caraway, coriander, and the sweet herbs of our own country, stimulate the stomach, promote its digestive powers, remove spasms arising from flatulency of food, and are antiseptic, moderating the putrid tendency of our food in the intestines. They ought only, says Cullen, to be used in the countries where they grow; they are introduced *here* unfitly, as any antiseptic virtue they have, would be overcome by their stimulant properties.

There are certain acrid or hot plants, as cresses, horseradish, mustard, &c., which have stimulant and other good properties. Garlic, shalots, &c., are of the same kind. They are diuretic and diaphoretic, that is, they promote urine and sweat.

The next thing to be considered, is, a maxim generally laid down by all authors on this subject; namely, that simplicity of food is more conducive to health than a variety; but experience teaches us the contrary. Milk, as we before observed, which affords great nourishment, is a mixture of three nutritive substances; and we may venture to affirm, that if an alderman was to eat as much of beef-steaks, as he does of other things, at a city feast, he would bring on sickness and vomiting. Put variety of grain before a hen, she will eat of what she likes best but, before the day is out, she will eat of the other. Instinct leads her to this, as most conducive to her health. The only danger in variety is eating too much ; if we can resolve against this, variety will not do harm, if of easy digestion.

Almost all food contains oil, and the stomach can better bear a variety of this oil, than a quantity of one particular sort. Besides, animal and vegetable food correct the ill qualities of one another. Animal food corrects the flatulency of vegetable ; and vegetable food, the putrescency of animal. But, a mixture of such foods as will disagree, viz. acids with milk, fish and milk is improper ; acids or fish coagulating milk too firmly for easy digestion ; but there is no rule without an exception.

Food may be very wholesome and nutritive in itself, yet when combined with other nutritive food, may be very injurious. Certain drinks may occasion what we have eaten to do harm. They may occasion fermentation in the stomach, or harden what we have eaten, and render it indigestible.

We shall now proceed to the properties of the different kinds of animal food. There are two substances in meat capable of nourishing ; mucilage and expressed oil.

Animal mucilages differ much from one another ; but considered as food, they do not. The only difference of consesequence is, as far as depends upon their texture. When the fibres of an animal are large, they are not easily dissolved ; of course, they are difficult of digestion. Beef is, on this account, more difficult of digestion than mutton ; the fibres of the one being larger than those of the other. On the same principle, when food is coagulated firmly, it is also difficult of digestion. The firmer the coagulum, that is, the less fluid it contains, the more difficult it will be of digestion. Animal food, whose fibres have but little fluid between them, that is, dry meat, is more indigestible than moist. Thus, lean animals are harder of digestion than fat ones ; and the lean part of fat meat is easier of digestion than the lean part of lean meat. By the same way of reasoning, meat roasted or boiled a great deal is not so digestible as when roasted or boiled but little ; for when the fluids are expelled by heat, the fibres approach closer to each other, and, when in the stomach, will not admit the juice of the stomach so readily to penetrate it; consequently, fermentation will not take place so soon. This also is the opinion of Dr. Cadogan, who recommends most persons, particularly weak persons, to eat their meat very little done.

The readier animal food dissolves in water, the more digestible it is. A flounder boiled in an equal quantity of water, is sooner dissolved than mutton; therefore, flounders are easier of digestion than mutton; the juice of the stomach being little else than warm water, helped by fermentation. But fish, though readily soluble in water, has a property in it that renders it indigestible, which is a certain glariness or viscidity; but, when the stomach is strong enough to digest it, it is easier of digestion than either flesh or fowl.

Meat apt in its nature to putrefy is sooner digested than such as is not. Pigeon will putrefy sooner than duck: of course, pigeon is easier of digestion than duck. Now, as the fluids in animal food tend to hasten putrefaction, by depriving it of those fluids, by long boiling or roasting, we render it harder of digestion. By boiling meat till it be free from gravy, we can keep it from corrupting for six months. A further proof that meat much dressed is less wholesome than such as is little dressed. Such meats, however, as putrefy the soonest, are injurious to weak stomachs, as this putrescency stimulates during the time of digestion.

It is with a view of rendering meat easier of digestion, that we keep it some time after it is killed, before we eat it, but the longer we keep it the less nutritive it is, losing its juices by drying. As soon as meat is killed, it begins to putrefy; and putrefaction is the most effectual breaker-down of animal substance, and a great assistant to solution, which is the immediate forerunner of digestion. But the length of time meat ought to be kept, should be proportioned to its tendency to putrefy, and the heat of the weather. It is eaten, for example, much sooner in summer than in winter. Let it be observed, at the same time, that though rendered easier of digestion, it is not so nourishing, as it loses some of its juices; and if any way tainted, it is still the worse.

But the property in which meats differ most is their viscidity or glariness. Such as are viscid, adhere to the sides of the stomach, and stimulate much. In quadrupeds, young animals have this property, such as veal, pig, fawn, and lamb; but in a smaller degree. Young birds have the same bad property, and all fish in a great degree; particularly shell-fish, which, on this account, has often proved poisonous and fatal to many. When these have proved fatal, it has been ascribed to the copper vessel in which they were dressed; but a little observation would show the contrary. When persons lose their lives by the ill effects of copper, sickness, vomiting, and purging, take place: but when poisoned by shell-fish, the head swells, the breast is oppressed, and stupor is the consequence.

Animal food dissolved in water, forms a gelatinous solution or jelly, which is of a viscid nature, and, in some degree, produces the same effect as viscid foods. It stimulates, but does not yield much nourishment. At the same time, it is difficult of digestion, and of course improper to be taken by diseased or weak stomachs. Jellies, though long prescribed to strengthen the system after a fever, have lately been found prejudicial, and the use of them is therefore exploded.

Essential oils, inherent in some animal food, render it difficult of digestion. The essential oils of vegetables are often agreeable to the stomach, and stimulate it so as to forward digestion; but those of animal food, though agreeable to the taste, are injurious. Pork, geese, ducks, salmon, &c., contain much of this oil, and are of course high-flavoured. They may be agreeable to the taste of those who have strong stomachs, but, if eaten in too great quantities, or if the stomach be too weak, they will disagree with it, and have the same effect with viscidity; that is, they will stimulate the system, and sometimes bring on a fever. Animal food, then, that is viscid, which contains much essential oil, or will not readily dissolve, is apt to remain too long in the stomach, and do harm. But that which will readily putrefy and dissolve, is retained but a short time in the stomach; and is of course easily digested: for digestion depending on the contraction of the stomach, if the stomach be so disordered as to lose any of its contractile powers, either by the oil or viscidity of the food, the food will be retained too long in it.

We seldom use animal food without some preparation.

These preparations are either exposing it to such heat as will coagulate the solids and fluids, or, after such coagulation, dissolving it in water. By coagulating any animal solid, we take off that viscidity which almost all have when raw, and the stomach consequently bears it much better. Thus we can digest twice the quantity of oysters roasted, that we can raw.

In coagulating animal substances by heat, we often expose them to a great fire, as in roasting; which coagulates the outer parts, forming a crust, as it were, round the inward fluids, and retaining them. This gives them an empyreumatic oil, offensive to the smell. In boiling, we avoid this empyreumatic oil, but then we take out the essential oil. In frying, we retain both oils, so that fried meat is more difficult of digestion than either roasted or boiled.

In baking, (particularly in baker's ovens, which contain variety of things,) whatever is evaporated from meats, &c. baked, is thrown down on them again by reverberation from the top of the oven, and gives them a very peculiar and unpleasant taste.

Dr. Cullen makes some judicious observations on our modes of cookery. The design of dressing meat, he says, is to render it soluble in the stomach for the purposes of digestion. Young animals are more soluble than old, but they are more viscid, and apt to cling to the coats of the stomach and do injury, unless eaten with sour sauces. It is for this reason lemon-juice is eaten with veal, mint-sauce with lamb, vinegar with lobster, &c. Viscid food is not so readily passed from the stomach. Persons are often more oppressed with a full meal of veal than of beef.

By boiling of meat we extract the juices from between the fibres, make the texture of that meat firmer and less soluble in the stomach and much more ready to putrefy. Those who throw away the broth of boiled meat, act very improperly. It is a fluid, not unpleasant to drink, and when drunk with our food, increases its solubility.

Roasting of meat retains those juices which boiling extracts, but the less meat is roasted the more soluble it is; raw meats are still more soluble: it is on this principle that Dr. Cadogan so warmly recommended meats very little roasted or boiled; but, at the same time, the less dressed they are, the more they are apt to putrefy in the intestines, an evil the other way.

Chicken, partridges, veal, &c., are more wholesome when roasted, than boiled. Mutton, beef, pork, &c., are easier digested when boiled.

All quadrupeds that feed on vegetables are used, somewhere or other, for food; such as the ox, the sheep, the deer, the goat, the hog, the hare, &c.

Birds also are made use of for food, except birds of prey, and all fish also have been eaten, and all shell-fish which have sufficient muscular flesh to render them worth eating.

Those birds that are not very putrescent in their nature, and are most free from essential oil, are the easiest of digestion. As for example, moor-game, poultry, partridges, pheasants, &c., and of quadrupeds, the deer, the sheep, the ox, &c. The older animals of this class are easier of digestion than the younger ones. Mutton, for instance, is easier of digestion than lamb; beef than veal; venison than fawn; and that on account of the viscidity of the flesh of young animals. Fish is more difficult of digestion than flesh, especially in weak stomachs. And of fish, those that have least flavour, that is, such as have least essential oil in them, are white, and have some degree of firmness, will digest much sooner than such as are of stronger flavour. Flounders, whitings, &c., are easier of digestion than salmon, soles, &c.

But still, quadrupeds afford more nourishment than either birds or fish; and those animals of stronger flavour, viz., pork, geese, duck, salmon, &c., afford more nourishment, and are fitter for such as labour or take a great deal of exercise, than animals of the same class, that are easier of digestion.

An equal quantity of liquid food is found to be more heavy than the same quantity of solid food; bread and flesh are light, wine and broths more heavy: a cup of wine is of greater weight than a piece of bread of thrice the bulk of the wine.

If a man feel himself lighter than in fact he is, it is an argument of a most healthful constitution.

NUTRITION IN GRAIN AND FLESH.

Vegetables contain a large portion of starch or sugar, which substances do not add to the nourishment of the body, but are embraced in the purposes of respiration, and maintain the animal heat. They are very necessary to the body.

Chemists agree that the substances of vegetables add to the organism, and are converted into the tissues of the body; are possessed of azotised, nitrogenised or nutritious principles; these are fibrin, albumen, and casein, and are denominated protein compounds. If we take wheat flour and knead it under water, the starch separates from it, and the *gluten* remains in the hand, which is insoluble in water. *Albumen* is coagulable by heat, and is, by this means, readily separated from the juices of many vegetables; as cauliflower, asparagus, or turnips, and is likewise abundant in certain seeds, as nuts or almonds. *Casein* is soluble in water; it does not coagulate with heat, but curds with acids; it abounds in peas and beans. Vegetable albumen and fibrin in the animal are found to be the same, and although grain contains much starch, yet the large quantity of albuminous matter is what renders it nutritious. The following table is given by Dr. R. D. Thomson, in his "Experimental Researches on the Food of Animals," &c.

	Albuminous, or Nutritive Matter, per Cent.		Albuminous, or Nutritive Matter, per Cent.
Bean meal	25·36	Hay	9·71
Linseed meal	23·66	Malt	8·71
Scotch oatmeal	15·62	Rice (East India)	8·37
Semolina	12·81	Sago	3·33
Canadian flour	11·62	South Sea Arrow-root	3·21
Barley	11·31	Tapioca	3·13
Maize	10·93	Potatoes	2·23
Essex flour	10·55 to 11·80	Swedish Turnips	1·32
E. Lothian flour	9·74 to 11·55		

Wheat.—The flour of wheat grown in the south of Britain contains more albumen than that of the north. That from warm climates possesses a greater portion of gluten. It is found in the flour of different grain that where one principle of nutrition is wanting others are increased or substituted.

Now, although the table already given may be strictly

correct in a chemical point of view, there are other considerations that mankind must take into account, in respect to themselves, before being satisfied with the apparent result; and that is, as to the digestibility of the articles, and their assimilation and conversion into animal organism.

On the nutritive properties of animal food Professor Brande writes:—"When the muscular parts of animals are washed repeatedly in cold water, the fibrinous matter which remains consists chiefly of albumen; and is in its chemical properties, analogous to the clot of blood. Muscle also yields a portion of gelatine; and the flesh of beef aud some other animals affords a peculiar substance, of an aromatic flavour, called by Thenard *osmazone*. Albumen and gelatine constitute the leading nutritive ingredients in the different kinds of flesh used as food, and it is curious that their relative proportions are not very dissimilar in quadrupeds, birds, and fishes, as shown in the following table. The water was determined by evaporation in a close-covered vessel, or at a temperature below 212.

100 Parts of Muscle of	Water.	Albumen or Fibrin.	Gelatine.	Total of Nutritive Matter.
Mutton	71	22	7	29
Chicken	73	20	7	27
Beef	74	20	6	26
Veal	75	19	6	25
Pork	76	19	5	24
Cod	79	14	7	21
Sole	79	15	6	21
Haddock	82	13	5	18

On looking at this table, we see it stated that chicken contains more nutritive matter than beef, and veal more than pork; yet we know from experience such a result does not take place in our own persons. And, again, on comparing the former with the latter table, we are aware that we should derive more nourishment from veal or pork than linseed-meal; hence, as we before observed, much depends on the suitability to the digestive organs, and the facility with which it combines with the animal organisation.

Professor Johnston has proved that bread perfectly white is not so nutritious as when mixed with the pollard or inner bran;

that this bran is richer in fatty matter, and nitrogenised principles than the grain itself. It contains more phosphate of lime, and is therefore more efficient in supplying the materials for building up the solid portions of the body. Brown bread should therefore be adopted, not merely on a principle of economy, but also as providing more of these ingredients, which are deficient in the better kind of flour.

It has been correctly ascertained that

112 lbs. of	Wheat flour	yield	154 lbs.	of bread.
Do.	Oatmeal	„	336	do.
Do.	Rice	„	450	do.
Do.	Maize	„	560	do.
Do.	Indian Meal	„	450	do.

But it is not to be supposed for one moment, that because Indian meal, by absorbing more water than wheat flour does, which merely causes it to swell into a greater bulk, that it contains more nutrition. Yet this property may serve as a recommendation to its use, by enabling us to obtain an equal weight of bread with a less consumption of flour, making up the deficiency by eating more of other and cheaper kind of vegetables.

HINTS IN EMERGENCIES.

Recovery of Persons apparently Drowned or Dead.

Recommended by the Royal Humane Society.

CAUTIONS.—1. Lose no time. 2. Avoid all rough usage. 3. Never hold the body up by the feet. 4. Nor roll the body on casks. 5. Nor rub the body with salt and spirits. 6. Nor inject tobacco smoke, or infusion of tobacco.

Restorative means, if apparently Drowned.

Send quickly for medical assistance ; but do not delay the following means :—

I. Convey the body CAREFULLY, with the head and shoulders supported in a raised condition, to the nearest house.

II. Strip the body, and rub it dry ; then wrap it in hot blankets, and place it in a warm bed in a warm chamber.

III. Wipe and cleanse the mouth and nostrils.

IV. In order to restore the natural warmth of the body:

1. Move a heated covered warming pan over the back and spine.
2. Put bladders, or bottles of hot water, or heated bricks, to the pit of the stomach, the armpits, between the thighs, and to the soles of the feet.
3. Foment the body with hot flannels; but, if possible,
4. Immerse the body in a warm bath as hot as the hand can bear without pain; as this is preferable to the other means for restoring warmth.
5. Rub the body briskly with the hand; do not, however, suspend the use of the other means at the same time.

V. In order to restore breathing, introduce the pipe of a common bellows, (where the apparatus of the Society is not at hand) into one nostril, carefully closing the other and the mouth; at the same time drawing downwards, and pushing gently backwards, the upper part of the wind pipe, to allow a free admission of air; blow the bellows gently, in order to inflate the lungs, till the breast be a little raised: the mouth and nostrils should then be set free, and a moderate pressure made with the hand upon the chest. Repeat this process till life appears.

VI. Electricity to be employed early by a medical assistant.

VII. Inject into the stomach, by means of an elastic tube and syringe, half a pint of warm brandy, or wine and water.

VIII. Apply sal-volatile or hartshorn to the nostrils.

If apparently dead from Apoplexy.

The patient should be placed in a cool air, and the clothes loosened, particularly about the neck and breast. Bleeding must be early employed by a medical assistant: the quantity regulated by the state of the pulse. Cloths soaked in cold water, spirits, or vinegar and water, should be kept applied to the head, which should be instantly shaved. All stimulants should be avoided. In cases of coup-de-soliel, or strokes of the sun, the same means to be used as in apoplexy.

If apparently dead from intense cold.

Rub the body with ice, snow, or cold water.—Restore warmth by slow degrees; and, after some time, if necessary, employ the means recommended for the apparently drowned. In these accidents, it is HIGHLY DANGEROUS to apply heat too early.

IF APPARENTLY DEAD FROM HANGING.

In addition to the means recommended for the apparently drowned, BLEEDING should early be employed by a Medical Assistant.

IF APPARENTLY DEAD FROM NOXIOUS VAPOURS, LIGHTNING, &C.

1. Remove the body into a cool fresh air.
2. Dash cold water on the neck, face, and breast frequently.
3. If the body be cold, apply warmth, as recommended for the apparently drowned.
4. Use the means recommended for inflating the lungs in Direction V.
5. Let Electricity (particularly in accidents from lightning) be early employed by a Medical Assistant.

TO PURIFY THE AIR.—Powdered nitre and oil of vitriol, six drachms each. Mix, by adding one drachm of vitriol at a time. The vessel must be placed on some hot substance, and the mixture stirred with a glass rod. Place in different parts of the room.

TO PREVENT INFECTION FROM TYPHUS FEVER.—Powdered nitre six drachms, sulphuric acid six drachms. Add one drachm of the acid at a time. Place the vessel on some hot substance, and stir with a glass rod or tobacco pipe; this to be placed in the sick room.

ANTIDOTES TO POISON.

The treatment of cases of poisoning must, of course, vary with the nature of the poison, the quantity taken, and the peculiarities of the individual. In almost all cases, copious vomiting should be excited as soon as possible by tickling the throat, and by emetics, such especially as sulphate of zinc, or ipecacuanha with emetic tartar; the former, however in ten-grain doses dissolved in a little warm water, and repeated every ten or fifteen minutes till it freely operates, is generally most effectual. The use of the stomach-pump should also be resorted to. The vomiting should be kept up, and the stomach washed out with bland albuminous or mucilaginous fluids, such as milk, barley-water, flour and water, or thin paste, etc.; sometimes sugar and water.

The following is a short summary of the antidotes which may be resorted to, in reference to particular poisons. They should, of course, be administered as speedily as possible.

EMETIC IN CASES OF POISON.—Two table-spoonfuls of made mustard in a pint of warm water; if taken immediately, this is a certain remedy, instantly producing violent vomiting. Administer large draughts of warm milk or water, mixed with oil, melted butter, or lard.

1. *Arsenic.*—Lime water, chalk and water, and the hydrated sesqui-oxide of iron, have each been strongly recommended; the last is decidedly the best.

2. For *Mineral Acids*, or *Acetic and Oxalic Acid.*—For this form of poison, give quickly large draughts of chalk, whiting, magnesia, soap and water, about as thick as cream; followed by albuminous diluents, such as milk, and white of egg mixed with water. Or, if these cannot be procured at once, warm water; and promote vomiting by tickling the throat.

3. *Alkalies, Soda, Potash, Ammonia*, etc.—Vinegar, or any mild acid and water, or even very dilute mineral acids, such as water acidulated by them; olive oil, almond oil.

4. *Corrosive sublimate.*—White of egg and water; milk and cream; decoction of cinchona; infusion of galls.

5. *Sulphate of Copper, and other poisons.*—Sugar and water; white of egg and water.

6. *Antimonial poisons.*—Warm milk, gruel, or barley-water: infusion of galls; decoction of cinchona.

7. *Nitrate of Silver.*—Copious draughts of warm salt and water.

8. *Sulphate of Zinc.*—Solution of carbonate of soda in water, with milk, and mucilaginous or farinaceous liquids.

9. *Acetate of Lead.*—Emetics, solution of sulphate of soda in water; milk, white of egg and water.

10. *Opium and its preparations.*—Emetics, strong coffee: dashing cold water upon the face and breast; preventing torpor by forced exercise.

11. *Prussic Acid.*—Ammoniacal stimulants cautiously applied to the nose; ammonia, or sal-volatile in repeated small doses of solution of chlorine in water; small doses of chloride of lime in water.

12. *Strychnia and vegetable alkaloids.*—Infusion of gall nuts; decoction of cinchona; emetics.

If apparently dead from Intoxication.

Lay the body on a bed, with the head raised: remove the neckcloth, and loosen the clothes. Obtain instantly medical assistance, as the treatment must be regulated by the state of the patient; but in the mean time apply cloths soaked in cold water to the head, and bottles of hot water, or hot bricks, to the calves of the legs and to the feet.

General Observations.

On restoration to life, a teaspoonful of warm water, should be given; and then, if the power of swallowing be returned, small quantities of warm wine, or weak brandy and water, warm; the patient should be kept in bed, and a disposition to sleep encouraged, except in cases of apoplexy, intoxication, and coup-de-soliel. Great care is requisite to mantain the restored vital actions, and at the same time to prevent undue excitement. The treatment recommended by the Society, is to be persevered in for *three or four hours.* It is an erroneous opinion that persons are irrecoverable because life does not soon make its appearance; and it is absurd to suppose that a body must not be meddled with or removed without the permission of a Coroner.

Remarkable instances of suspended Animation.

At the annual Meeting of the Bristol Humane Society, the Society's silver medal was presented to Dr. Fairbrother, of Clifton, for his exertions in recovering a boy who had been under the water in the floating harbour a quarter of an hour;

and another quarter of an hour had elapsed before the Doctor could operate upon the body. The most remarkable feature in this case is the new mode by which Dr. Fairbrother succeeded in his laudable object; namely, by closing the mouth with his finger, sucking off the foul air from the lungs through the nostrils, and promoting respiration by pressing on the abdominal muscles on the sides. The usual method is to inflate the lungs, but it is very seldom that persons are recovered by this method if they have been under water more than a few minutes.

J. W., a seaman belonging to a packet-ship from New York to Havre, fell over the side into the dock, where the water was from 12 to 16 feet deep. Some stragglers saw the accident, and gave the alarm. Two men, who had not perceived it, jumped in at hazard, but were unsuccessful in finding him, owing to his having sunk in the mud. A grappling iron was obtained, and the man hauled up. He was carried to the guard-house, nearly fronting the vessel, and from thence he was conveyed to the Stranger's Hospital, a distance of half a mile. On his been brought in, fourteen minutes after the submersion occurred, as stated by Dr. Douglass, Physician to the Hospital, he was immediately stripped and laid on a bed. It was then ten minutes past three P. M. There was not the slightest appearance of animation. Whilst water was being heated, and bags of hot salt got ready, Dr. Douglass says, "I desired 4 of the men to commence rubbing the body with dry flannel cloths. These men were relieved every half-hour by 4 of their ship mates, and constant friction was thus kept up. Bags of hot sand, placed round the body, and lavements of hot water, to which were added spirits of turpentine and tincture of assafœtida, formed the whole treatment. I was frequently on the point of abandoning all hope; but I saw, or thought I saw, slight convulsive twitchings in the right interior eyelid and around the mouth. This animated me. The relays worked on well; and at a quarter after eleven at night we perceived respiration, *eight hours and a half from the time of immersion.* Before twelve o'clock he swallowed a tea-spoonful of warm brandy and water. It required for some time great care to keep up the feeble spark that animated the frame; but it was two days before intelligence was restored. Within twenty-four hours, re-action set in so violently, I was obliged to order four leeches for each temple, and to take six ounces of blood from the arm. It was well blood was abstracted so cautiously, for the pulse suddenly fell, and became almost imperceptible, the respiration becoming greatly hurried; stimulants were instantly had rescourse to. Typhoid symptoms supervened, which we had to combat for six weeks; however, he was discharged cured from the hospital."

NOTES ON NURSING THE SICK.

No one has done more to elevate nursing to what it really should be—a social science than Miss Nightingale, whose efforts are gradually bearing fruit in hospitals and infirmaries all over the kingdom. Her experience has been embodied in an earnest and interesting pamphlet, entitled "Notes on Nursing," a real and practical hand-book for the household, from which we extract the following useful hints:—

There are not a few popular opinions, in regard to which it is useful at times to ask a question or two. For example, it is commonly thought that children must have what are commonly called "children's epidemics," "current contagions," &c.; in other words, that they are born to have measles, hooping-cough, perhaps even scarlet fever, just as they are born to cut their teeth, if they live. Now, do tell us why a child must have measles—and it must take them—and it is safer that it should. But why must other children have measles? And if they have, why must yours have them too? If you believed in and observed the laws for preserving the health of houses which inculcate cleanliness, ventilation, white-washing, and other means, and which, by the way, *are laws*, as implicitly as you believe in the popular opinion, for it is nothing more than an opinion, that your children must have children's epidemics, don't you think that upon the whole your child would be more likely to escape altogether?

Is it not living in a continual mistake to look upon diseases, as we now do, as separate entities, which must exist, like cats and dogs, instead of looking upon them as conditions, like a dirty and a clean condition, and just as much under our own control; or rather as the reactions of kindly nature against the conditions in which we have placed ourselves? I was brought up both by scientific men and ignorant women, distinctly to believe that small-pox, for instance, was a thing of which there was once a first specimen in the world, which went on propagating itself, in a perpetual chain of descent. Since then I have seen with my eyes and smelt with my nose small-pox growing up in first specimens, either in close rooms or in overcrowded wards where it could not by any possibility have been "caught," but must have begun. Nay, more, I have seen diseases begin, grow up, and pass into one another. I have seen, for instance, with a little overcrowding, continued fever grow up; and with a little more, typhoid fever, and with a little more, typhus, and all in the same ward or hut. Would it not be far better, truer, and more practical, if we looked upon disease in this light? For diseases, as all experience shows, are adjectives, not noun substantives.

A few words upon bedsteads and bedding; and principally as regards patients who are entirely, or almost entirely, confined to bed. Feverishness is generally supposed to be a symptom of fever—in nine cases out of ten it is a symptom of bedding. How can it be otherwise? Look at the ordinary bed in which a patient lies. If I were looking out for an example in order to show what *not* to do, I should take the specimen of an ordinary bed in a private house; a wooden bedstead, two or even three mattrasses piled up to above the height of a table; a valance attached to the frame—nothing but a miracle could ever thoroughly dry or air such a bed and bedding. The patient must inevitably alternate between cold and damp *after* his bed is made, and warm damp *before*, both saturated with organic matter, and this from the time the mattrasses are put under him till the time they are picked to pieces, if this is ever done. A nurse will be careful even to fidgetiness about airing the clean sheets from the damp. Airing the dirty sheets from noxious damp will never occur to her. Besides this the most dangerous effluvia we know of are from the excreta of the sick —these are placed, at least temporarily, where they must throw their effluvia into the underside of the bed, and the space under the bed is never aired, it cannot be with our arrangements. My heart always sinks within me when I hear the good housewife, of every class, say, "I assure you the bed has been well slept in," and I can only hope it is not true. What! is the bed already saturated with somebody else's damp? Has it not had a single chance to be aired? No, not one. "It has been slept in every night."

When I see a patient in a room nine or ten feet high, with his head, when he is sitting up in bed, actually within two or three feet of the ceiling, I ask myself, is this expressly planned to produce that peculiarly distressing feeling common to the sick—namely, as if the walls and ceiling were closing in upon them, and they becoming sandwiches between floor and ceiling, which imagination is not, indeed, here so far from the truth. If, over and above this, the window stops short of the ceiling, then the patient's head may literally be raised above the stratum of fresh air, even when the window is open. Can human perversity any farther go in unmaking the process of restoration which God has made? I need scarcely say the old four-post bed with curtains is utterly inadmissible, whether for sick or well.

Never use anything but light Witney blankets as bed covering for the sick. The heavy cotton impervious counterpane is bad, for the very reason that it keeps in the emanations from the sick person, while the blanket allows them to pass through. Weak patients are invariably distressed by a great weight of bed-clothes, which often prevents them getting any sound sleep whatever. Every weak patient, be his illness whatever it may, suffers more or less from difficulty in breathing. To take the weight of the body off the chest, which is hardly up to its work as it is, ought therefore, to be the object of the nurse in arranging his pillows.

Another extraordinary fallacy is the dread of night air. What air can we breathe at night but night air? The choice is between pure night air from without and foul night air from within. Fully one half of all the disease we suffer from is occasioned by people sleeping with their windows shut. An open window most nights in the year can hurt no one. I could better understand in towns shutting the windows during the day than during the night, for the sake of the sick. The absence of smoke, the quiet, all tend to making night the best time for airing the patient. Often the night air is the best and purest in the twenty-four hours. Always air your room, then, from the outside air if possible.

SARRACENIA PURPUREA.

A NEW REMEDY FOR THE SMALL POX.—The *Sarracenia Purpurea*, or Indian cup, a native plant of Nova Scotia, the specific used by the Indians against the small pox, bids fair to realise the expectations entertained by medical men of its efficacy. In a letter addressed to the *American Medical Times*, Dr. Frederic W. Morris, president physician of the Halifax Visiting Dispensary, states that this *Sarracenia*, a papaveraceous plant, will cure small pox in all its forms within twelve hours after the patient has taken the decoction. "However alarming and numerous the eruptions," he says, "or confluent and frightful they may be, the peculiar action of the medicine is such that very seldom is a scar left to tell the story of the disease. If either vaccine or variolous matter is washed with the infusion of the *Sarracenia*, they are deprived of their contagious properties. So mild is the medicine to the taste that it may be mixed with tea and coffee, and given to connoisseurs in these beverages to drink without being aware of the admixture. The medicine has been successfully tried in the hospitals of Nova Scotia, and its use will be continued."—*Galignani.*

"We are now favoured with the following particulars respecting this valuable plant. The *Sarracenia Purpurea*, or *Indian cup*, a native plant of Nova Scotia, found in swamps and moss bogs, has the wonderful reputation among the Mic-Mac Indians of curing Small Pox; and of being as great a specific in this disease as quinine for ague. It is supposed to act by neutralizing the virus in the blood, rendering it inert and harmless; and that this is its action may be gathered from the fact that if either vaccine or variolous matter be washed with the Infusion of the Sarracenia, it is deprived of its contagious property. Moreover the eruption, even if confluent, on its disappearance, leaves no trace behind. The root of the plant is the part employed. The dose, when reduced to powder, is about a dessert-spoonful, simmered in a pint of water down to half a pint; this is usually divided into two doses, to be taken during the day. Sugar should not be used with it."

MEDICAL RECEIPTS

BOTANICAL, ALLOPATHIC, & HOMŒOPATHIC.

ACETOUS CATAPLASM, OR POULTICE.—This is made with vinegar and bran only, or with the addition of oatmeal, or bread crumbs. It is a simple poultice, but very useful for sprains and bruises. As it becomes dry, it should be moistened with vinegar.

AIR:—COUNTRY SUPERIOR TO TOWN AIR.—"If you examine," says M. Pouchet, "the bodies of animals, who live in our towns, and in our houses, you will be astonished at the enormous quantity of starch contained in their respiratory organs. In birds you will find it even in the middle of their bones. Particles of soot, filaments of the different kinds of textures of which our clothes are made, are also found there in great abundance. But the further the animal lives from a town, the more scarce become these bodies. In animals and birds living in the midst of forests, you will scarcely find any at all of them; in their case the respiratory apparatus is, on the contrary, filled with a large quantity of vegetable *debris*, *chlorophyllæ*, &c. I have found in the lungs of man the same atmospheric corpuscles as in animals. I found two persons who died in one of our Hospitals—a man and a woman—and whose lungs I inspected, a notable quantity of fecula, normal, or after panification, particles of silica, and fragments of glass; fragments of painted wood of a beautiful red colour; *debris* of clothes, and a larvæ of a microscopic *arachnis* still alive."

APERIENT, INFANTS'.—Take of rhubarb, five grains; magnesia, three grains; white sugar, a scruple; manna, five grains; mix. Dose, varying from a piece half the size of a sweet-pea to a piece the size of an ordinary pea. Magnesia is a useful remedy in *acidity* of the *stomach and bowels*, particularly of children, and proves to them a suitable and efficient purgative, when combined, as above, with Rhubarb. It may be mixed with a little Aniseed Water, which will tend to expel wind, a common ailment of Infants.

APERIENTS, SPRING, FOR CHILDREN.—Nothing is better than:—1. Brimstone and treacle; to each teacupful of this, when mixed, add a tea-spoonful of cream of tartar. As this sometimes produces sickness, the following may be used.—2. Take of tartrate of soda one drachm and a half, powdered jalap and powdered rhubarb, each fifteen grains; ginger, two grains: mix. Dose for a child above five years, one small tea-spoonful; above ten years, a large tea-spoonful; above fifteen, half the whole, or two tea-spoonfuls; and for a person above twenty, three tea-spoonfuls, or the whole, as may be required by the habit of the person. This medicine may be dissolved in warm water, common or mint tea. This powder can be kept for use in a wide-mouthed bottle, and be in readiness for any emergency that may occur.

APERIENT, TONIC.—Take of Epsom salts one ounce, diluted sulphuric acid one drachm, infusion of quassia chips, half an imperial pint, compound tincture of rhubarb two drachms. Half a wine-glassful for a dose—to be taken twice a day.

ASCARIDES, OR SEAT-WORMS TO DESTROY.—A tea-spoonful of flowers of sulphur, in a wine-glassful of Gin, or Brandy, in a morning fasting. The addition of a small quantity of Aloes will render it more effectual.

ASTHMA.—Take of the Milk of Gum Ammonia, six ounces; syrup of squills, four ounces and a half; mix. A spoonful to be taken when relief is required. It greatly relieves by copious expectoration.

BALSAM, FRIAR'S.—The old monks knew what was good. This balsam was used by them. Gum Benzoin, 3½ ounces; Strained Storax, 2½ ounces; Balsam of Tolu, 10 drachms; Aloes, 5 drachms, rectified spirits, 2 pints; let it stand 14 days, shaking well occasionally; and always before using. It is very useful in confirmed Asthma, catarrhs, and consumption, with a languid circulation. Dose, half a drachm in mucilage, or dropped on lump sugar. Applied to wounds, it stimulates gently, and nicely heals them.

BARLEY WATER.—Carefully clean two table-spoonfuls of pearl barley, put it into a quart jug, adding a very little salt, and lump sugar to taste. Fill up with boiling water, and keep stirring for ten minutes. Cover, and let cool. It will be fit for use in ten or twelve hours. Finely shred lemon peel, or a little calf's feet jelly, greatly improves it.

BITE OF A MAD DOG.—Wash well with a strong decoction of tobacco, and then bind wetted tobacco on the wound.——Or, take a pound of salt, dissolve in a quart of water. Squeeze, bathe, and wash the wound with this liquid for one or two hours; then bind some salt upon it for ten or twelve hours.

BITTERS, OR A TONIC.—Take Gentian root two ounces, dried orange peel two ounces and a half, cochineal, in powder, half a drachm, proof spirit or brandy, two pounds; let them stand ten or twelve days, and decant off what is clear for use.

BLACK DRAUGHT.—Take of senna leaves six drachms, bruised ginger half a drachm, sliced liquorice-root four drachms, boiling water half an imperial pint. Keep this standing on the hob, or near the fire for three hours, then strain, and after allowing it to grow cold, add of sal volatile one drachm and a half, of tincture of senna and of tincture of cardamoms, each half an ounce. (This mixture will keep a long time in a cool place.) Dose—a wine-glassful for an adult; two table-spoonfuls for young persons above fifteen years of age. It is not a suitable medicine for children.

BREATH, FŒTID.—Many persons suffer from fœtid breath, without this being attributable to the presence of bad teeth, or the want of attention to the mouth, the gums and mucus membrane being also quite healthy. The smell may proceed from the lungs or the stomach, but in nine cases out of ten it originates in the stomach, and the following is then a simple and prompt remedy:—Three hours after a meal take a large tea-spoonful of a solution of six parts of chlorate of potash in 120 parts of sugared water, and at the same time rinse out the mouth well with the same solution.

BURNS AND SCALDS. See SPANISH FLIES.—If the clothes have caught fire, wrap the person in a shawl, coat, blanket, &c. very tightly, to extinguish the flames; or when these are not at hand, roll the person on the floor. Then gently disengage the clothes from around the burned surface. If any part of the dress should stick to the burned part, do not remove them, but cut the clothes from around that part.

The treatment for burns is applicable to scalds. *If the injury is merely superficial*, saturate a piece of cotton wool, or wadding, &c. with Tincture of Spanish Flies, largely diluted with water, and apply it over the burned or scalded part, and cover it with folded cotton or linen, &c. to exclude the atmospheric air. Saturate with the liniment as the cloth dries.——*If the wound is deep*, use the Arnica Lotion, (See plant Leopard's Bane,) instead of Cantharis. When the burning pain ceases, apply simple cerate spread on a linen rag, and cover well up. During this process three drops of Arnica Liniment, should be taken every quarter of an hour, to compose the excited nervous system. Liniments are better than Lotions, as they contain soap dissolved in spirits of wine, both curative of burns, &c. To be obtained from any Homœopathic Chemists.

When the afore-mentioned liniments are not at hand, Cotton Wool, or a Linen rag may be well saturated in oil and soap lather, and applied. In scalding of the mouth, soap liniment, may be advantageously used, which is made by dissolving soap in spirits.

"A most primitive, yet very effectual remedy in the treatment of burns and scalds is *cow-dung;* and from its being so rich in phosphorus, it must exert a specific, and a mechanical action to cure injuries resulting from fire."

Some persons will object to the treatment of burns and scalds by Spanish Fly Liniment. But of late years has come into practice the use of irritating substances in preference to the injurious method of treatment with ice, cold water, and other refrigerants. The treatment now recommended is *not* the old treatment by *contraries;* but that "likes should be treated with likes."

Burns and Scalds.—A few raw potatoes are to be peeled, and finely beaten in a mortar; add a drachm or two of laudanum; apply to the affected parts, like a poultice. It is very efficacious in the cure of burns or scalds, and other inflamed parts.

Charcoal Medicine.—This is extensively used in Mexico, and in many parts of South America, where few drugs are procurable, save those "simples" which the ingenuity and experience of the *Indian Herbalists* have devised. Freshly-burnt Charcoal, reduced to powder and given in water, is in great repute. Within a few hours of taking, it removes offensive odours from intestinal and renal discharges, and purifies the breath, also offensive exhalations from the feet, any part of the body, either given in water, or in the form of pills, made up in wheat flour, or gum mucilage. It removes those local pains about the right shoulder which are usually attributed to obstructions of the liver, and this within forty-eight hours. As an antiacid, either alone, or combined with rhubarb, and carbonate of soda, it speedily and permanently removes heartburn. Charcoal is a powerful antiseptic, removing, or checking decay, and must be very valuable in the incipient stages of consumption.

CHILBLAINS.—To cure chilblains, simply bathe the parts affected in the liquor in which potatoes have been boiled, at as high a temperature as can be borne. On the first appearance of this ailment, indicated by inflammation and irritation, this bath affords almost immediate relief. In the more advanced stages, repetition prevents breaking out, followed by a certain cure; and an occasional adoption will operate against a return.

COLD, A, HOW TO CURE.—The following plan is very effectual in curing most colds, but not all:—Let a man eat nothing for two days, provided he is not confined to bed, because by taking no carbon into the system by food, and by consuming the surplus which caused his disease, by breath he soon carries off his disease by removing the cause. This will be found more effectual if he adds copious water draughts to protracted fasting. By the time a person has fasted one day and night, he will experience a freedom from disease, and a clearness of mind, in a delightful contrast with mental stupor, and physical pain caused by colds. How infinitely better is this method of breaking up colds than by medicines.

COLD, CURE FOR.—One handful of Yarrow, half an ounce of Ginger root, bruised, or a teaspoonful of Cayenne Pepper, and about three pints of water. Boil to one pint. Add a little sugar if you like. Take a good dose at bed-time, and your cold will be cured by the next morning; if not, repeat the dose.

COLD, TO AVOID CATCHING.—Accustom yourself to the use of sponging with cold water every morning on first getting out of bed. It should be followed with a good deal of rubbing with a wet towel. It has considerable effect in giving tone to the skin, and maintaining a proper action in it, and thus proves a safeguard to the injurious influence of cold and sudden change of temperature. Sir Astley Cooper said, "The methods by which I have preserved my own health are—temperance, early rising, and sponging the body every morning with cold water, immediately after getting out of bed; a practice which I have adopted for thirty years without ever catching cold."

COLTSFOOT WINE TO MAKE EQUAL TO SHERRY.—Take twenty pounds of Coltsfoot, and twenty-two quarts of cold water, let it stand three days, drain the coltsfoot well from the liquor through a sieve; put three and a half pounds of *brown* sugar, three lemons, three sweet and one bitter orange to each gallon of liquor, then put the whole in a tub, with a few spoonfuls of yeast; let it work two or three days, stirring it frequently; drain through a sieve again, and put into a barrel; when done fermenting, add half an ounce of isinglass, bung the barrel well up, let it stand six months, then add a bottle of brandy, and bottle it.

CONSUMPTION, USEFUL DRINK FOR.—Coltsfoot, two ounces; Horehound, one ounce, and the same of Rue. Boil in three quarts of water down to two quarts. Strain, and to the liquor, add of figs and sugar, of each four ounces, and boil fifteen minutes. Take a wine-glassful three or four times a day.

CORNS, A POSITIVE CURE FOR.—The strongest acetic acid, applied night and morning with a camel's hair brush. In one week the corn will disappear—soft or hard corns.

CORPULENCY.—Mr. Alfred William Moore, sent the following communication to the *Medical Times*:—"Fat is a necessary ingredient of the body. Nature, however, is sometimes too liberal in its supply; it then becomes burdensome, and subjects the objects of its prodigality to much ridicule. The discovery of a certain remedy, under these circumstances, may prove a boon. The following experiment, or systematic plan of treatment, adopted by myself, who am constitutionally fat, will clearly show that abstaining from bread and fermented liquors will remedy this inconvenience in an incredible manner: —Weighing 15½ stone, I reduced myself in three months to 12½ stone, by strictly adhering to the following plan of dieting myself: — Breakfast early, consisting of 2oz. of biscuit, 1 egg, two cups of tea or coffee; then fasted till five; my dinner consisting of animal food, &c., but no bread; likewise avoiding bread at my tea or supper.

Cough.—Two table-spoonfuls of Linseed, four ounces of Liquorice root, or Spanish Juice, four ounces of Elecampane root, water three quarts; boil down to three pints. Dose, a wine-glassful four or five times a day.

Cough.—Powder of tragacanth, one drachm; syrup of white poppies, two drachms; laudanum, forty drops; water, four ounces. Shake the powder in the water till it is dissolved, then add the others. Dose:—A teaspoonful three times a day.

Cough—Asthmatic.—Take two good handfuls of Coltsfoot leaves, one ounce of Garlic, and two quarts of water. Boil down to three pints. Strain, and to the liquor add eight ounces of sugar, boil gently for ten minutes. Take half a cupful occasionally.

Cough, Consumption, &c. Cure for.—The following is a most valuable recipe:—Of Sanctuary, Horehound, Barberry Bark, two pennyworth of each; and of Agrimony, Raspberry Leaves, Clevers, and Ground Ivy, one pennyworth; Extract of Liquorice, 4 oz.; and half a tea-spoonful of Cayenne pepper. Gently simmer in two gallons of water for half an hour.

Cough, Cure for Dry.—Take of powdered gum-arabic, half an ounce; liquorice juice, half an ounce. Dissolve the gum first in warm water; squeeze in the juice of a lemon; then add of paregoric, too drachms; of syrup of squills, one drachm. Cork all in a bottle, and shake well. Take one teaspoonful when the cough is troublesome.

Deafness Cured by Ether.—A poor French governess, Madlle. Cléret, has succeeded in partially curing several persons afflicted with deafness and loss of speech. The French Academy have awarded the Monthyon Prize for the discovery, which was accidental, and has been proved perfectly innocuous. The method consists in introducing sulphuric ether into the aural conduit, in doses of four to eight drops a day for about twenty days, when the application is suspended for a short time, and again recommenced. Since the publication of this fact numerous applications from persons suffering from deafness have been received by physicians, and a certain number of cases have been made public. A gunner's mate, aged 51, had been attacked six months before with acute rheumatism, which at length became chronic and complicated, with deafness in the left ear, and difficulty of hearing in the right one. There was frequent singing in both ears, but no otorrhœa; and the deafness used to increase and diminish with the rheumatic pains. At the first, a few drops of ether were instilled into both his ears, when he immediately experienced a feeling of expansion within, accompanied by a slight pain, and from that moment he could distinguish sounds less confusedly. On the following morning he declared he could hear with his right ear quite as well as before his illness; the instillation was therefore only repeated in the left ear, and on the fourth day he declared himself quite cured. Another case, similar to this, is reported by Dr. Berlemont, of Joncourt; and Dr. Coursier, of Honnecourt, announces that he has been treating six patients, between five and fifteen years of age, for some time with ether, to their manifest advantage. In one of these cases, however, the application was productive of much local pain.

Diarrhœa.—Blackberry Cordial.—To one quart of blackberry juice add one pound of white sugar, one tablespoonful of cloves, one of allspice, one of cinnamon, and one of nutmeg. Boil all together fifteen minutes; add a wineglass of whisky, brandy, or rum. Bottle while hot, cork tight and seal. This is almost a specific in diarrhœa. One dose, which is a wineglassful for an adult—half that quantity for a child—will often cure diarrhœa. It can be taken three or four times a day if the case is severe.

Drink for the Sick.—Take half an ounce of sugar-candy, quarter of an ounce of cream of tartar, and a few lemon and orange chips; pour upon them one quart of boiling water. When cold pour off

EYES, GOOD FOR THE.—To give brilliancy to the eyes, shut them early at night, and open them early in the morning; let the mind be constantly intent on the acquisition of benevolent feelings. This will scarcely ever fail to impart to the eyes an intelligent and amiable expression.

EYE-LID, REMOVING FOREIGN BODIES FROM BENEATH THE.—M. Renard, in the case of small moveable bodies which become entangled beneath the upper eyelid, recommends the following simple procedure, which will often dispense with all others. Take hold of the upper eyelid near its angles with the index finger and thumb of each hand, draw it gently forwards and as low down as possible over the lower eyelid, and retain it in this position for about a minute, taking care to prevent the tears from flowing out. When, at the end of this time, you allow the eyelid to resume its place, a flood of tears washes out the foreign body, which will be found adhering to, or near to, the lower eyelid.

EYE POULTICE.—Stir two drachms of powdered alum in the whites of two eggs till a coagulum be formed. Place it between a piece of soft linen rag, and apply it. Very applicable for inflamed eyes attended with a purulent discharge, and for chilblains.

EYE-WATER.—Half a pint of the best brandy, two pints of spring water, and sugar of lead, one ounce; mix. This is a good eye-water.

EYE-WATER AN EXCELLENT.—Take six ounces of Rectified Spirits of Wine, dissolve in it one drachm of Camphor, then add two small handfuls of dried Elder Flowers; infuse twenty-four hours. Bathe the forehead, over your eyes, and each temple, several times a day; meantime, dip a soft rag in stale small beer, new milk warm, and bathe each eye a few times gently morning and evening. If it is a watery humour, wet the eyelids two or three times, but be sure to shut your eyes, or it will make them smart and burn excessively.

It is also a good remedy for the Toothache, or swelled face, bruises, &c., used as a rubefacient.

FRAGRANT ODOUR, TO DIFFUSE A.—A few drops of oil of

sandal wood dropped on a hot shovel, will diffuse a most agreeable balsamic perfume throughout the room.

GRAVEL OR STONE.—Take one ounce of the spirits of sweet nitre, two drachms of liquid laudanum, and half an ounee of the oil of juniper. Take a tea-spoonful in a cup of linseed tea sweetened with honey. This has performed wonders.

GRAVEL, EXCELLENT FOR THE.—Take of Dandelion and Marsh Mallows roots, of each two ounces, Agrimony a small handful, to three quarts of water; boil to two quarts. Dose—a wineglassful every three or four hours.

HARD AND SWELLED BREASTS.—An excellent remedy is made of Camomile Flowers, and bruised Marshmallow roots, each one ounce; boil in one quart of water down to one pint. Foment with the liquor, as hot as can be borne; and then place the flowers and roots in a cloth, and apply as a cataplasm or poultice.

HEAD ACHE.—One scruple turbith mineral, half a drachm of powdered ginger, one scruple of powdered nutmeg, three drops of the oil of rosemary, all mixed, and snuffed up the nose.

HEAD-ACHE.—Take a small handful of Centaury, and as much Feverfew, and one ounce of Camomile Flowers, to two quarts of water; boil to one quart; then add while hot half an ounce of rhubarb, and stir well. Dose—a wine glassful three times a day.

HOOPING COUGH.—Dissolve a scruple of salt of tartar in a quarter of a pint of water; add to it ten grains of cochineal; sweeten it with sugar. Give to an infant a fourth part of a tablespoonful four times a day; two years old, half a spoonful, from four years a table-spoonful.

HOOPING COUGH. Take flower of Benjamin, and strained opium, of each two drachms, camphire, two scruples, essential oil of aniseeds, half a drachm, rectified spirit of wine, one quart, four ounces of powdered liquorice, and four ounces of honey: then digest and strain off the elixir. Or,

Take of the musk juleps, six ounces, paregoric elixir, half

an ounce, volatile tincture of valerian, one drachm, mix them, and take two spoonfuls three or four times every day.

HYDROPHOBIA.—Immediately wash the bitten part with clear water; then take good tobacco, (leaf tobacco, if possible; if not, strong manufactured cut tobacco) and make a bandage for the place, changing it three or four times a day for a week. This effectually absorbs every thing poisonous.

INDIGESTION.—Take of Gentian and Columba roots (bruised) and Camomile Flowers, of each one ounce, to three quarts of water; boil to three pints. Dose—two or three teacupfuls a day.

JAUNDICE, YELLOW.—Burdock root, one ounce, Agrimony one ounce, water, two quarts; boil down to three pints. Dose, a wine-glassful two or three times a day.

JELLY FOR THE SICK.—Mix one ounce each of rice, pearl barley, sago, and hartshorn shavings, in three pints of water; boil till reduced to one, and strain. When required for use, dissolve in milk, wine, or broth.

LINIMENT, VOLATILE.—Spirit of hartshorn, one ounce; olive oil, one ounce and a half. Shake them well in a bottle. If a drachm or two of laudanum be added, it will make it more efficacious. Rub the affected part with it, apply afterwards a rag saturated with it. It removes pains and swellings.

LOTION VALUABLE.—Camphor, five drachms, cut it into small pieces, and dissolve in half a pint of spirits of wine in a closely corked bottle; when fully dissolved, add half a pint, or more, of oxgall, which can be bought of any butcher, and about fifty or sixty drops of laudanum. Shake it well, and bottle for use.—This has been a patent medicine, and is very efficacious in the cure of fresh wounds, cuts, bruises, swellings, sores, and inflamed and pained parts. It ought to be kept in every house ready for need, as a Domestic Embrocation.

MARIGOLDS.—Their virtues have been lost sight of. The juice, or a strong decoction, with (or without) a very small portion of spirits of wine, is a rare application for healing lacerations, bruises, cuts, both pain and bleeding being immediately arrested. By its use in severe wounds Erysipelas is prevented. It seldom leaves a cicatrix, or mark, behind it. It has a tendency to contract the mouths of the small arteries, when directly cut across, and where they have been slit longitudinally. The Tincture may be purchased of the Homœopathic Chemists; and largely diluted with water, it is a first-rate remedy.

MEASLES.—This disease prevails extensively in cities during the winter season, and will usually cure itself, if only protected against adverse influences. The older persons are, the less likely they are to recover perfectly from this ailment, for it very oft leaves some life-long malady behind it. The most hopeless forms of consumptive disease are often the result of ill-conducted or badly-managed measles. In nine cases out of ten, not a particle of the medicine is needed. Our first advice is, always, and under all circumstances, send at once for an experienced physician. Meanwhile, keep the patient in a cool, dry, and well-aired room, with moderate covering, in a position where there will be no exposure to draughts of air. The thermometer should range at about 65 degrees where the bed stands, which should be moderately hard, of husk, straw, or curled hair. Gratify the instinct for cold water and lemonade. It is safest to keep the bed for several days after the rash has begun to die away. The diet should be light, and of an opening and cooling character. The main object of this article is to warn persons that the greatest danger is after the disappearance of the measles. We would advise that for three weeks after the patient is well enough to leave his bed, he should not go out of the house, nor stand or sit for a single minute near an open window or door, nor wash any part of the person in cold water or warm, but to wipe the face and hands with a warm damp cloth. For a good part of this time the appetite should not be wholly gratified; the patient should eat slowly of light nutritious food. In one case, a little child, almost entirely well of the measles, got to playing with its hands in cold water; it gradually dwindled away and died. All exercise should be moderate, in order to prevent cooling off too quickly afterwards, and to be in danger of exposure to draughts of air, which by covering the surface causes chronic diarrhœa if it falls on the bowels, deafness for life if it falls on the ear, or incurable consumption if it falls on the lungs.

MILK, TO KEEP SWEET.—A correspondent informs us, that he has practised a peculiar method with much success of preserving milk sweet in the pans. It simply consists in placing a piece of new hammered iron, or three twelve-penny nails, in each tin pan, then pouring the warm milk on them. He believes that electricity has something to do with producing the result. He had tried many experiments before he hit on this one, which he found to preserve the milk sweet for a longer time than other plans tried by him.

OINTMENT, CHILBLAIN.—Two ounces of lard, half an ounce of turpentine, and a quarter of an ounce of camphor, melted together.

OINTMENT FOR BROKEN CHILBLAINS OR CHAPPED HANDS, &c. Sweet oil, one pint; Venice turpentine, three ounces; hogs' lard. half a pound; bees' wax, three ounces. Put all into a pipkin over a slow fire, and stir it with a wooden spoon till the bees' wax is melted, and the ingredients simmer. It must be spread very thin on soft rag, or (for chaps or cracks) rubbed on the hands when you go to bed.

OINTMENT, SPERMACETI.—Take Spermaceti, one ounce; white wax, two drachms; olive oil, three ounces. Melt over a slow fire; when cool it is fit for use. It is good for healing blisters, excoriations, and abrasions of the skin.

PAINS IN THE HEAD AND FACE.—Take half a pint of rose water, two tea-spoonfuls of white vinegar, and form a lotion. Apply it to the affected part three times a day. It requires fresh linen and lotion each application; this will, in two or three days, gradually take the pain away.

PAINS IN THE JOINTS.—Make a poultice of the young leaves of Rag-wort, and put on as hot as can be borne.

PILLS FOR A BAD COUGH.—Compound ipecacuanha powder, half a drachm; fresh dried squills, ten grains; sulphate of ammoniacum, ten grains; sulphate of quinine, six grains; treacle, sufficient quantity to make a mass. Divide into twelve pills; one to be taken night and morning.

PILLS, USEFUL APERIENT.—Take of compound rhubarb pill a drachm and one scruple, of powdered ipecacuanha six grains, and of extract of hyoscyamus one scruple. Mix and beat into a mass, and divide into twenty-four pills. Take one, or two, or, if of a very costive habit, three at bed time. For persons requiring a more powerful purge, the same formula, with ten grains of compound extract of colocynth, will form a good purgative pill. The mass receiving this addition must be divided into thirty, instead of twenty-four pills.

RHEUMATISM AND ITS REMEDIES.

To those who dwell in damp districts, or damp houses, and are hence subject to rheumatism, coughs, colds, &c., the free use of lemom juice (when strained and where it does not disagree with the stomach) is a most effectual preventive as well as a remedy! I have found the regular use of a wine-glassful or two a day so to strengthen a very delicate constitution, liable to colds on the slightest occasions, that it in a short time defied not only damp, but every inclemency, and all exposure.

Rheumatism, Cure for.—A Correspondent of the *Medical Circular* vouches for the relief he has experienced in the liberal use of lime (fresh lemon) juice, whilst labouring under the paroxysms of rheumatism. By repeated indulgence in the above simple acid, for the space of three days, avoiding all stimulating liquids, the most confirmed rheumatism will, he says, relax, and the tone of the muscular and nervous system will be restored to its usual character. The fact was first established by the circumstance of the Jews being as a general body, scarcely ever affected with the above disease, and this particular exemption from the malady under consideration, as affecting the disciples of the Hebrew persuasion, was, and has been, attributed to the very free indulgence which the above people exercise in their dietary consumption of lemon-juice.

When lemon juice disagrees, either of the two following formulæ may be substituted :—R—Lemon juice (strained or filtered) and treacle, equal parts; powdered sugar candy, q. s.; mix intimately—a table spoonful three or four times a day.

Second Recipe.—R.—Powdered rhubarb, 2 drachms; acetate of potash, 1 ounce; guaiacum, 1 drachm; sulphur, 2 ounces; 1 nutmeg, grated very fine; treacle, 16 ounces.

Mix—take two teaspoonfuls night and morning.

The seat of rheumatism is in the muscles—electro galvanism must be used; it is generally the best plan to begin with currents of the weakest power, and gradually to increase their strength so long as the application causes no pain. Dumb bells should be used above all, every day; they should never exceed in weight one pound for ladies and four for men. Silk is the best nonconductor of cold we have, and it is affirmed that those of the fair sex who wear tight fitting sleeves to their silk dresses are not so subject to rheumatism; males should wear thick silk sleeves to all their waistcoats; they can be easily taken off, and tacked or sewn on to another vest; besides the above precautions, flannel must be worn summer and winter by day, "but never by night," next the skin: at night a small flannel spencer or jacket should be worn over the night dress.

Tailors and milliners have much to answer for in introducing such modern inventions as the wide sleeves, and in like manner "the apology of a bonnet," this last the cause of tic doloreux, rheumatism, &c.

Embrocation for rheumatism:—R.—Olive oil, 2 ounces; water of ammonia, 2 drachms; oil of rosemary, 10 drops; oil of cloves, 5 drops. Mix and keep tightly corked.

Rheumatism.—Take a large handful of Buckbean, four ounces of White Mustard Seeds, and one of Lignum Vitæ, or Wood of Life, to two quarts of water; boil to three pints. Dose—three tea-cupfuls a day. Use also the following *Liniment.* Take of Sal Volatile three ounces; oil, one ounce, Camphor, quarter of an ounce, Laudanum one ounce. Rub the part affected with this liniment three times a day.

Rheumatic Pains.—Take opodeldoc, one ounce; tincture of cantharides, three drachms; spirits of sal ammoniac, three drachms; rectified oil of amber, three drachms. This forms a liniment, wherewith frequently to rub the painful part. Wrap up in fine, soft flannel, and keep warm.

Rheumatic pains and aches in the bones and joints, a remedy for.—Take friar's balsam and tincture of myrrh of each one ounce, spirits of turpentine two ounces, and good old strong ale dregs three ounces; mix all of them well together, and bathe the afflicted part with the same.

SALVE, FAMILY.—Take the root of yellow dock and dandelion, equal parts; add a good proportion of celandine and plantain. Extract the juices by pressing or steeping. Strain carefully and simmer the liquid with sweet cream, or fresh butter and mutton tallow, or you may take sweet oil and mutton tallow. Simmer together until no appearance of the liquid remains. Before it is quite cold, put it into boxes as you may desire. This is one of the most soothing and healing preparations for burns, scalds, cuts, and sores of every description that can be produced.

SALVE FOR ALL WOUNDS.—Take one pound of hog's lard, three ounces of white lead, three ounces of red lead, three ounces of bees' wax, two ounces of black rosin, and four ounces of common turpentine; all these ingredients must be put together in a pan, and boil three quarters of an hour; the turpentine to be put in just before it is done enough, and give it a gentle boil afterwards. This is an excellent cure for burns, sores, or ulcers, as it first draws, then heals afterward; it is excellent for all wounds.

SCRATCHES, HINTS ABOUT.—Trifling as scratches often seem, they ought never to be neglected, but should be covered and protected, and kept clean and dry, until they have completely healed. If there is the least appearance of inflammation, no time should be lost in applying a large bread-and-water poultice, or hot flannels repeatedly applied, or even leeches in good numbers may be put on at some distance from each other.

SCURF IN THE HEAD.—This is a simple and effectual remedy. Into a pint of water drop a lump of fresh quick-lime, the size of a walnut; let it stand all night, then pour the water off clear from sediment or deposit, add a quarter of a pint of the best vinegar, and wash the head with the mixture, wetting only the roots of the hair. It is perfectly harmless.

SCURVY.—Dandelion roots, and field Daisies, of each two ounces, in three quarts of water, boil to two quarts. Take a tea-cupful night and morning.

SCURVY IN THE GUMS.—Make strong sage tea and dissolve therein a little alum, dip a cloth therein and rub your gums with the same. If you wish to make your teeth white, mix a little burnt alum with six spoonfuls of honey, and two spoonfuls of the juice of celandine, and rub your teeth with the same.

SMALL-POX, PREVENTION OR PITTING IN.—Mr. Startin, the senior surgeon to the Gurney Hospital for Diseases of the Skin, has communicated to the *Medical Times* a very important plan, which he has adopted during the last fourteen years, for preventing pitting in small-pox, and which, he states, has always proved successful. The plan consists in applying the *acetum cantharidis* or any vesiccating fluid, by means of a camel-hair brush, to the apex of each spot or pustule of the disease, on all the exposed surfaces of the body, until blistering is evidenced by the whiteness of the skin in the parts subjected to the application, when the fluid producing it is to be washed off with water or thin arrowroot gruel. The pain attending the application of the vesiccating fluid is very slight and transient.

SORE THROAT, CURE FOR A.—Pour a pint of boiling water upon twenty-five or thirty leaves of common sage; let the infusion stand for half an hour. Add vinegar sufficient to make it moderately acid, and honey according to the taste. This combination of the astringent and the emollient principle seldom fails to produce the desired effect. The infusion must be used as a gargle several times a day. It has this advantage over many gargles—it is pleasant to the taste, and may be swallowed occasionally, not only without danger, but with advantage.

SPANISH FLIES; *(Greek, Cantharis;)*—TINCTURE OF.—Take of Spanish Flies, reduced to a fine powder, 2 ounces; spirit of wine, one pint; infuse for two or three days, and then strain. It is an acid stimulant for external use. It will prevent the formation of blisters in cases of burns or scalds, and chilblains are cured by a weak solution of the Tincture. In burns or scalds it is very important to protect the injured surface from the air, for which purpose cotton wool, or cotton of close texture, is the best. It is very efficacious for chafed skin, and for frost-bites *especially*.

Tea and Coffee, Substitute for.—Substitute for Tea as follows:—Take a small handful of Agrimony, one handful of Blackberry leaves, and a few Raspberry leaves, and a very small quantity of Balm or Mint, according to taste; put it into a jug that will hold three pints, then pour on boiling hot water, let it stand about five minutes, then sweeten to palate; for a change, you may use Avens in the same way and manner as Agrimony.

Substitute for Coffee. Take six or eight pounds of Dandelion roots, cut off the tops, then wash the earth from them. After which, hang them up to dry; when dried take one of the roots and grate it like Ginger. Grate about a teaspoonful and a half, put it in a pot that will hold a pint and a half. Let it stand for five minutes, then use it.

Teeth, Cements for Stopping the.—M. Vagner recommends the following:—A drachm of gutta percha, softened by hot water, is to be worked up with catechu powder and tannic acid, of each half a drachm, and with a drop of essential oil. For use, a morsel is to be softened over the flame of a spirit lamp, introduced while warm into the cavity of the tooth, and adapted properly. The mass becomes hardened, and even after several months exhibits no traces of decomposition. M. Pouton states that we may also obtain an excellent cement by dissolving one part of mastic in two of collodion. Having well dried out the cavity, a small ball of cotton soaked in some drops of the solution is to be introduced. It soon solidifies, and will remain *in situ*, seeming also to exert an influence on the further progress of the caries.

Tobacco, British Herb.—The principal ingredient in this compound is *dried* coltsfoot leaves, to which a smaller portion of thyme, wood betony, eye-bright, rosemary, and yarrow are added.

Tumours, Cure of.—Dr. Simpson, of Edinburgh, has been experimenting on the removal of tumours by a method novel in this country. He introduces a hollow acupuncture needle, or very fine trocar, into their tissue, and injects in a few drops of some irritant liquid, such as a solution of chloride of zinc, perchloride of iron, or creosote. The effect has been to destroy the vitality of the tumours so treated, and they have been separated by a process of enucleation. We have seen a somewhat similar plan adopted in Paris by M. Maisonneuve. He had slender stylets, made of a paste composed of flour, water, and chloride of zinc. These are baked. A puncture is made in the tumour, the caustic stylet is inserted, broken off, and left. We saw several malignant tumours treated in this manner, and some cases in which a healthy granulating surface was left, after the separation of tumours which had been destroyed in this manner.

VINEGAR, AROMATIC.—Dissolve one ounce of camphor in a pound of the strongest acetic acid (vinegar), and add one ounce each of the oils of lemon, cloves, and lavender.

WARTS.—The juice of Marigolds frequently applied is effectual in removing warts.

WHITLOWS.—A lady who had been troubled some time with a whitlow on her finger, gives a simple remedy, from which she experienced great relief, and which enabled her to obtain sleep after many restless nights. It is, to cut a hole in a lemon, and wear it on the finger like a thimble—the whitlow being encased in the fruit.

WIND IN THE STOMACH.—Take a large handful of Feverfew, and Cummin seeds and Ginger, one ounce of each, to three quarts of water ; boil to three pints. Dose—three or four wine-glassfuls a day.

WIND IN THE STOMACH.—Take oil of Juniper, tincture of myrrh, lavender water, sweet nitre, equal quantity of each : shake them in a bottle. Dose :—One teaspoonful in a cup of cold water. The above is a dose for an adult.

WORM LOZENGES.—Jalop, quarter of an ounce ; powdered rhubarb, quarter of an ounce ; gamboge, two drachms ; syrup of bear's-foot, sufficient to make it into paste ; then make it into ordinary sized lozenges. Dose :—For a child three years old, half a lozenge ; six years, one lozenge ; and so on, according to years.

INDEX OF DISEASES

WHICH THE PLANTS IN THIS HERBAL ARE ADAPTED TO RELIEVE AND TO CURE.

DEFINITION OF TERMS.

Amaurosis—Loss of sight proceeding from paralysis of the optic nerve.

Anodyne.—Medicines which assuage pain.

Anthelmintics.—Medicines which expel worms.

Antispasmodic.—Medicines which abate or remove spasms.

Antiseptic.—Medicines which prevent putrefaction.

Antidote.—Medicines opposed to any disease.

Astringent.—Remedies which act by contracting the animal fibres, and rendering the solids denser and firmer.

Cachexia, Cachectic.—A bad habit of the body—an unhealthy state of system resulting from want of nutrition, bad air, &c.

Carminatives.—Remedies which allay pains, and expel flatulency, or wind.

Cataplasm.—A poultice.

Catarrh.—Inflammation of the mucous membrane of the nostrils, or bronchial passages, &c.

Cathartics.—Laxative, purgative, or drastic medicines which open the bowels.

Cephalics.—Remedies for diseases of the head.

Chlorosis.—The green sickness.

Chronic.—Diseases of long standing.

Cicatrix.—A scar or mark left by a wound.

Collyrium.—A wash for the eye.

Constipation,—Habitual confinement of the bowels.

Demulcents.—Medicines which have softening and soothing properties.

Deobstruent. - Medicines which remove obstructions from any part of the body.

Diaphoretic.—Medicines which increase the natural exhalations of the skin, or perspiration.

Discutient.—Medicines which disperse the morbid matter of tumours, &c.

Diuretic.—Medicines which increase the urinary discharge.

Emetic.—Medicines which cause vomiting.

Emmenagogue.—Medicines to promote the monthly discharge.

Emolient.—Medicines which relax and soften the animal fibre.

Empiric.—Formerly, an experimenter in medicine; but now a vender of nostrums—a quack.

Enema.—A clyster, lavement, or injection.

Expectorants.—Medicines which promote a discharge of mucous or other matters from the trachœa and its branches.

Febrifuge.—A medicinal agent used for the reduction of fever.

Flatulence.—Wind in the intestines.

Gangrene.—The first stage of mortification.

Hæmoptysis.—A flow of blood from any part of the body.

Hœmorrhage. A flow of blood from any part of the body.

Hydrophobia.—Canine or dog madness.

Hydrops.—Dropsies.

Lethargy.—Profound and continuous sleep.

Leucorrhœa.—The Whites.

Nausea.—Sickness at the stomach; loathing.

Phthisis.—A disease produced by tubercles on the lungs, called Consumption.

Styptic.—Medicines which stop bleeding.

Sudorifics.—Medicines which promote perspiration or sweating.

Suppuration.—The formation of matter in abscesses &c.

Tenesmus.—Powerful and frequent straining at the rectum, to procure stool, ending in discharge of mucous only.

Tetanus.—Contraction of the muscles of voluntary motion, in which a part or the whole of the body becomes rigid.

Tetters.—Skin eruptions, consisting of clusters of vesicles seated upon inflamed patches of irregular size and form.

Vulnerary.—Herbs, medicines, &c. which have the power to heal wounds.

Whitlow.—An inflammation at the end of a finger or thumb, painful, having a tendency to suppurate.

GENERAL INDEX.

WILLIAM NICHOLSON, PRINTER,

Published by

Facsimile Publisher
Ashok Vihar, Delhi-110052 (India)
Website. www.facsimilepublisher.com

Distributed by

Gyan Books Pvt. Ltd.
5, Ansari Road, Daryaganj, New Delhi-110002 (India)
E-mail: books@gyanbooks.com, Website: www.gyanbooks.com

2 222000 008390